THE LOWER FEMALE GENITAL TRACT

A Clinicopathologic Approach

THE LOWER FEMALE GENITAL TRACT
A Clinicopathologic Approach

DEBRA S. HELLER, MD
Associate Professor of Pathology and Laboratory Medicine
University of Medicine and Dentistry of New Jersey—New Jersey Medical School
Newark, New Jersey

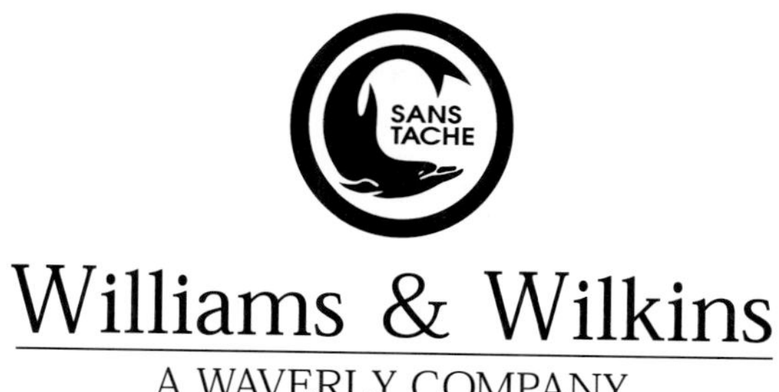

Williams & Wilkins
A WAVERLY COMPANY

BALTIMORE • PHILADELPHIA • LONDON • PARIS • BANGKOK
BUENOS AIRES • HONG KONG • MUNICH • SYDNEY • TOKYO • WROCLAW

Editor: Charles W. Mitchell
Managing Editor: Keith Rhett Murphy
Marketing Manager: Lori Smith
Production Coordinator: Pete Carley
Project Editor: Lisa J. Franko
Design Coordinator: Mario Fernandez
Illustration Planner: Lorraine Wrzosek
Typesetter and Digitized Illustrations: Maryland Composition Co., Inc.
Printer/Binder: Edwards Brothers, Inc.

351 West Camden Street
Baltimore, Maryland 21201-2436 USA

Rose Tree Corporate Center
1400 North Providence Road
Building II, Suite 5025
Media, Pennsylvania 19063-2043 USA

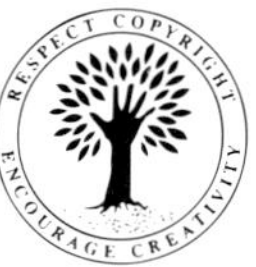

Accurate indications, adverse reactions, and dosage schedules for drugs are provided in this book, but it is possible that they may change. The reader is urged to review the package information data of the manufacturers of the medications mentioned.

Printed in the United States of America

Library of Congress Cataloging-in-Publication Data

Heller, Debra S.
    The lower female genital tract : a clinicopathologic approach/Debra S. Heller.—1st ed.
      p.   cm.
    Includes bibliographical references and index.
    ISBN 0-683-30340-6
    1. Generative organs, Female—Cytopathology. 2. Generative organs, Female—Diseases—Cytodiagnosis. 3. Generative organs, Female—Precancerous conditions. I. Title.
    [DNLM: 1. Genital Diseases, Female—pathology. WP 141 H477L 1998]
RG107.H44 1998
618.1'07—dc21
DNLM/DLC
for Library of Congress
                                                97-40571
                                                 CIP

The publishers have made every effort to trace the copyright holders for borrowed material. If they have inadvertently overlooked any, they will be pleased to make the necessary arrangements at the first opportunity.

To purchase additional copies of this book, call our customer service department at **(800) 638-0672** or fax orders to **(800) 447-8438.** For other book services, including chapter reprints and large quantity sales, ask for the Special Sales department.

Canadian customers should call **(800) 665-1148,** or fax **(800) 665-0103.** For all other calls originating outside of the United States, please call **(410) 528-4223** or fax us at **(410) 528-8550.**

Visit Williams & Wilkins on the Internet: **http://www.wwilkins.com** or contact our customer service department at **custserv@wwilkins.com.** Williams & Wilkins customer service representatives are available from 8:30 am to 6:00 pm, EST, Monday through Friday, for telephone access.

                                                98 99 00
1 2 3 4 5 6 7 8 9 10

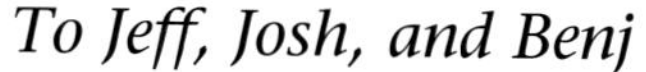

To Jeff, Josh, and Benj

FOREWORD

M. Leon Tancer, MD
Professor Emeritus of Clinical Obstetrics and Gynecology
College of Physicians and Surgeons
Columbia University
New York, New York

The clinicopathologic approach to diseases of the female genital tract in a single compact text is a useful addition to the library of the busy practicing obstetrician-gynecologist and pathologist. It will permit them to review each particular disease area without recourse to broad, special texts on each subject at hand.

Such a volume requires that discussions of the various disease areas be expressed by individuals with special competence in each disease field. Thus, cutaneous diseases of the vulva are discussed by Alex Young, a dermatologist with a special interest in vulvar disease; lower genital tract cytology by Ruth Kreitzer and Diane Hamele-Bena, two cytopathologists; clinical aspects of lower genital tract neoplasia are reviewed by Daniel Smith, a gynecologic oncologist; molecular pathology as it applies to the lower genital tract is addresssed by Tamara Kalir, a gynecologic pathologist and researcher; and DES-related conditions are analyzed by Stanley Robboy, who did much of the seminal work in the area. He is joined by colleagues with an interest in gynecologic pathology, Drs. Bentley, Krigman, and Anderson.

Discussions on the pathology of benign and malignant diseases of the lower genital tract will be the province of the editor, who is both a board-certified pathologist with special interest and training in gynecologic pathology and a board-certified obstetrician-gynecologist with a practice background in obstetrics and gynecology.

This unique text will stir the interest and provide information to the clinician and the pathologist in a readily available manner.

PREFACE

Debra S. Heller, MD

The purpose of this volume is to enhance care to the female patient by furthering communication between the gynecologist and the pathologist. By providing input by authors who are both clinicians and pathologists, this book seeks to help each specialty acquire insight into the point of view of the other, leading to the best care for the patient.

The first part of the book discusses clinical aspects of diseases of the lower female genital tract. As clinical history often does not accompany specimens submitted to pathology laboratories, this section provides insight into the thinking of the clinician and an understanding of how and why clinicians perform procedures that result in the specimens we receive.

The second part of the book discusses the pathology of the lower genital tract. A practical rather than exhaustive discussion, this section emphasizes recognizing the "horse" that is likely to be seen in daily practice rather than the rare "zebra." This should serve not only the pathologist, but also the clinician, who needs to understand the pathology report he or she receives.

Hopefully, this approach will prove useful to both the gynecologists and pathologists who provide care for female patients.

CONTRIBUTORS

MALCOLM C. ANDERSON, FRCOG, FRCPath
Honorary Consultant Gynaecological
Pathologist
Department of Pathology
University Hospital
Queens Medical Centre
Nottingham, England

REX C. BENTLEY, MD
Department of Pathology
Duke University Medical Center
Durham, North Carolina

DIANE HAMELE-BENA, MD
Assistant Professor of Pathology
College of Physicians and Surgeons of
Columbia University
New York, New York

DEBRA S. HELLER, MD
Associate Professor of Pathology and
Laboratory Medicine
University of Medicine and Dentistry of
New Jersey—New Jersey Medical School
Newark, New Jersey

TAMARA KALIR, MD, PhD
Assistant Professor of Pathology
Mount Sinai School of Medicine
New York, New York

RUTH KREITZER, MD
Associate Professor Emeritus
Mount Sinai Medical Center
New York, New York

HANNAH R. KRIGMAN, MD
Department of Pathology
Division of Surgical Pathology
The University of Texas Medical Branch
at Galveston
Galveston, Texas

STANLEY J. ROBBOY, MD
Department of Pathology
Department of Obstetrics and
Gynecology
Comprehensive Cancer Center
Duke University Medical Center
Durham, North Carolina

DANIEL SMITH, MD
Associate Professor of Clinical Obstetrics
and Gynecology
Director, Gynecologic Oncology
College of Physicians and Surgeons of
Columbia University
New York, New York

ALEX W. YOUNG Jr, MD
Clinical Professor of Dermatology
Director, Cutaneous-Vulvar Service
College of Physicians and Surgeons of
Columbia University
New York, New York

CONTENTS

CHAPTER 6

Benign Diseases of the Vagina **165**
Debra S. Heller, MD

■

CHAPTER 7

Malignant Diseases of the Vagina **179**
Debra S. Heller, MD

■

CHAPTER 8

Benign Diseases of the Cervix **197**
Debra S. Heller, MD

■

CHAPTER 9

Malignant Diseases of the Cervix **223**
Debra S. Heller, MD

■

CHAPTER 10

Diethylstilbestrol (DES) and the Lower Genital Tract   **271**

Stanley J. Robboy, MD, Rex C. Bentley, MD, Hannah R. Krigman, MD, and Malcolm C. Anderson, FRCPath, FRCOG

■

CHAPTER 11

The Role of Molecular Pathology in Diseases of the Lower Female Genital Tract   **305**

Tamara Kalir, MD, PhD

■

EXAMINATION OF THE VULVA AND VAGINA
The Evaluation of Vulvar Cutaneous Disorders

Alex W. Young, Jr, MD

■

Patient's History
Examination of a Patient with a Vulvar Cutaneous Disease
Vaginal Discharge and Its Relation to Vulvar Cutaneous Disease
Diagnostic Tests: Office and Laboratory
Office Procedures and Tests
Cytodiagnosis
Culture: Viral, Fungal, and Bacterial
Biopsy

The diagnosis of vulvar disease is based on history, morphologic examination, and diagnostic procedures as indicated.

Obtaining a history from a patient with a cutaneous vulvar problem requires extensive patience and time, and an unusual degree of tactfulness on the part of the physician. In many instances, the patient is reluctant to discuss her problem while simultaneously being fearful that a serious condition may exist or that successful treatment is hopeless. Many patients at the time of presentation have already consulted a host of physicians without experiencing improvement in their condition, and they even may have used medication that resulted in a worsening of the complaint.

Examination of a patient with a vulvar complaint or disorder is not limited to observing the vulvar area alone but must include a close inspection of the glabrous skin of the hands and feet, axillae, and scalp as well as the mucous membranes of the mouth. One must remember that the vulva is subject to both gynecologic and dermatologic disorders, and the expertise of both specialties may be required to reach a diagnosis and institute appropriate management.

Diagnostic office and laboratory procedures are often necessary to determine whether vaginitis or vaginosis plays a primary part in the presenting vulvar condition. Not all vaginal discharges appearing at the vulva indicate a pathologic condition; some are physiological.

PATIENT'S HISTORY

SIGNIFICANCE OF SYMPTOMS AS DESCRIBED BY THE PATIENT

A number of disorders of the vulva are characterized by a specific set of symptoms that may point to a diagnosis. The course and development of the complaint, whether it is an intermittent or persistent symptom, and its relation to **exercise, types of clothing, menstrual cycles, sexual intercourse,** and **time of most severity over a 24-hour period** are important elements to note in the patient's history. These features may provide early clues to the diagnosis and directions to be followed for further investigation. The following are significant presenting complaints:

1. **Acute onset of sharp and disabling pain.** Infection (viral—herpes simplex, herpes zoster; bacterial—furuncle, abscess, chancroid), trauma, and on occasion, self-inflicted injury are the major considerations.
2. **Burning vulva syndrome (vulvar vestibulitis).** Focal discomfort, burning, coital pain, and pain elicited just anterior to the hymenal ring by touching it with a cotton swab are characteristic. The symptoms may have occurred for months or even years, and the patients have often already undergone a variety of treatments, some of which may have worsened the condition.
3. **Ill-defined discomfort, ache, and persistent burning.** This may occur in patients over the age of 50 years. No clinical signs of inflammation, vaginitis, or vaginosis are present, and a biopsy of the involved area is nonspecific. In such cases, a provisional diagnosis of **essential vulvodynia** can be made. One must keep in mind, however, that lichen sclerosus may be preceded by such symptoms and that the patient should be followed for the development of this condition.
4. **Intractable, severe pain, and pruritus.** Persistent and disabling pruritus coupled with pain and scratching can produce lichenification (thickening of the folds of the skin). The condition is usually diagnosed as **lichen simplex** and may be extremely difficult to manage. Taking a careful history is necessary to uncover the underlying aspects of the condition.
5. **Persistent soreness and burning.** This is a nonspecific complaint frequently seen in obese patients and commonly occurring during warmer weather. Heat, moisture, and friction induce intertrigo, which is frequently complicated by a secondary candidiasis. In patients with this condition, diabetes should always be ruled out.

Comment

By the time the patient presents herself for consultation, symptoms related to the vulvar problem frequently have been present over some period of time without response to therapy. At this point, overwhelming concern has been focused upon the vulvar area. Establishing a good rapport with the patient is important as is adequately explaining the disorder, the diagnosis, and the options for management once a diagnosis has been firmly established. The patient should be assured that some help can be offered.

Chief Symptom and Present Illness

Because disorders of the vulva cross many medical disciplines, namely dermatology, gynecology, general medicine, and infectious disease medicine,the history obtained must be inclusive but flexible enough to focus specific attention on the areas of special concern to the patient.

The patient's description of her symptoms is particularly significant and may suggest a diagnosis or special areas to be investigated in depth. The date of onset of the symptoms; the duration of the symptoms; and the characteristics of the symptoms, whether sudden and acute, progressive, continuous, or intermittent, are initial questions. What relieves or aggravates the condition and how the condition is affected by coitus, type of sexual practices, pressure from clothing, stress, anxiety, fatigue, and the menstrual cycle are additional questions to be asked.

Obtaining information regarding the past and current treatment, previous test results, and diagnoses from the referring physician is important. Having the patient bring all her previous medications with her on her first visit and having her describe how the condition responded to treatment is a wise course of action.

Contributing History

For completion, a vulvar history must include inquiry concerning **vulvar hygiene** (use of douches; menstrual hygiene and protection; use of soaps, powders, sprays, perfumes, and detergents; and types of clothing materials worn), **contraceptive practices, genitourinary symptoms,** and **obstetrical history.**

Past History
A history of dermatologic and gynecologic problems may be helpful in providing clues concerning the diagnosis of the presenting situation. Histories of eczema (atopic dermatitis), acne, psoriasis, urticaria, seborrheic dermatitis, contact sensitivity, infections, hay fever, or asthma in the family or patient should be noted as these conditions may contribute to the diagnosis.

Family History
This history includes the points enumerated in the previous section.

General Medical History
This section of the complete history includes information concerning the most recent physical examination and laboratory values, past hospitalizations, current medical diagnoses, and current medications. Histories of diabetes, anemia, gastrointestinal problems, and urological problems are areas to discuss with the patient.

Comment

Although many of the points or items described in a vulvar history may appear to be repetitious, one must realize that many of the same or similar questions should be asked in different ways and at different times during the course of history-taking in order to minimize omissions.

EXAMINATION OF A PATIENT WITH A VULVAR CUTANEOUS DISEASE

The glabrous (nonhairbearing) skin of the hands and feet as well as the axillae and scalp should be examined. Any evidence of cutaneous disease should be noted, with particular attention to pigmented lesions, such as nevi, and the presence of papules and nodules. A breast examination and palpation of both axillary and inguinal-femoral areas for abnormal lymph nodes, whose presence might suggest a neoplastic, inflammatory, or systemic disorder, are in keeping with a complete examination. Inspection of the oral mucosa should not be overlooked.

With the patient in stirrups and suitably draped, the vulva and surrounding areas including the mons pubis, medial aspects of the upper thighs, anus, perianal area, and distal portion of the intergluteal fold are exposed for examination using a proper light source. With gloved hands, the physician should inspect the skin surfaces, hairs, and hair follicles for any abnormalities such as inflammation or plugging. The intertriginous areas of the interlabial sulci and labial-crural folds require special attention to detect erythema, scaling, discharge, or other residuum. To conduct a thorough examination, a magnifying lens may be a useful tool. The use of vital stains such as toluidine blue or acetic acid (aceto-whitening) is rare at this time because of difficulties in interpreting the results.

Inspection of both surfaces of the labia minora is best achieved by gently stretching them outward. The presence (absent in lichen sclerosus), number, size, and distribution of Fordyce spots (sebaceous glands) should be noted at this time. Exposure of the glans clitoris is accomplished by retraction of the prepuce using very modest pressure because this may be painful to the patient or impossible (phimosis) if the patient suffers from lichen sclerosus.

The vestibule is that portion of the vulva external to the hymen that extends from the clitoris to the fourchette and is medial to Hart's line. The vagina, ducts of the Bartholin's glands, Skene's ducts, and the urethra open into the vestibule. Minor vestibular glands (mucous) and Fordyce spots are found within this structure.

No matter how small or large the lesion—whether an inflammatory dermatitis, ulcer, papule, nodule, or mass—palpation is necessary to determine whether it is soft or firm, fluctuant, cystic or solid, tender or nontender, and defined or ill-defined. Sensitivity of the lesion may be determined by probing with a cotton swab. A focus of tenderness is especially to be noted just anterior to the hymenal ring in vulvar vestibulitis. Palpation of the Bartholin glands, urethra, and paraurethral ducts is an essential part of the vulvar examination.

If histories of sexually transmitted disease, urinary tract infection, dysuria, or urinary incontinence have been noted, milking the paraurethral ducts and urethra in an attempt to obtain material for culture and testing for antibiotic sensitivity should be attempted.

Finally, consideration should be given to obtaining a photograph of the presenting condition, if permission is given, in order to record the presenting condition and its response to treatment. This is particularly helpful when prolonged follow-up is required as in the nonneoplastic epithelial disorders of the vulva, pigmented lesions, and lesions of vulvar intraepithelial neoplasia. If the patient wishes to return to her referring gynecologist or dermatologist, the presenting photograph and record of her consultation should be forwarded to him or her.

Once the patient has been properly informed, the examining physician should insert an appropriately sized speculum into the vagina to look for the presence of any discharge, noting the color of the walls of the vagina, general appearance, consistency, odor, and any suggestion of vaginitis or vaginosis.

The cervix should be inspected for discharge, polyp, acute or chronic inflammation, ectropion, or ulceration. The speculum examination of the cervix may reveal small petechial-like hemorrhages, so-called "strawberry spots," which characterize trichomonas vaginitis. Cultures of any abnormal vaginal discharge are obtained, pH of the vagina is taken, and an estrogen maturation index and a Papanicolaou smear are also obtained. A bimanual pelvic and rectal examination complete the investigation. A sample examination form and letter to the referring physician are shown in Figures 1.1 and 1.2.

Following the examination, a few minutes spent showing the patient the structures of the vulva using a hand mirror and explaining the nature and morphology of the disorder will help her understand the problem and promote compliance. Using this technique, the proper application of local medication can be demonstrated. Frequently, using a diagram of the vulva after the clinical examination when the patient is seen in the consultation room helps detail future management and underscore the clinical findings.

If a biopsy or surgical procedure is required, a detailed explanation is provided and the patient is reassured that the procedure is necessary, that no mutilation will occur, and that her sexual feelings will not change.

VAGINAL DISCHARGE AND ITS RELATION TO VULVAR CUTANEOUS DISEASE

Not all vaginal discharges appearing at the vulva indicate a pathological condition. Some are physiological and arise from the cervix at the time of ovulation. Others may be more chronic in character and arise from the use of oral contraceptive pills or estrogens, which perhaps had been prescribed for the treatment of menopausal symptoms. In some cases, an annoying and constant but otherwise asymptomatic vaginal discharge requiring the use of a protective panty shield may become a major concern to the patient.

Judging the amount and character of discharge can be entirely subjective on the part of the patient. An asymptomatic, watery, and sometimes blood-tinged discharge may appear at the vulva, especially in elderly patients, without being noticed. This may signify a malignancy in the fallopian tube, uterine cavity, cervix, or vagina and will require careful investigation. Most discharges seen on the vulva arise from a vaginitis or vaginosis, which upon reaching the vulva, may or may not irritate the tissues to produce erythema, soreness, itchiness, a burning sensation, or a combination of these. The discharge may be odorous; white, grayish-yellow, or pink in color; and creamy, thick, or watery in consistency.

When a discharge is perceived or judged to be a factor in producing or exacerbating the presenting vulvar condition, study of the discharge is mandated. This may include the following: vaginal pH; normal saline and KOH microscopic preparations; culture for bacterial, viral, and fungal organisms; and Tzanck smear for exfoliative cytology.

DIAGNOSTIC TESTS: OFFICE AND LABORATORY

The initial step in making a diagnosis of a vulvar disorder is compiling a history that focuses on the dermatological and gynecological aspects of the presenting complaint

CUTANEOUS-VULVAR PROGRAM

**COLUMBIA UNIVERSITY, COLLEGE OF
P&S**

VULVAR CONSULTATION

NAME:_________________________ **DATE:** ____________ **AGE:**______

CHIEF COMPLAINT: _____________________________________

____

PAST/CURRENT THERAPY: _______________________________

____

PAST HISTORY (Med., Derm., Gyn-parity, Surg., Allergy, Drug): _______________

____

VULVAR EXAMINATION:

VAGINAL: _______________________ GLABROUS:____________

PELVIC: ____

IMPRESSION: _____________________________________

TREATMENT: _____________________________________

____

SIGNATURE: _______________________ MD

and the influence other systems may play in causing the condition or altering its course. This program is followed by a cutaneous, vulvar, and gynecological examination and the determination of which routine or special laboratory tests are indicated to aid in the diagnosis or confirm the impression. These tests are performed at the time of examination and, for the most part, are office procedures. Depending upon the need for more sophisticated techniques, the use of outside laboratory facilities may be required.

OFFICE PROCEDURES AND TESTS

Common office procedures include **normal saline wet-mount vaginal smears** (for *Trichomonas, Gardnerella, Mobiluncus,* and *Lactobacillus*) and **potassium hydroxide (KOH)** (for *Candida albicans* and *Candida glabrata* [*Torulopsis*]) (Fig. 1.3).

A drop of fresh normal saline is placed on a clean glass slide and mixed with a specimen obtained from the speculum using the end of a cotton-tipped applicator. A cover slip is applied, and the preparation is examined under the microscope. The active, ovoid-shaped flagellated trichomonads are easily identified by their active motility. The "clue cells" of *Gardnerella vaginalis* may also be identified in this preparation. Clue cells are recognized as clusters of coccobacilli on the surface of desquamated epithelial cells. When clue cells are seen in the presence of a pruritic vulvitis, a "fishy" odor is present, and a vaginal pH test indicates a level of 5.0 or 6.0, the diagnosis of *Gardnerella* (bacterial vaginosis) can be made.

Mobiluncus mulieris and *curtissi* are characterized by curved rods with corkscrew mobility and are frequently seen in bacterial vaginosis in association with *Gardnerella vaginalis.* An increase in *Lactobacilli* (*Doderlein bacilli*), which are pleomorphic; aerobic bacteria; or facultative anaerobic non–spore forming bacteria is associated with cytolytic vaginosis (1). The condition is characterized by the absence of *Trichomonas, Gardnerella,* or *Candida;* a paucity of white blood cells and evidence of cytolysis; and pH ranges from 3.5 to 4.5.

Candida, which is responsible for the majority of vulvo-vaginal infections, is easily identified in a 10% KOH preparation by identifying the candidal hyphae and spores. Most of the cellular material and debris are dissolved by this preparation. When a large number of spores alone are seen, *Candida (Torulopsis) glabrata* infection is suggested. The technique requires mixing a drop or two of KOH with a drop of vaginal secretion and viewing the specimen under lowered stage light.

CYTODIAGNOSIS

The Tzanck test (2), an exfoliative cytology test, was developed by Arnault Tzanck and is helpful in identifying herpes simplex virus (HSV). In evaluation of possible HSV,

FIGURE 1.1.   History and examination sheet from the Cutaneous-Vulvar Program, Columbia University, College of Physicians and Surgeons outlines the essential features to be included in working up a vulvar problem, with a diagram of the vulvar area to be completed by the examiner. To be added to this outline are relevant history, including the relation of the symptoms to the menstrual cycle, preferred methods of contraception and menstrual hygiene, pregnancies and their outcomes, clothing material usually worn, and possible relation to contacts, such as soaps, sprays, etc.

COLUMBIA-PRESBYTERIAN DERMATOLOGY ASSOCIATES
16 EAST 60TH STREET
NEW YORK, N.Y. 10022
TEL. (212) 326-8465
FAX (212) 326-8567

Date: _________________________

Dear

Thank you for giving us the privilege of seeing your patient
_________________________________ in consultation. She was examined by our
group on _____________________ .

Her history and clinical findings strongly suggest a diagnosis of
____ .

According to our current protocol, we have prescribed the following treatment
plan and will see her in four to six weeks. At this time, we will re-evaluate her clinical
progress and symptoms and possibly change or adjust her medication.

Initial Treatment/Management Plan:
1.

2.

3.

4.

Thank you for referring this interesting patient to our service. Should you have
any questions, please don't hesitate to call me during telephone hours on Tuesday,
Wednesday, or Thursday from 1:00 to 1:30 at (212) 326-8450.

Sincerely yours,

Alexander W. Young, Jr., MD
Director, The Cutaneous-Vulvar Service

FIGURE 1.2. Sample consultation, a brief note to be sent to the referring physician.

examining a new lesion, either a vesicle or pustule, is the most productive method. The
lesion is wiped with alcohol and allowed to dry, following which the vesicle is unroofed
and a scraping of the base of the vesicle is obtained, smeared on a glass slide, and allowed
to air dry. A variety of stains, including toluidine blue, are commonly used to identify
the multinucleated giant cells with homogeneously stained "ground glass" nuclei that
characterize HSV infection; intranuclear viral inclusions (Lipschutz or Cowdry) may be

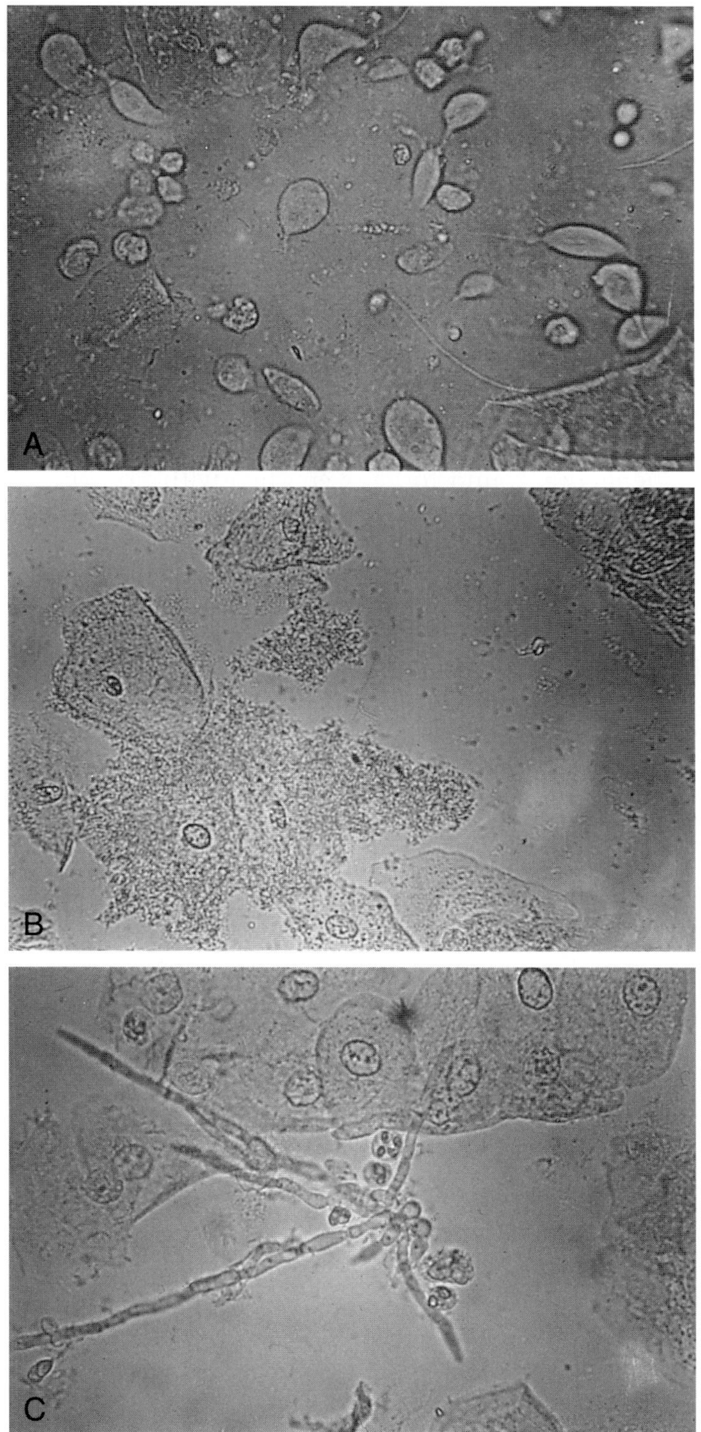

FIGURE 1.3.   Wet smears. **A.** Normal saline preparation showing trichomonas. **B.** Normal saline preparation showing the "clue cells" of *Gardnerella vaginalis*. **C.** KOH preparation showing *Candida*.

seen with dyes containing eosin. The Tzanck test may also reveal malignant cells or acantholytic cells suggestive of bullous dermatoses.

CULTURE: VIRAL, FUNGAL, AND BACTERIAL

When deemed appropriate, cultures are generally taken at the time of the initial examination in conjunction with the wet mount and Tzanck test as indicated. The material is obtained in the same manner as the other two tests.

A viral culture is an essential step in the diagnosis and management of one of the various clinical types of HSV infections and in differentiating these from a host of ulcerative conditions that may affect the vulva. A positive culture for HSV is more reliable than the Tzanck test; however, both must be done within a reasonable time after onset of the infection, preferably within 1 to 3 days.

Cultures of the vaginal discharge other than for fungi detection are of limited use because they are frequently found to be overgrown with nonpathogenic organisms. They may, however, be of value since a report of "normal genital flora" can rule out other complicating organisms.

Superficial (cutaneous) fungi are evidenced as a slightly scaling, sometimes erythematous, plaque-like lesion having an active scaling border located on the inner thighs. *Candida* infection appearing in the crural area and inner thighs is red, well defined, with satellite vesicopustules. A scraping of the periphery of this type of lesion with a #15 scalpel blade is easily done; the material collected is placed on a glass slide, a drop of KOH is added, and a cover slip is applied. The slide is then gently heated to dissolve any keratinous material and examined under the microscope for hyphal elements. Culture of this material on Sabouraud's dextrose agar with cyclohexamine and chloramphenicol to inhibit contaminant growth is routinely recommended.

BIOPSY

A biopsy should be taken whenever doubt concerning the nature of the lesion exists and confirming the clinical impression is necessary. Concern for the possibility of malignancy is always present in cases in which a diagnosis is not apparent. Two types of cutaneous biopsies are available; both require local anesthesia and are performed as office procedures.

PUNCH BIOPSY

A simple punch biopsy may be performed at the time of the first visit without undue apprehension on the part of the patient if one takes the time to explain the purpose of the procedure and its simplicity. A disposable Keyes cutaneous punch is the most satisfactory tool for performing a biopsy (Fig. 1.4). The 3 mm or 4 mm size is my usual choice. After preparing the site with an alcohol wipe and injecting subcutaneously 3 to 6 cc of a 2% lidocaine (Xylocaine) solution with or without epinephrine, the tissue for biopsy is gently compressed between the thumb and index finger and the punch is firmly pressed through the dermis into the subcutaneous fat. Thereafter, a cylindrical plug of tissue can be raised and cut away from the underlying tissue with a fine pair of conjunctival scissors. As a rule, no sutures are required; however, a 3–0 gut chromic suture can be used. The application of a few drops of Monsel's

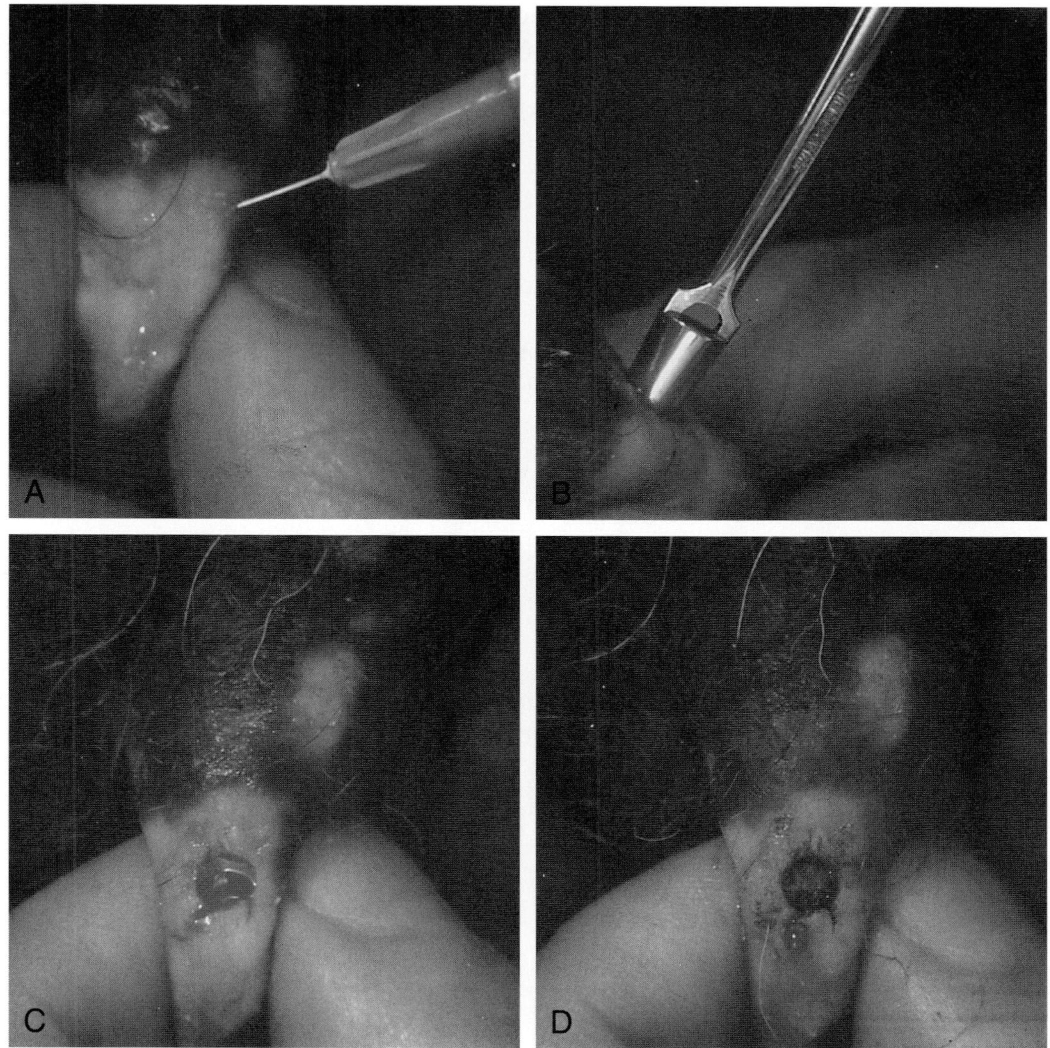

FIGURE 1.4.   Keyes punch biopsy technique. **A.** Induction of local anesthesia. **B.** 4 mm Keyes punch biopsy. **C.** Biopsy site. **D.** Biopsy site after application of Monsel's solution. Reprinted with permission from Chapman & Hall, New York.

solution or 50% solution of aluminum chloride applied with a cotton-tipped applicator may suffice for hemostasis.

In selected cases, it may be reasonable to admit the patient to an ambulatory surgical pavilion when multiple biopsies are indicated, as is necessary for long-standing, nonresponsive vulvar nonneoplastic epithelial disorders, multifocal carcinoma-in-situ, or suspected neoplasia.

EXCISIONAL BIOPSY

A number of conditions are best managed by excisional biopsies, including adnexal tumors, nevi, pigmented lesions, papules, nodules, and other conditions that can be removed using a #15 Bard-Parker scalpel blade. Care must be taken to make an elliptical incision perpendicular to the skin surface, not slanted. The length should be 2.5–3 times the required width and preferably located in a skin crease. The incision is closed with a single layer of interrupted sutures using a fine, synthetic, absorbable, monofilament suture material on an atraumatic cutting needle. The patient is instructed to use ice packs and warm sitz baths three or four times daily for 3 or 4 days. Healing should occur within the week.

REFERENCES

1. Cibley LJ, Cibley LJ. Cytologic vaginosis. Am J Obstet Gynecol 1991;165(4pt2):1245–1249.
2. Solomon AR. The Tzanck smear. Int J Dermatol 1986;25:169–170.

2

DIAGNOSTIC AND THERAPEUTIC PROCEDURES IN THE TREATMENT OF LOWER FEMALE GENITAL TRACT PATHOLOGY

Daniel Smith, MD

■

Diagnosis and Colposcopy
Therapy
Human *Papillomavirus* (HPV)
Summary

Interest in the origins of invasive malignancies of the lower female genital tract has led investigators to develop techniques and procedures that have dramatically affected the care and outcome of women with all degrees of preinvasive conditions of the lower genital tract. The combination of physical examination, Papanicolaou screening, colposcopy, directed biopsies, and selective treatment methods allows the patient the most surety, safety, and best expected outcome. Despite these advances in diagnosis and treatment, patients must continue to have careful, periodic evaluations for possible recurrence or associated conditions.

Care of women with potentially preinvasive conditions of the lower genital tract has evolved from methods of "nonspecific" screening to techniques of "directed" diagnosis and treatment. The Papanicolaou smear was initially developed as a method of assessing the phase of a woman's estrous cycle. Incidentally, it was noted that malignancies could also be detected using this same technique. Refinements of sample acquisition and slide evaluation have resulted in a powerful tool for screening not only for cervical cancer but also for other conditions of the lower genital tract and other areas. Currently, the Bethesda System of reporting the Papanicolau smear is the standard for characterizing the cervical smear (Tab. 2.1). Automated reading systems are now competing with skilled visual "readers" to maximize the accuracy of interpreting the samples taken.

TABLE 2.1.   The Bethesda System

I. Adequacy of the specimen
  A. Satisfactory for evaluation
  B. Satisfactory for evaluation by limited by...(specify reason)
  C. Unsatisfactory for evaluation...(specify reason)
II. General categorization
  A. Within normal limits
  B. Benign cellular changes
  C. Epithelial cell abnormality
III. Descriptive diagnoses
  A. Benign cellular changes
    1. Infection
    2. Reactive changes
  B. Epithelial cell abnormalities
    1. Squamous cell
      a. Atypical squamous cells of undetermined significance
      b. Low grade squamous intraepithelial lesion
      c. High grade squamous intraepithelial lesion
      d. Squamous cell carcinoma
    2. Glandular cell
      a. Endometrial cells (postmenopausal)
      b. Atypical glandular cells of undetermined significance
      c. Endocervical adenocarcinoma
      d. Endometrial adenocarcinoma
      e. Extrauterine adenocarcinoma
      f. Adenocarcinoma, NOS
    3. Other malignant neoplasms
    4. Hormonal evaluation

Modified from Sherman ME. Cytopathology. In Kurman RJ, ed. Blaustein's Pathology of the Female Genital Tract. 4th ed. New York: Springer-Verlag, 1994:1098.

Nevertheless, the Papanicolaou smear report is still a "screening" method, and it still depends on the clinician to sample the area in question properly and completely.

DIAGNOSIS AND COLPOSCOPY

Ironically, a much more specific system of cervical (as well as vulvar and vaginal) evaluation was developed long before the Papanicolaou smear. In 1925, Hans Henselman pioneered a method of examination of the cervix called colposcopy, in which the cervix was essentially examined by a portable, low-power microscope. Cataloguing his findings, Henselman developed a complex system of terminology that correlated visual surface patterns on the cervix with pathologic degrees of preinvasive disease. Terminology of the visual patterns seen, as well as the names of the pathologic and cytologic diagnoses, have greatly changed. However, this system of correlating visual surface patterns with pathologic diagnosis has allowed directed investigation and directed therapy of women with suspected lesions of the lower genital tract epithelium.

The colposcope, in essence, is a mobile, binocular microscope of low magnification (approximately 8–18×). Additions, such as multiple levels of magnification, mobile holder, and video/photographic equipment are often added (Fig. 2.1). The light source is included in the head of the microscope and can be either a tungsten bulb or a fiber-optic source. A green filter is placed between the light source and the target to highlight the vascular patterns of the dysplastic epithelium.

An average clinician should be able to perform a colposcopic examination in only a few minutes. In addition to the colposcope, the clinician should have appropriate speculae (assorted vaginal and endocervical), materials for performing a PAP smear, large cotton swabs, 3% acetic acid solution, and other instruments necessary for diagnosis (biopsy—ectocervical and endocervical) and therapy (chemo-ablation, cryosurgery, cautery, loop electrosurgical excision procedure). The procedure should be carefully explained to the patient, and an informed consent must be obtained. A medical assistant should be present to position the patient and to handle and label all specimens obtained. (Tab. 2.2, Tab. 2.3) (Figs. 2.2–2.8).

Whether having the vulva, the vagina, or the cervix examined, the patient will be best examined in the lithotomy position. There is little variation in technique of colposcopy for lesions of any part of the lower genital tract; however, each site will need slightly differing attention.

For the vulva, careful examination of the entire vulva may be time-consuming, but it is necessary to evaluate a patient with suspected vulvar neoplasia. Leukoplakia (a hypertrophic condition), particularly common on the vulva but also seen throughout

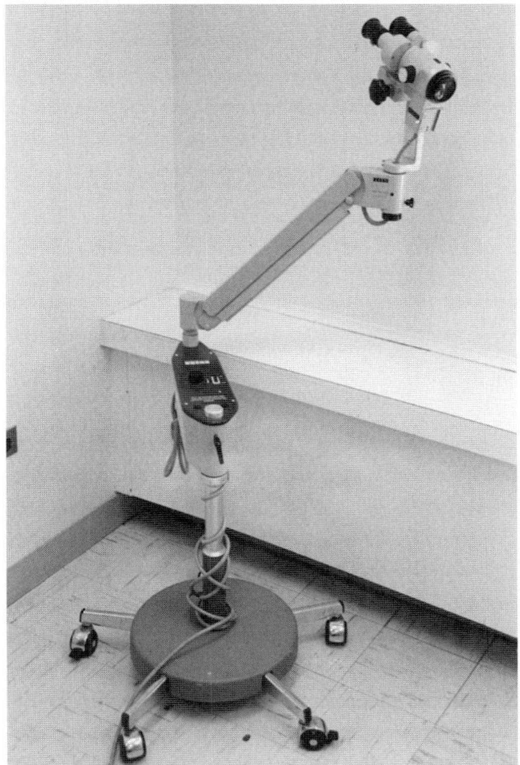

FIGURE 2.1. The colposcope is essentially a low-magnification microscope.

TABLE 2.2. Equipment for Performing Colposcopy

Colposcope
Appropriate speculae
  Vaginal
  Endocervical
Large cotton swabs
3% acetic acid
Cyto brush
Ayre spatula
Biopsy instruments
Hemostasis articles
  Silver nitrate sticks
  Monsel's solution
Slides
Fixative
Labels
Identification markers
Cytology/Pathology slips

TABLE 2.3. Abnormal Colposcopic Findings

          Findings
Condyloma
  Planum
  Accuminata
White epithelium
  Before 3% acetic acid
    Keratosis
    Leukoplakia
  After 3% acetic acid
    Metaplasia
    Punctation
    Mosaicism
    Atypical vessels
Other
  Inflammation
  Trauma
  Polyps
  Invasive lesions-cancer

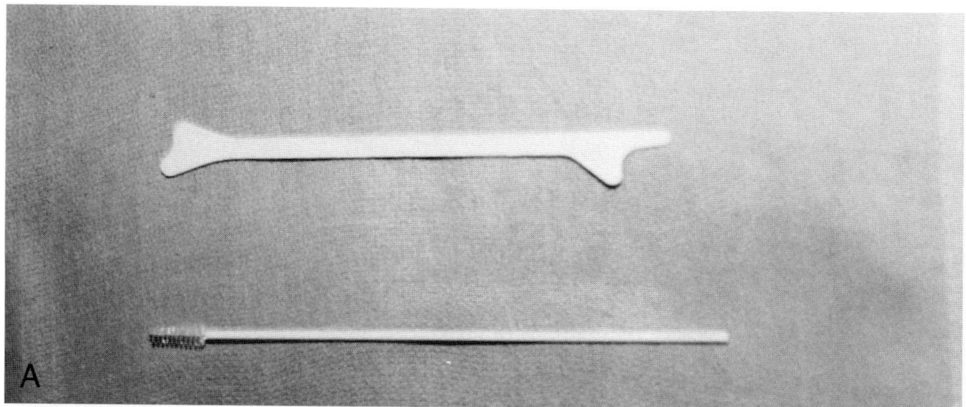

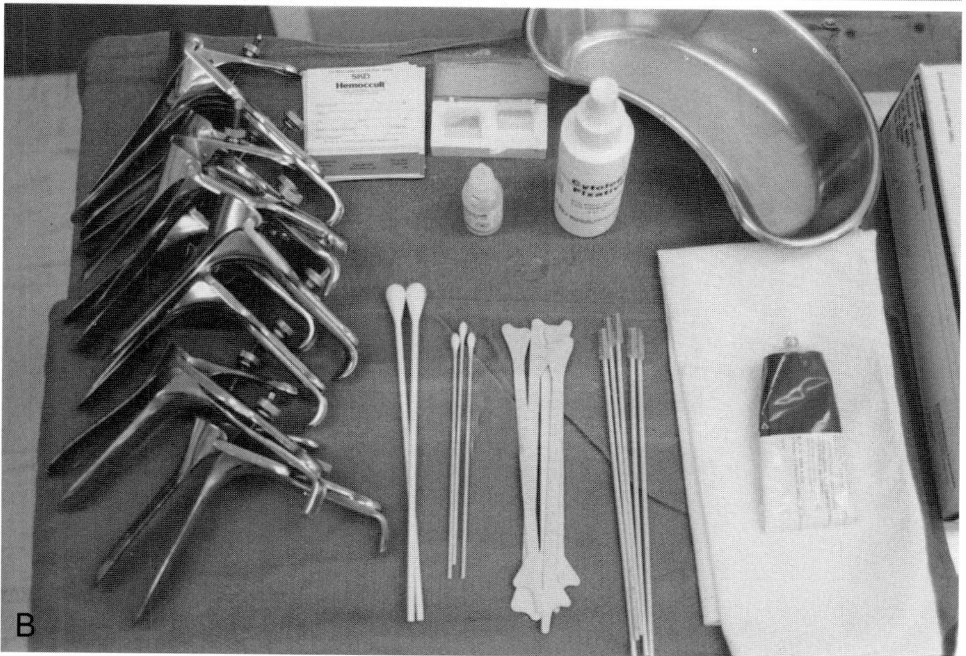

FIGURE 2.2.   **A.** Pap smears may be obtained with an Ayre spatula for ectocervical sampling (top), with endocervical sampling performed with the cytobrush (bottom). **B.** Tray setup for a gynecological examination with speculuae and pap smear equipment.

the lower genital tract epithelium, cannot be evaluated by colposcopy and will always need biopsy and/or excision. Atrophic areas, by contrast, may be well-evaluated by colposcopy and will need biopsy only if there is evidence of atypia or dysplasia.

The vagina has the lowest incidence of dysplasia in the lower genital tract epithelium, but the vagina is also the most difficult to examine. While invasive lesions of the vagina are reportedly more frequent in the posterior fornix, preinvasive lesions can occur in almost any region of the vaginal epithelium. The tangential view of the more proximal vagina makes colposcopy of this region most difficult. However, if a lesion is suspected distally or examination of this area is necessary, careful use of standard vaginal speculuae and additional special retractors will usually allow for a satisfactory examina-

FIGURE 2.3. An endocervical speculum may be used for improved visualization of the endocervical canal.

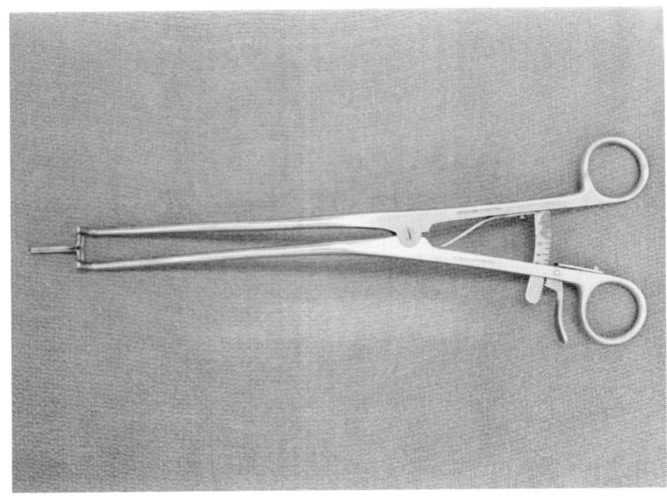

FIGURE 2.4. **A.** An endocervical curette is used to obtain tissue from the endocervical canal. **B.** Directed cervical biopsies are obtained with the punch biopsy instrument.

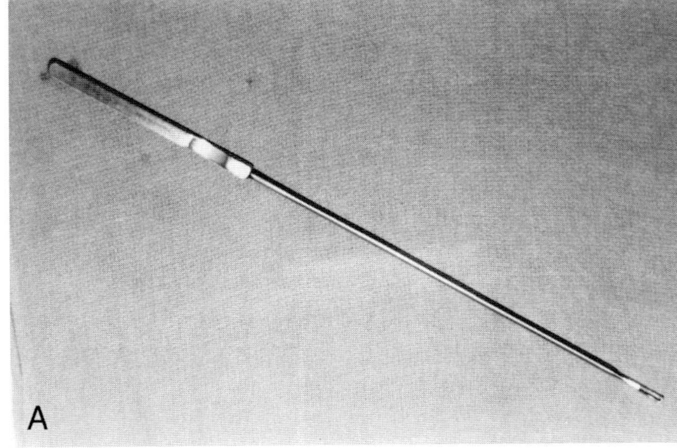

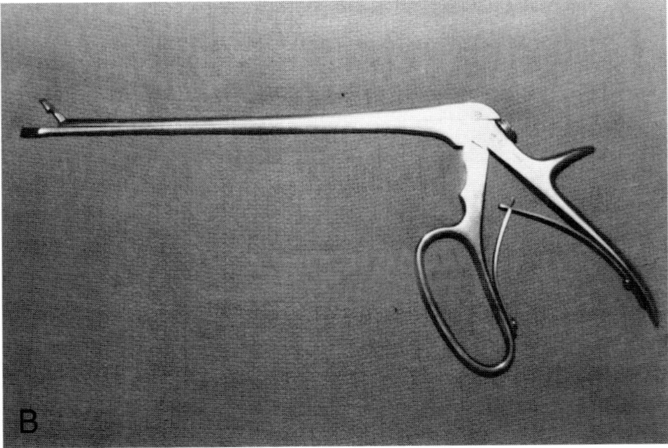

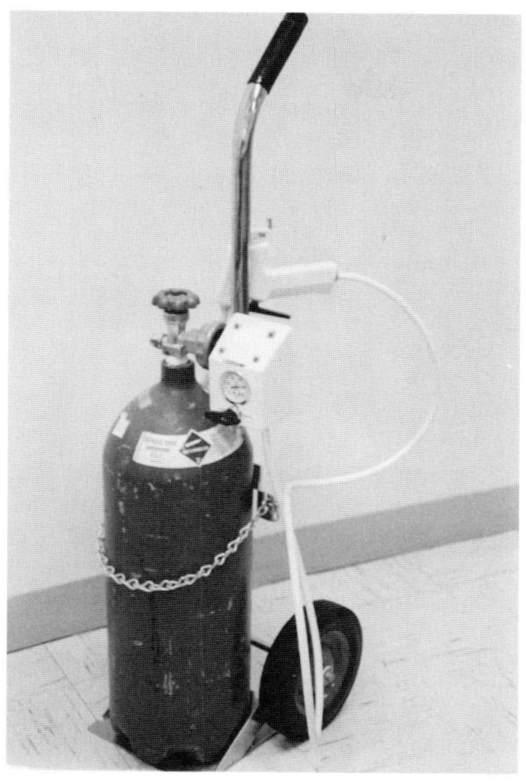

FIGURE 2.5. Cryounit, consisting of nitrous oxide tank connected to applicator.

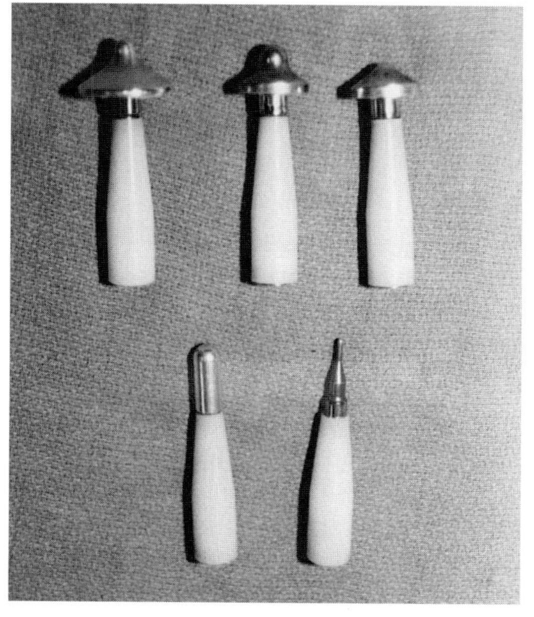

FIGURE 2.6. A variety of cryotips is available.

FIGURE 2.7. CO_2 laser unit.

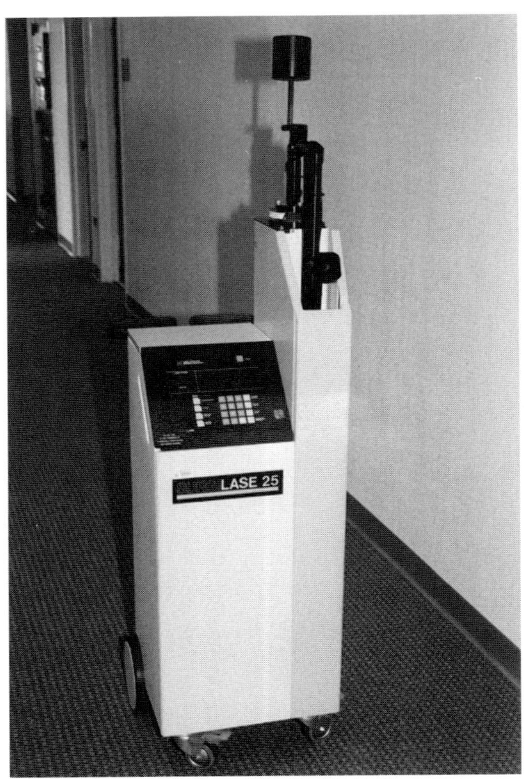

tion. The discomfort of the retraction and vaginal sensitivity may, nevertheless, make biopsy without anesthesia an unsatisfactory option.

In the case of cervical examination, following the placement of a suitable vaginal speculum, the cervix is inspected for gross lesions and another PAP smear is obtained, using a cytobrush for the endocervical specimen and an Ayre spatula for the ectocervical specimen (Fig. 2.2). Both samples are then placed on a single slide, which is then immediately treated with a fixative. The cervix is cleansed with a 3% acetic acid solution for approxiately 3–5 minutes. The solution acts as a mucolytic to cleanse the cervix of mucous and debris. It also causes transient cellular whitening, more pronounced with dysplastic than normal epithelium. The resultant patterns of white epithelium are correlated by the examiner with degrees of premalignant and possible malignant changes in the cervix noted (Fig. 2.9). Specific diagnosis is confirmed by biopsy.

The apparent site of beginning dysplastic changes in the cervix is the squamocolumnar junction. In most menstrating women, this junction of squamous and columnar epithelium is readily identifiable. Dysplastic changes, if present, will occur around this junction. When the entire extent of the squamocolumnar junction can be seen, the colposcopy is said to be "satisfactory." Rarely, a special endocervical speculum will be necessary to open the os of the cervix so that this important area can be identified (Fig. 2.3). With cervical maturity, the process of metaplasia can change the cervix so that the squamocolumnar junction is quite high in the endocervical canal—a condition often encountered in postmenopausal women. An examination where the entire squamocolumnar junction is not visualized is classified as "unsatisfacory" and is noted on

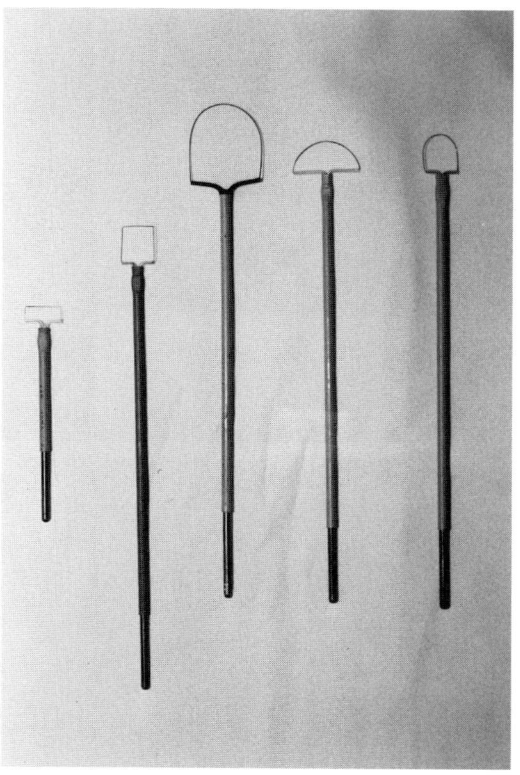

FIGURE 2.8. Loops for LEEP (loop electrosurgical excision procedure).

the patient's chart. Whether the examination is satisfactory or unsatisfactory, an endocervical curettage is performed to sample the endocervical canal. An instrument is used to collect the bloody mucous at the os and include this with the curettings. Ectocervical biopsies are then performed on the most striking or suspicious areas of white epithelium (Fig. 2.4). While anesthesia (e.g., paracervical block) is rarely needed, local hemostatic measures such as silver nitrate sticks or Monsel's solution are sometimes necessary. The accumulated information from physical examination, PAP smear, colposcopy, endocervical curettage, and colposcopically directed biopsies will then be used to determine the treatment according to accepted guidelines.

THERAPY

Therapy of lower genital tract epithelial lesions varies greatly with the location, severity, and extent of the lesions. Invasive cancer should be treated by established protocols and will not be discussed further in this chapter. Preinvasive lesions can basically be treated in the following three ways: 1) observation, 2) ablative methods, and 3) excisional procedures.

Observation is now becoming a recognized and often recommended method of care for many patients with atypical findings or findings with low malignant potential. Not only is the skill of the observer and the completeness of the examination important, but also patient reliability for follow-up care is necessary for good outcome using this method. An adjunct to observation is treatment of coexisting conditions that may nega-

FIGURE 2.9. A. Colpophotograph. An abnormal pattern is present in this colpophotograph of an invasive carcinoma. **B.** Cervicogram. Cervicography has been introduced as a screening procedure requiring less expertise than colposcopy. In cervicography, the cervix is photographed, and the cervicograph is analyzed. This large white lesion was a high-grade squamous intraepithelial lesion on biopsy. Photograph courtesy of T. Wright, Jr, MD.

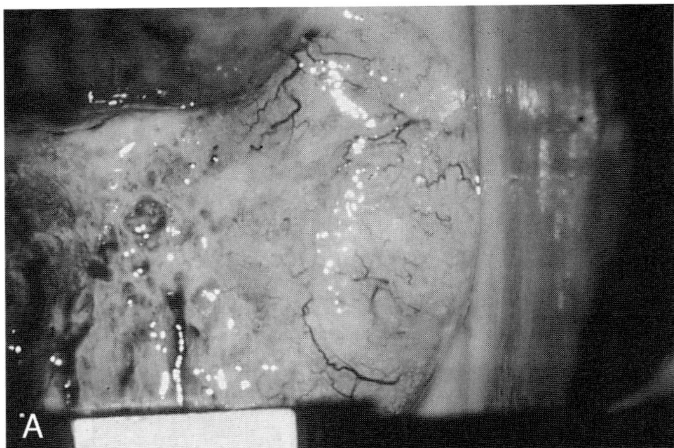

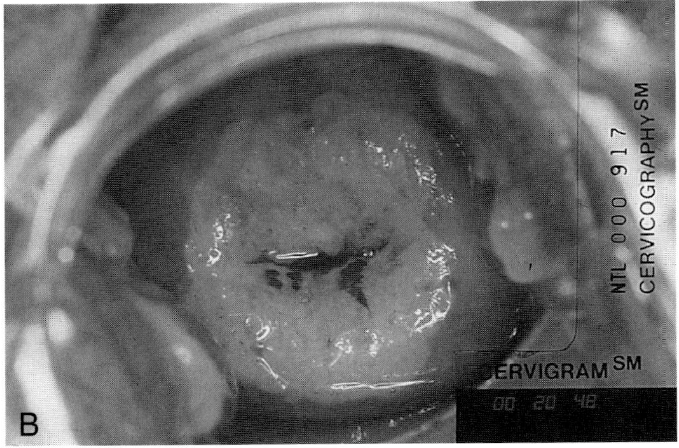

tively affect observations, e.g., inflammation, infection, or atrophic changes. Observation and re-examination following treatment of vulvitis, cervicitis, or atrophic epithelium may result in resolution of lesions initially thought to represent low-grade preinvasive lower genital tract pathology. However, failure of resolution or increasing abnormalities during observation mandate proceeding to other diagnostic and treatment modalities.

Ablative techniques can be effectively and properly used only if one is sure that no invasive malignant disease is present. All areas of suspect lesions must be examined, and multiple, ample samples must confirm the premalignant, noninvasive nature of the lesion. Any significant discrepancy between physical examination (plus colposcopy when indicated), PAP smear, and biopsies would suggest that excision techniques would be preferred to ablation.

Available ablative techniques include chemo-ablation (e.g., trichloracetic acid, podophyllin, 5-fluorouracil cream), cryosurgery (Figs. 2.5, 2.6), cryocautery (rarely used in this country), and LASER (CO_2 LASER) therapy (Fig. 2.7). Appropriate use of each technique depends upon site and extent of the lesion. When depth of therapy is important, ablative procedures may not be as easy to gauge as excisional methods.

Excision of a lower genital tract epithelial lesion is preferred when discrepancies in evaluation exist or when exact depth and clear margins are necessary. Simple excision of any lesion of the vulva, vagina, or cervix has long been a common method of therapy. Cone biopsy of the cervix, in particular, has remained a standard of care for women with cervical lesions that are incompletely seen by colposcopy or have evidence of possibly invasive disease. A variation of the cone biopsy, the loop electrosurgical procedure (commonly called LEETZ or LEEP) (Fig. 2.8) has been applied to therapy of all sites in the epithelium of the lower genital tract—cervix, vagina, and vulva. Often used in an office setting with local anesthesia, loop excision has increased the use of excision as a method of therapy. Excisions of more extensive lesions may necessitate using an operating room. Occasionally, concerns about hemostasis may indicate the need for hospital-based procedures, loop or not, instead of office surgery.

For the vulva, lesions can normally easily be seen. Observation is rarely used to follow vulvar lesions because of the accessibility of the lesion for evaluation, diagnosis, and treatment. Certain ablative techniques (5FU cream, LASER) are useful but can cause extensive pain and discomfort and should be reserved for patients with multifocal premalignant changes and with contraindications to other methods of care. For patients with extensive lesions of the vulva, the most satisfactory procedures for the patient and her physician are either ablative (LASER) or excision, including partial/skinning vulvectomy procedures performed under brief general or regional anesthesia. Following extensive LASER treatment to the vulva, a specific care plan for analgesia and wound care must be implemented to ensure patient comfort and proper healing. The use of oral analgesics, Sitz baths, and liberal applications of Silvadene cream have proved most effective.

Treatment of preinvasive vaginal lesions is more difficult than at other sites mainly because of difficulties in adequately viewing and mapping lesions. The vagina is a corrugated and distensible tube that requires careful and methodical inspection for complete evaluation. Standard vaginal speculae will block views of the anterior and posterior walls near the introitus. The speculum must, therefore, be turned sideways or special vaginal wall retractors should be used for complete viewing. Having described the difficulties in defining lesions, it follows that treatment may also be difficult. The vaginal mucosa is sensitive; thus, cautery, LASER, and loop excision all can cause considerable pain. Local anesthesia is awkward to apply, and often is incomplete. Even cryosurgery may cause significant discomfort and be difficult to use in a specific locale without touching other unaffected areas. For a discrete, localized lesion, operative ablation using the LASER or excision methods (both in the operating room with appropriate anesthesia) may be the most efficacious method of care. For women with multifocal or extensive preinvasive lesions, the use of 5 gm of 5-fluorouracil (5FU) cream nightly for five nights is often recommended. The patients should be cautioned to apply the 5FU cream high in the vagina at night and to douche and wash the vulva thoroughly in the morning. Even with the recommended care, vulvar irritation is common and difficult to ease except with local hygiene and oral analgesics. Although the method is effective in cure, all patients should be counseled and prepared for the painful side effects of this treatment.

The various methods used for treatment of preinvasive cervical epithelium include many new techniques and reapplications of older ones. All of the methods have been studied, and each can have a specific or selective advantage. Ablative techniques, whether chemo-ablative, cryosurgery, or CO_2 LASER treatment, must be selectively used only in those patients in whom the lesions are well defined, completely evaluated, and found to be without any evidence of invasive disease. Use of chemo-ablative material (e.g., 5FU cream) can be useful in patients with multifocal, low-grade lesions often also affecting the vaginal surfaces. The same precautions and complications of therapy apply as with treating primary vaginal lesions. Cryosurgery of the cervix has generally replaced electrocautery due to safety and patient comfort. Cryosurgery can be performed in the case of a preinvasive lesion of the ectocervix with satisfactory colposcopy and a negative endocervical curettage. The instrument is readily available in most clinical settings and uses a nitrous oxide coolant (Figs. 2.5, 2.6). A soluble lubricant is applied to a tip selected to cover the entire lesion when applied (Fig. 2.6). The patient has been counseled about the procedure and has signed a consent. In the lithotomy position, the cervix is again colposcoped. Seeing the lesion and protecting the vagina, the operator applies the tip and begins cooling. An ice ball rim will emanate from the tip and should extend 4–5 mm from the edge of the instrument onto the cervix. With proper coolant pressure, this should occur in 2–4 minutes with moderate cramping felt by the patient. The cervix is allowed to thaw for about 5 minutes, and the freezing is again repeated (freeze-thaw-freeze technique). The patient will experience moderate, watery vaginal discharge for approximately 10–14 days following treatment. An alternative to cryocautery is CO_2 LASER ablation (Fig. 2.7). Criteria for treatment and patient preparation are the same as for cryotherapy. With LASER ablation, however, established safety measures for the patient and attending personnel must be observed (e.g., special nonreflective instruments, eye protection, etc.). Particular attention must be paid to avoiding contact of the LASER beam to the vaginal wall during therapy. Before commencing treatment, most clinicians recommend infiltrating the cervix in the four quandrants with 1% lidocaine with epinephrine. This local injection will provide anesthesia and help with hemostasis. The technique of CO_2 LASER ablation is completely described elsewhere. Briefly said, it accomplishes tissue vaporization of the lesion/transformation zone to a depth of 7 mm. Hemostasis is facilitated by the liberal use of Monsel's solution in the crater following treatment. A LASER cone biopsy has been generally supplanted by other methods of excision.

Excisional therapy for preinvasive cervical lesions provides both adequate therapy and complete pathologic confirmation of the lesion. Cold-knife conization remains the standard of care for patients with possibly invasive lesions, positive endocervical canal curettings, or unsatisfactory colposcopic examination with significant ectocervical lesions. However, the procedure generally includes the following: (1) general or regional anesthesia, (2) an operating room, (3) recovery from anesthesia, and (4) significant concern about hemostasis. While cone biopsy is necessary for the above-mentioned indications, the loop electrosurgical excision procedure (LEEP, LEETZ) is useful in management of less-advanced lesions and can often be safely performed in the practitioner's office. Indications for loop excision are generally those explained for cryocautery. In selected cases, patients with either a positive endocervical curettage or an unsatisfactory colposcopy can be treated/examined by loop excision using additional endocervical passes of the loop. Patient preparation is again similar to that of cryotherapy or LASER treatment. Local anesthesia (with epinephrine) to the cervix is recommended. Using commercially available electrosurgery units, a selected loop (Fig. 2.8) (selected for the size and location of the lesion and the size of the cervix) is used to remove the lesion and the transformation zone. In special cases, a second pass using a more narrow loop is used to further assess the endocervical canal. A separate tip (ball) is used to cauterize the bed of the excision to secure hemostasis. Monsel's solution is again applied to the bed for further hemostasis protection. Patients may experience some posttreatment cramping, which is generally alleviated with nonsteroidal antiinflammatory medications.

TABLE 2.4. Human *papillomavirus* (HPV) Associated Cervical Lesions by Frequently Associated Type

Lesion	HPV Type
Condyloma accuminata	6, 11
Low-grade squamous intraepithelial lesions (SIL)	6, 11, 16, 18, 31, 33, 35, 39, 42, 43, 44, 45, 51, 52, 56
High-grade SIL	16, 18, 31, 33, 35, 39, 45, 51, 52, 56
Invasive carcinoma of cervix	16, 18, 31, 33, 35, 39, 45, 51, 52, 56

* Modified from Wright TC, Jr., Kurman RJ, Ferenczy A. Precancerous lesions of the uterine cervix. In: Kurman RJ, ed. Blaustein's Pathology of the Female Genital Tract. 4th edition. New York: Springer-Verlag, 1994: 235.

HUMAN *PAPILLOMAVIRUS* (HPV)

Human *papillomavirus* is currently implicated as a causative factor in many lower genital tract dysplastic lesions. (Tab. 2.4). Certainly, the virus can also manifest itself in patients with condyloma acuminata of all sites—vulva, vagina, and cervix. Diagnosis of these presumed viral lesions must be confirmed by tissue sampling. Histologic studies will characterize the dysplasia or possibly more severe lesions. Special tissue testing can further categorize the lesions according to human *papillomavirus* subtypes—each with a relatively recognized potential association with benign, premalignant, or malignant changes. Treatment of condyloma can be performed using the guidelines previously described for premalignant lesions of the vulva, vagina, or cervix. Since these lesions are usually associated only with mild to moderate dysplastic changes, treatment is usually by office techniques rather than operative procedures. Altering treatment of dysplastic lesions based upon HPV subtype is currently not suggested. However, the role of HPV subtyping of mild to moderate dysplastic lesions in order either to limit care of nonprogressive lesions or to identify lesions requiring vigorous removal is being studied. It is, in fact, these clinical studies of visual appearance, histologic characterization, and molecular biologic specification that form the exciting frontier in the diagnosis and therapy of preinvasive lower genital tract epithelial abnormalities.

SUMMARY

Despite the many advances in diagnostic techniques and treatment procedures, vigilance in follow-up care is also important for a successful outcome. Treatment failure or recurrent disease can usually be successfully treated. A careful and methodical plan for patient evaluation must be outlined for the patient by the physician. Equally important is patient diligence in attending posttreatment visits. When patients with premalignant lesions of the lower genital tract epithelium are identified, current diagnostic techniques should quickly define the nature and extent of the lesion. Directed procedures can then provide effective therapy. Diligence in follow-up by the patient and physician is necessary to maintain a successful outcome.

Bibliography

Brodman M, Port M, Friedman F. Jr. et al. Operating room personnel morbidity from carbon dioxide laser use during preceptored surgery. Obstet Gynecol 1993;81(4):607–609.

Burke L, Antonioli DA, Ducatman BS. Basic & Advanced Colposcopy: Text and Atlas. Norwalk: Appleton and Lange, 1991.

DiSaia PJ, Creasman WT. Clinical Gynecologic Oncology. St. Louis: Mosby, 1993.

Gage AA. Cryosurgery in the treatment of cancer. Surg Gynecol Obst 1992;174(1):73–92.

Hatch K. Colposcopy of vaginal and vulvar human papillomavirus and adjacent sites. Obstet and Gynecol Clin North America 1993;20(1):203–215.

Kaufman RH. Intraepithelial neoplasia of the vulva. Gynecol Oncol 1995;56(1):8–21.

Mathevet P, Dargent D, Roy, M. et al. A randomized prospective study comparing three techniques of conization: cold knife, laser, and LEEP. Gynecol Oncol 1994;54(2):175–179.

Nuovo GJ. Cytopathology of the Lower Female Genital Tract. Baltimore: Williams & Wilkins, 1994.

Richart RM. The patient with an abnormal PAP smear: screening techniques and management. N Engl J Med 1980;302:332–334.

Sammarco MJ, et al: Local anesthesia for cryosurgery on the cervix. J Repro Med 1993;38(3): 170–172.

Stafl A. Cervicography: A new method for cervical cancer detection. Am J Obstet Gynecol 1988;139:815–825.

Townsend DE, Levine RU, Crum CP, et al. Treatment of vaginal carcinoma in situ with carbon dioxide laser. Am J Obstet Gynecol 1982;143:565.

Townsend DE, Richart RM. Cryotherapy and carbon dioxide laser management of cervical intraepithelial neoplasia: a controlled comparison. Obstet Gynecol 1983;61:75.

3

CYTOLOGY OF THE LOWER FEMALE GENITAL TRACT

Ruth Kreitzer, MD and Diane Hamele-Bena, MD

■

Cytology of Inflammatory and Infectious Processes
The Vulva
The Vagina
The Cervix

The intention of this chapter is to present a comprehensive overview of the basic cytological findings of studies of the vulva, vagina, and cervix using the Pap smear and all it encompasses. Occasionally, if a lesion is easily accessible and palpable, fine needle aspiration biopsy may be used to obtain a cytologic sample. We must emphasize that, although at times diagnostic, the Pap smear is best viewed as a mass screening test. False negative reports may occur due to errors in sampling, screening, and interpretation. The rate of false negatives is directly related to the following factors:

- The experience and technical skill of the clinician obtaining the sample (collection technique, instruments used, proper fixation)
- The accessibility and differentiation of the lesion (obesity or location of a lesion high in the cervical canal preventing visibility, necrotic tumors yielding few or nonviable cells, and well-differentiated neoplasms appearing benign)
- The individual laboratory used (staining, cytotechnology staff, cytopathologist)

A problem with any one or any combination of these elements may ultimately result in an inaccurate diagnosis. Therefore, finding a very large range of false negatives reported in the literature (1.1% to 69%) is not surprising (24, 61). In contrast, a positive cytology report is more reliable. Even though the Pap smear has known limitations, many important diagnostic entities are detected with this inexpensive and easily performed procedure. Early detection by Pap smear followed by the appropriate clinical management has greatly reduced the rate of invasive cervical carcinoma in countries worldwide that routinely use Pap smears.

CYTOLOGY OF INFLAMMATORY AND INFECTIOUS PROCESSES

The vaginal epithelium is responsive to various hormonal, traumatic, infectious, and physiological influences that ultimately affect vaginal squamous cell maturation and pH (8, 45). These factors, in turn, are critical to the composition of the bacterial flora and may influence the growth of pathogens. Although predominantly composed of *Lactobacilli* (Fig. 3.1), the endogenous vaginal flora is polymicrobial (8). An overgrowth of a nonspecific mixed flora (including *Gardnerella, Bacteroides, Prevotella, Mobilunucus, peptococci,*and *peptostreptococci*) is reported according to the Bethesda system (TBS) as *"predominance of coccobacilli consistent with shift in vaginal flora (37); findings are c/w bacterial vaginosis"* (8, 23, 76). Previously, identification of specific organisms was suggested if characteristic changes were present, e.g., "clue cells" of *Haemophilus vaginalis* (*Gardnerella*) (Fig. 3.2). Identification of clue cells is one of the criteria used for diagnosing bacterial vaginosis; however, in a comparison study, Platz-Christensen and colleagues (65) found that detection of clue cells in Pap smears had a sensitivity of only 88.2% and a specificity of 98.6% when compared with the clinical diagnosis of bacterial vaginosis, as compared to 100% and 97.3% for Gram's stains and 100% and 95.9% for wet smears. Therefore, in rendering a diagnosis of bacterial vaginosis, the Pap smear should be used in conjunction with the clinical presentation and wet mount preparations, Gram's stains, and specific microbiologic isolation as indicated.

The lower female genital tract may be infected directly (e.g., *Chlamydia*, human

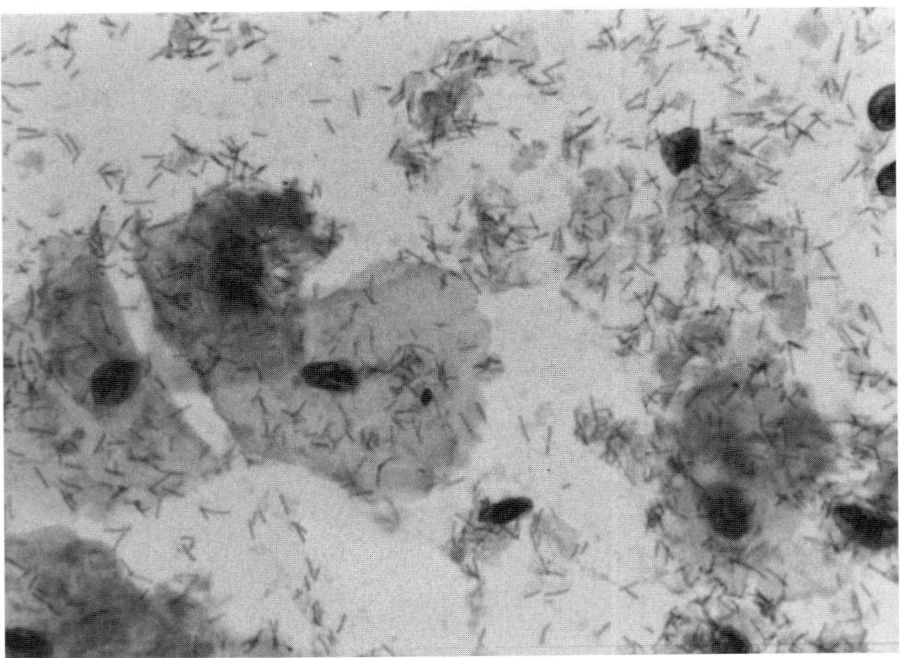

FIGURE 3.1. Lactobacilli (*Doderlein bacilli*) are Gram-positive rods commonly seen amongst intermediate cells in the late luteal phase, pregnancy, and early menopause. The extensive cytolysis (cytoplasmic fragments and naked intermediate cell nuclei) present is secondary to the organisms. (40x)

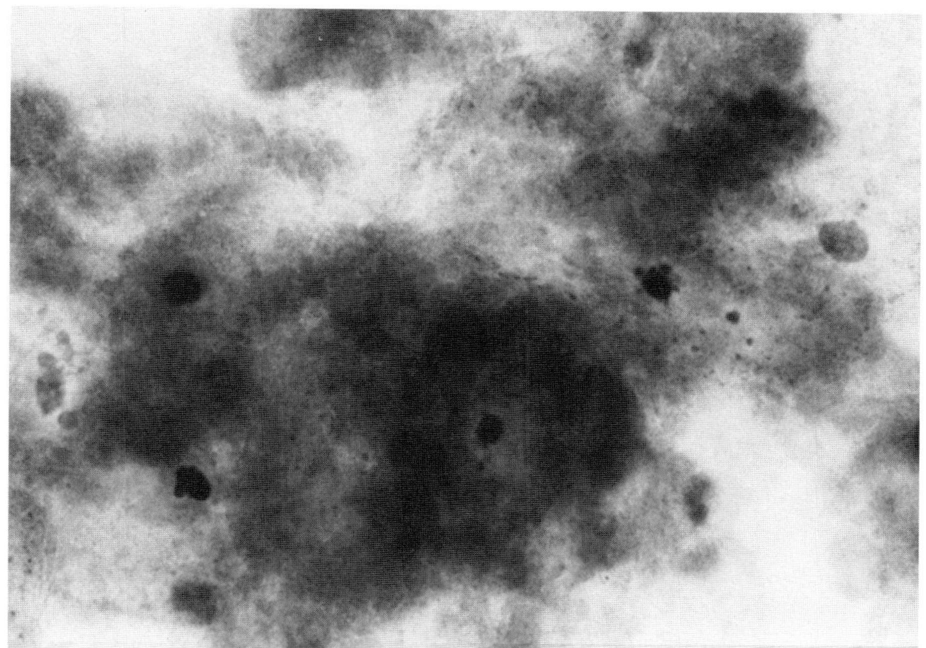

FIGURE 3.2. *Gardnerella vaginalis* (*Haemophilus vaginalis, Corynebacterium vaginalis*). The coccobacillary organisms cover and obscure squamous cells and their margins, creating "clue cells." Clinically, a malodorous discharge may be noted. (40x) (8)

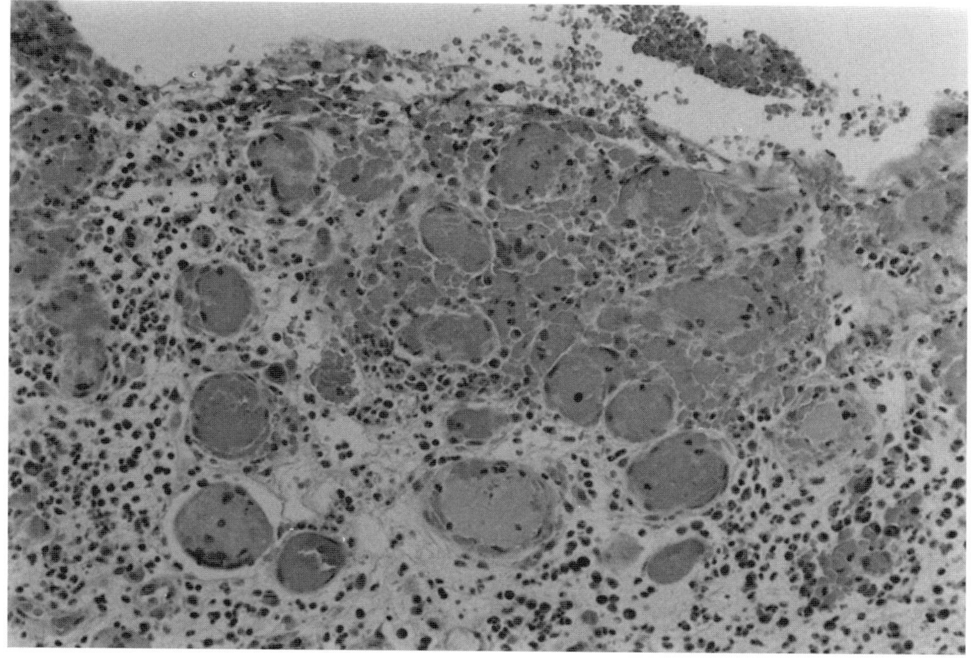

FIGURE 3.3. Cervical biopsy with surface ulceration and underlying exuberant granulation tissue formation (newly formed blood vessels and fibroblastic proliferation) with associated marked acute inflammatory response. (10x)

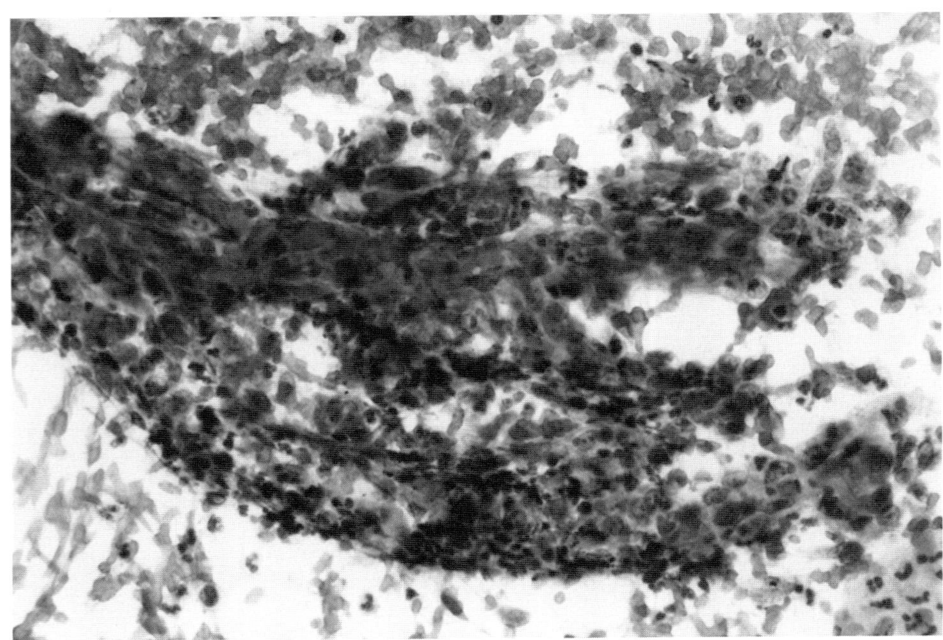

FIGURE 3.4. Pap smear of the same patient as in Figure 3.3 showing delicate capillaries (seen along their long axis) and an intense neutrophilic infiltrate. (20x)

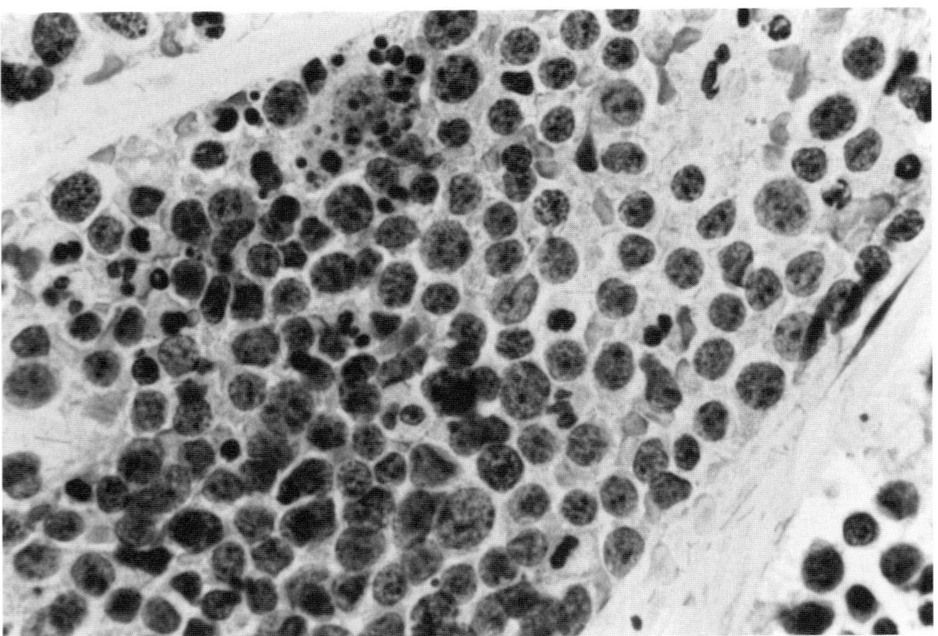

FIGURE 3.5. Follicular cervicitis. A dispersed, heterogenous population of lymphocytes (mature and immature) and tingible-body macrophages are present. Half of the patients with this finding have associated *Chlamydia* infections. Differential diagnoses include nonspecific chronic inflammation and lymphoma/leukemia. (40x) (45)

Papillomavirus [HPV]), by extension from contiguous organs (local abscess), or by a hematogenous route (e.g., tuberculosis) (45). The direct route is the path most commonly encountered, obviously because of the proximity of the organs to the body's exterior. Infected patients may be totally asymptomatic or may present with symptoms specific to the underlying causative agent. For instance, a patient with herpes simplex virus type 2 may be asymptomatic or may present with constitutional symptoms followed by mucosal vesicular lesions and ulcerations causing pain, dysuria, and discharge (8), whereas a patient infected with *Candida albicans* may have no symptoms or may present with intense vulvar pruritus and a white cheesy discharge (8). Whether a patient is symptomatic following exposure depends on her current immune status, hormonal influences, and epithelial and cellular responses.

The covering layer, or epithelium, of the vulva, vagina, and cervix may undergo reactive, degenerative, or dysplastic changes in response to specific organisms or stimuli. **Reactive changes** include ulceration followed by surface repair and stromal healing (granulation tissue) (Figs. 3.3 and 3.4), acute and chronic inflammatory responses (Fig. 3.5), hyperplasia, metaplasia, hyperkeratosis (Fig. 3.6), and parakeratosis (Fig. 3.7). Reactive cellular changes include increased nuclear/cytoplasmic ratio, nucleolar prominence, multinucleation (Fig. 3.8), chromatin smudging or clearing, cytolysis (Fig. 3.1), pseudoeosinophilia, and "syncytial" arrangements (Fig. 3.9). Many cellular alterations are diagnostic of the underlying infection, such as the classic viral inclusions present in

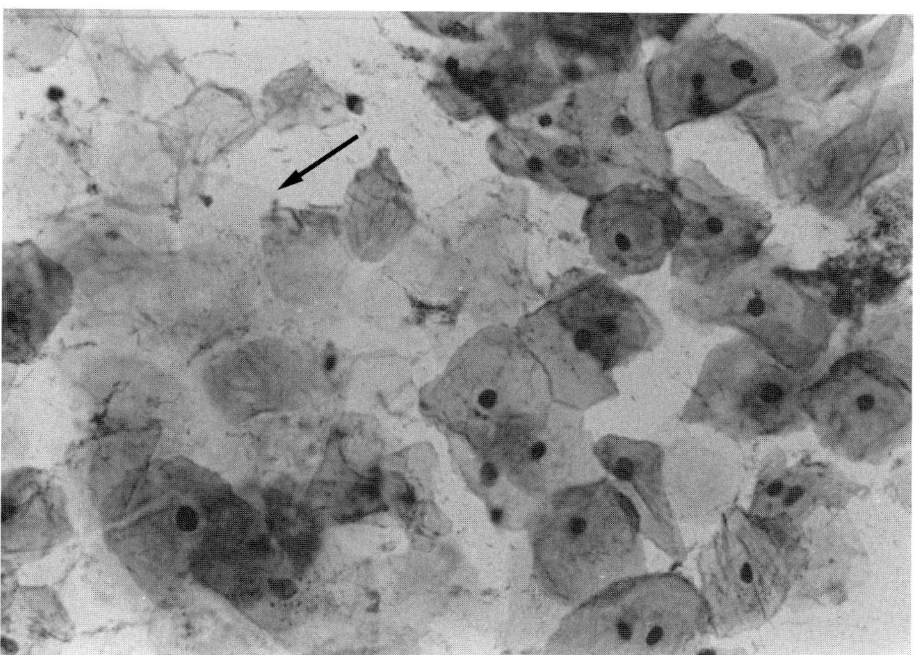

FIGURE 3.6.   Hyperkeratosis. This is a nonspecific finding consisting of plaques and single anucleated squamous cells, which appear yellow-orange in a Pap smear. Clinically, a white patch (leukoplakia) may be seen secondary to excessive surface keratin formation. Hyperkeratosis may be associated with diaphragm or pessary use, *Gardnerella* infection, uterine prolapse, or an underlying squamous lesion; however, often no other pathological finding is noted. (20x)

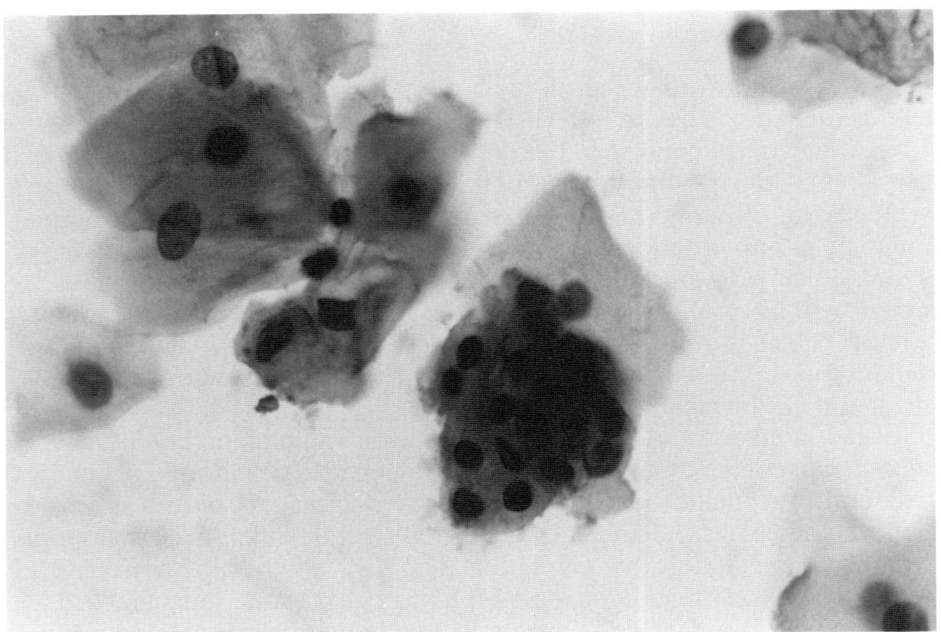

FIGURE 3.7. Parakeratosis. This is another nonspecific finding, consisting of tiny squamous cells with uniform, hyperchromatic nuclei and orangiphilic cytoplasm, which may or may not be keratinized. Parakeratosis may be found in many conditions, including acanthosis (thickened epithelium) and hyperkeratosis, in association with a squamous lesion, or as an isolated finding. (40x)

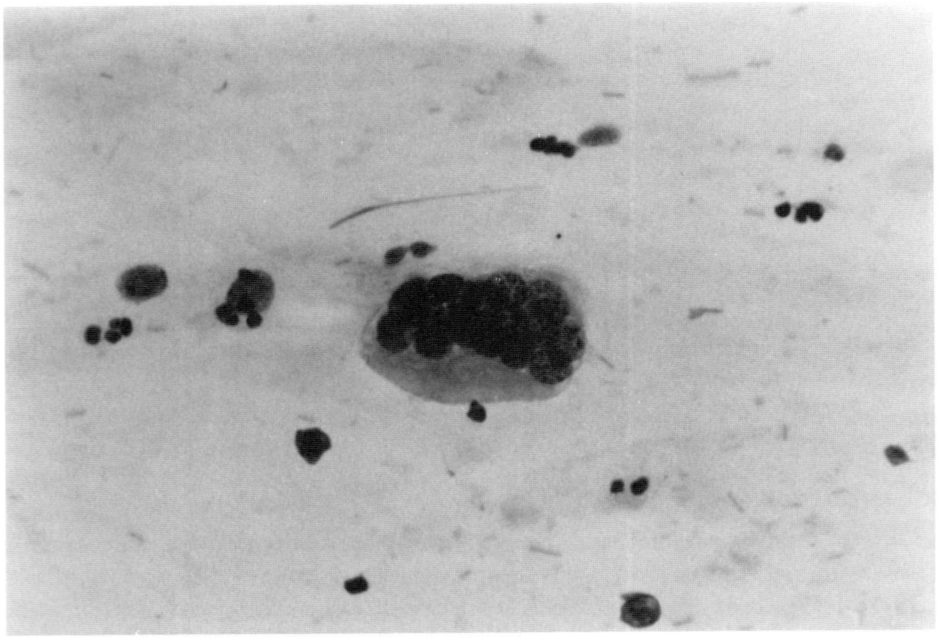

FIGURE 3.8. Reactive multinucleated endocervical cells. The columnarity of the cells is retained and the nuclei are still polarized toward the basal portion of the cells. (40x)

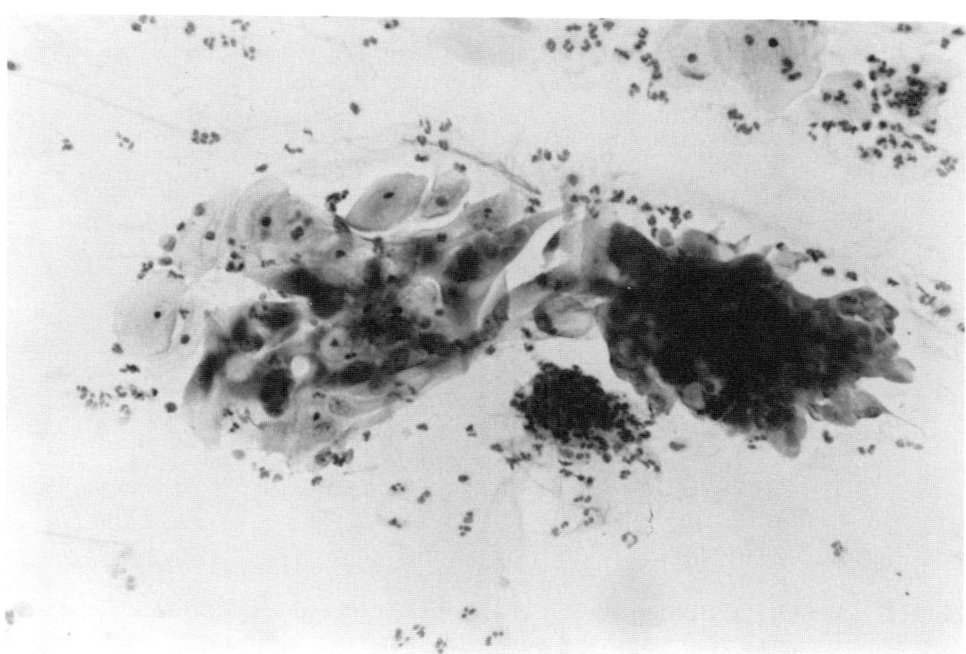

FIGURE 3.9.   Reparative change. "Syncytial" cellular sheets as shown here are typical of reparative change. Note the indistinct cell borders between the cells and the pulled or stretched edges of the sheet. The nuclei are enlarged with open chromatin, prominent nucleoli, and occasional mitoses. (10x)

cytomegalovirus (CMV) infections (Fig. 3.10). Reactive responses may also be observed following exposure to exogenous stimuli. For instance, one may observe syncytial cellular sheets, karyomegaly, cytomegaly, bizarre cells, spindle cells, and a foreign body giant cell reaction following radiation therapy (Figs. 3.11 and 3.12). Foreign materials can induce cellular responses, such as a foreign body giant cell (granulomatous) response with acute or chronic inflammation secondary to suture material (Fig. 3.13). Examining the slide under polarized light may help the detection of foreign material (5). Hyperkeratosis may be present secondary to diaphragm (40) and pessary use, and cytoplasmic vacuolization with or without associated nucleolar prominence may be noted following placement of an interuterine device (IUD). Tissues may also respond to stimuli by proliferating (hyperplasia) or by changing cell type (metaplasia).

Degenerative changes are important to recognize and differentiate from cellular changes that occur in reactive and dysplastic processes. Degenerative changes may involve the cytoplasm, nucleus, or both. Cells undergoing degeneration may exhibit ill-defined perinuclear halos, as in *Trichomonas* infection (Fig. 3.14), which must be differentiated from the perinuclear clearings as seen in koilocytotic atypia secondary to HPV infection. Koilocytes have broad, sharply demarcated perinuclear halos; nuclear atypia; thickened, undulating cytoplasmic borders; and frequent binucleation (Fig. 3.15). Intracytoplasmic vacuoles are another cytoplasmic degenerative change. This finding alone is nonspecific and may be seen in many conditions, including radiation (Fig. 3.16), adenocarcinoma (Fig. 3.17), IUD use (45), and *Chlamydia* (Fig. 3.18) (30). Degenerative processes may also involve the nucleus, resulting in pyknosis (nuclear condensation)

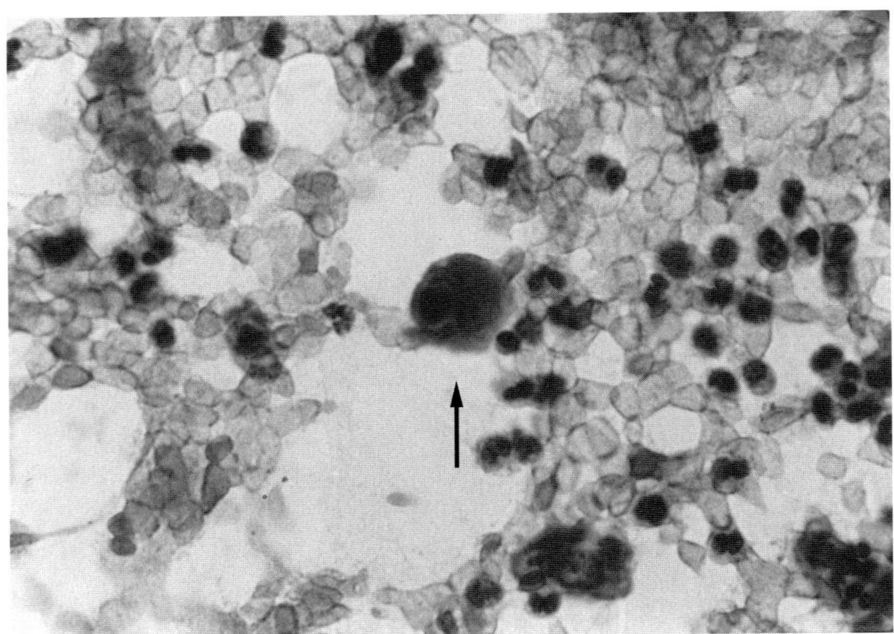

FIGURE 3.10. Cytomegalovirus. Rare, poorly preserved endocervical cells with changes diagnostic of CMV infection are seen in this smear in a background of acute inflammation and fresh blood. The characteristic large intranuclear inclusion is surrouded by a distinct broad halo. Closer inspection reveals fine punctate basophilic inclusions in the cytoplasm. (40x) (8)

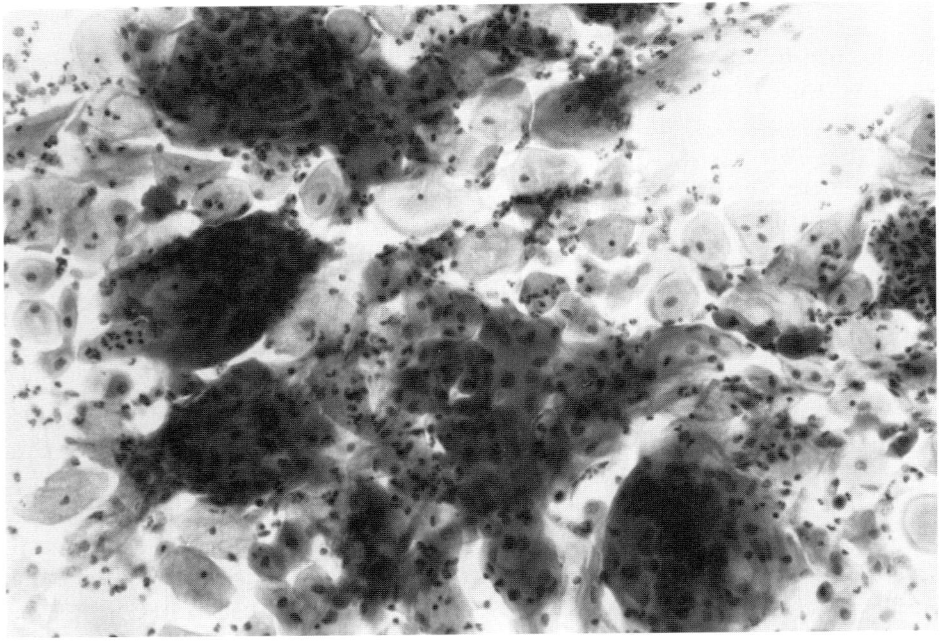

FIGURE 3.11. Radiation effect. One characteristic finding following radiation therapy is the presence of multinucleated foreign body giant cells. In this field, these cells encircle a syncytial sheet of squamous cells. (20x)

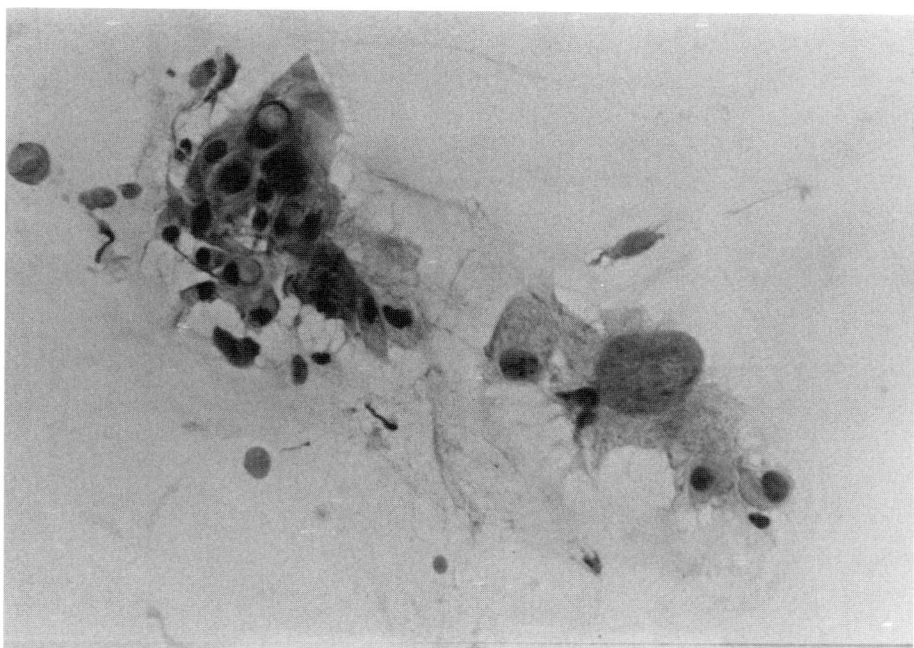

FIGURE 3.12. Endocervical cells displaying radiation changes. One cell shows marked nuclear enlargement without any chromatin changes or nuclear membrane irregularities. Compare this to the adjacent cluster of endocervical cells, which appear normal in size. (20x)

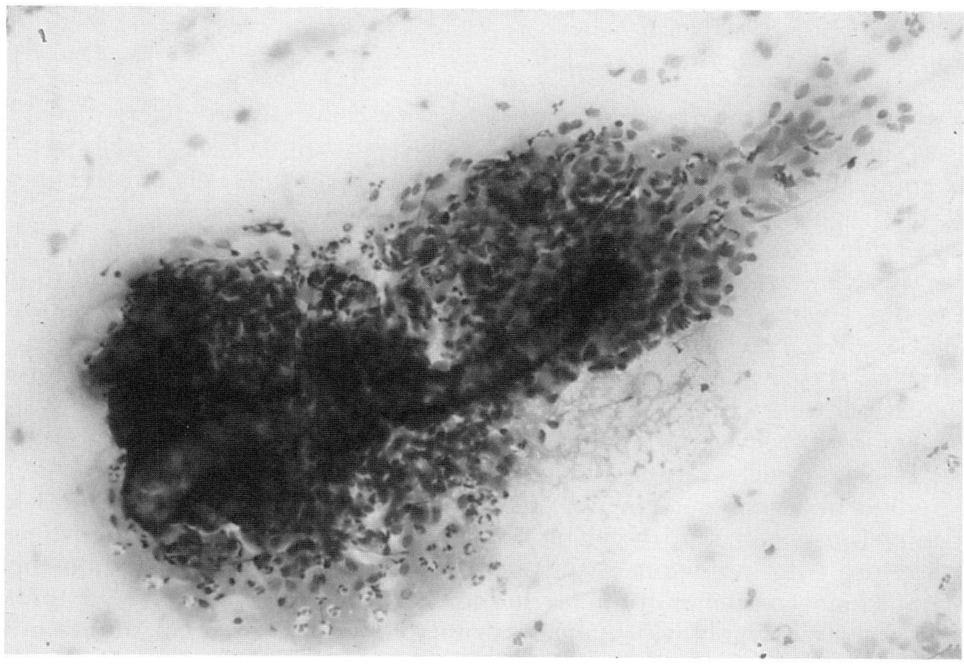

FIGURE 3.13. Granulomatous reaction induced by foreign material. (40x)

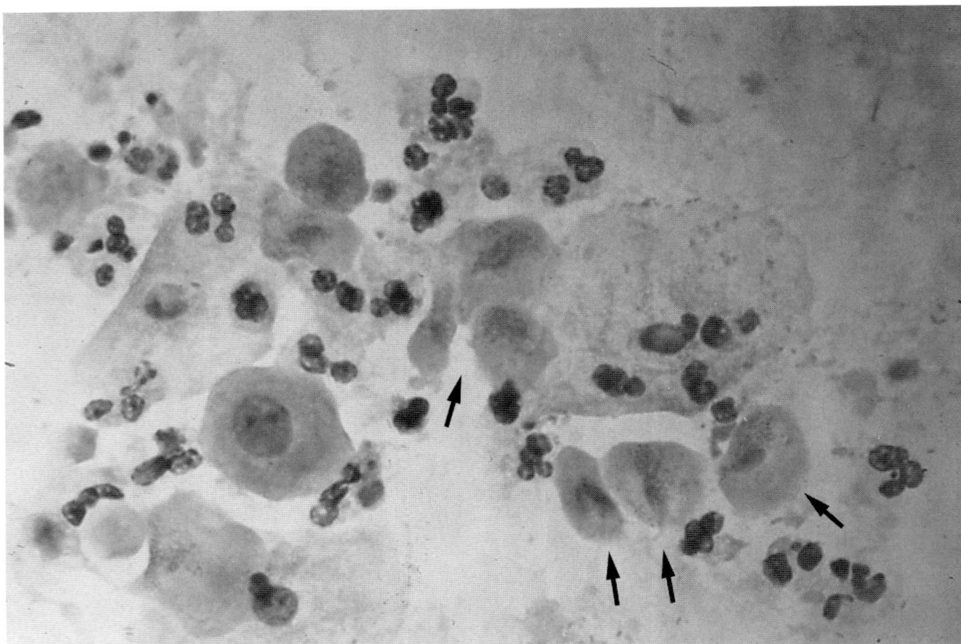

FIGURE 3.14. Trichomoniasis. The organisms are blue-grey and round or shield-shaped, vary considerably in size, contain an eccentric, elliptical nucleus, and display fine, red cytoplasmic punctation. (40x). Filamentous organisms (Leptothrix) coexist with *Trichomonads* in most cases (not shown). Characteristic squamous cell alterations include a narrow and indistinct degenerative perinuclear halo, cytoplasmic pseudoeosinophilia, and nuclear enlargement. Clinically, a thick yellow malodorous discharge or strawberry-appearing cervix/ vagina may be seen. (8, 45)

and karyorrhexis (nuclear fragmentation). Pyknotic cells must be differentiated from atypical cells and parakeratotic cells—both of which also display darkly staining nuclei. For example, the orangiphilic, pyknotic, degenerated parabasal cells usually found in smears of atrophic vaginitis (Fig. 3.19) may be confused with parakeratotic cells. The finding of other degenerative changes in the same smear may aid identification of the cellular alterations as degenerative in nature. These changes include breakdown in the nuclear membrane, cytoplasm, or both; nuclear chromatin clumping or beading; and the presence of fragmented cellular debris in the background.

Nuclear atypia may be present following exposure to various infectious and external agents, following recent local procedures (surgery, cryotherapy, etc.), and sometimes in association with severe inflammation, repair, or dryness. Mild glandular and squamous metaplastic nuclear atypia is often associated with *Chlamydia* infections (30). If a more significant degree of atypia is present, a diagnosis of dysplasia must be considered. Human *Papillomavirus* has now been proven to be the agent related to squamous intraepithelial lesions (SIL), condylomas, squamous cell carcinomas, adenocarcinoma-in-situ (AIS), and adenocarcinomas of the uterine cervix (8, 37, 45, 58). Infected cells may or may not display morphologic changes secondary to the virus. Viral studies used in conjunction with a Pap smear increase the accuracy rate of HPV detection. Postradiation and/or postchemotherapy smears may show cytologic atypia, which is generally charac-

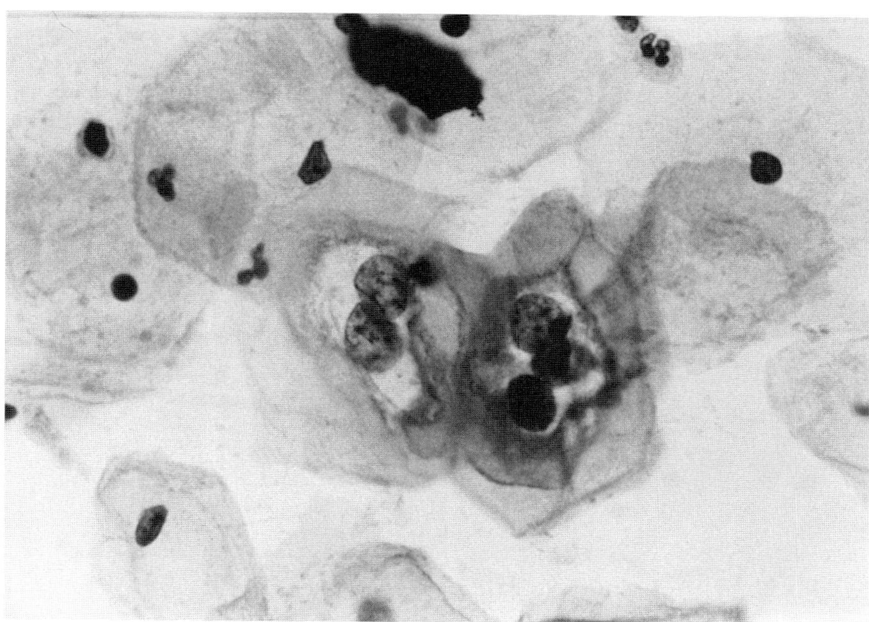

FIGURE 3.15.   Koilocytosis. Koilocytotic atypia is a HPV-related change occurring in squamous cells. Two classic koilocytes are present in the center of the field. In contrast to the degenerative perinuclear halos seen in Figure 3.14, koilocytes have characteristic broad, sharp perinuclear halos. Other features include multinucleation; nuclear molding; altered chromatin pattern; nuclear enlargement; and crisp, thick cytoplasmic outlines bordering the halos. (40x)

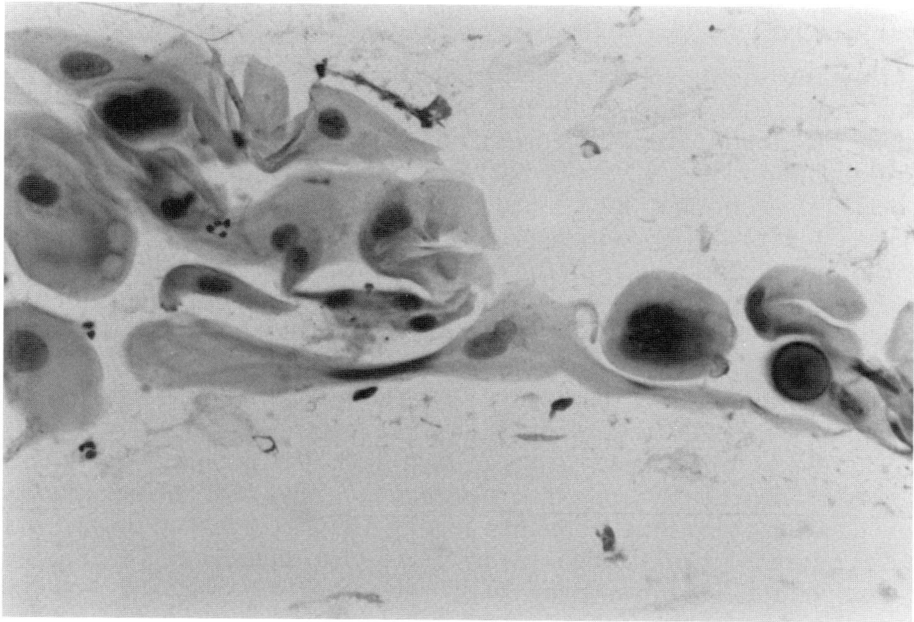

FIGURE 3.16.   Cytoplasmic vacuoles secondary to radiation. Often, neutrophils infiltrate the vacuoles. Additional radiation changes depicted in this photograph include bizarre cellular shapes, multinucleation, and syncytia. (20x)

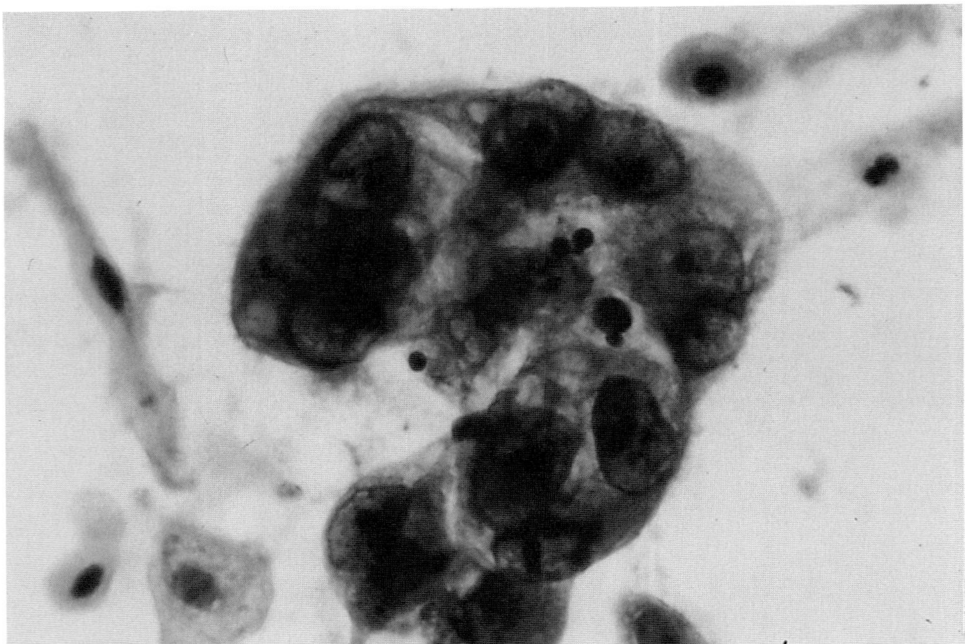

FIGURE 3.17. Adenocarcinoma. The cytoplasmic vacuoles often contain mucin; in some types of adenocarcinomas, they may displace the nucleus peripherally, forming a crescentric "signet" shape. This case is metastatic ovarian carcinoma present in a Pap smear. (40x) Another feature of some adenocarcinoma cells with vacuoles is the presence of neutrophils within the vacuoles.

teristic of the treatment. On rare occasions, determining whether the cellular atypia is secondary to the treatment or reflective of recurrent or residual disease may not be possible. In this situation, the differential diagnosis is stated as such, and further clinical investigation should follow. Severe reparative atypia can be quite alarming and is best interpreted in the context of the clinical scenario (cervical polyp, recent surgery, etc.). Squamous cell atypia in the setting of atrophy often requires the cytopathologist to exercise caution. In atrophic smears, plump parabasal cells are often distorted or degenerated secondary to vaginal dryness, and their nuclei may appear enlarged and hyperchromatic. A brief trial with estrogen therapy eliminates these artifacts and allows their differentiation from a significant lesion on a subsequent Pap smear.

The specific **organisms** that infect the lower genital tract can be classified into bacterial, fungal, parasitic, and viral. **Bacterial** infections may be nonspecific (see the previous discussion) or may be due to a particular organism, such as *Gonococcus, Staphylococcus, Tuberculosis, Gardnerella, Actinomycosis* (Fig. 3.20), and *C. granulomatis.* Cytologic identification of these organisms may be suggested by Pap smear, but confirmation by culture is recommended. For instance, a Pap smear containing granulomas (aggregates of epithelioid histiocytes), Langhans-type giant cells, lymphocytes, and necrotic material may be suggestive of the diagnosis of tuberculosis; however, the organisms are not visible on Pap-stained smears. If extra smears are available, acid-fast stains may be employed for diagnostic confirmation. Another example is the venereal disease Gonorrhea. *Gonococcal* organisms are Gram-negative diplococci found adherent to squa-

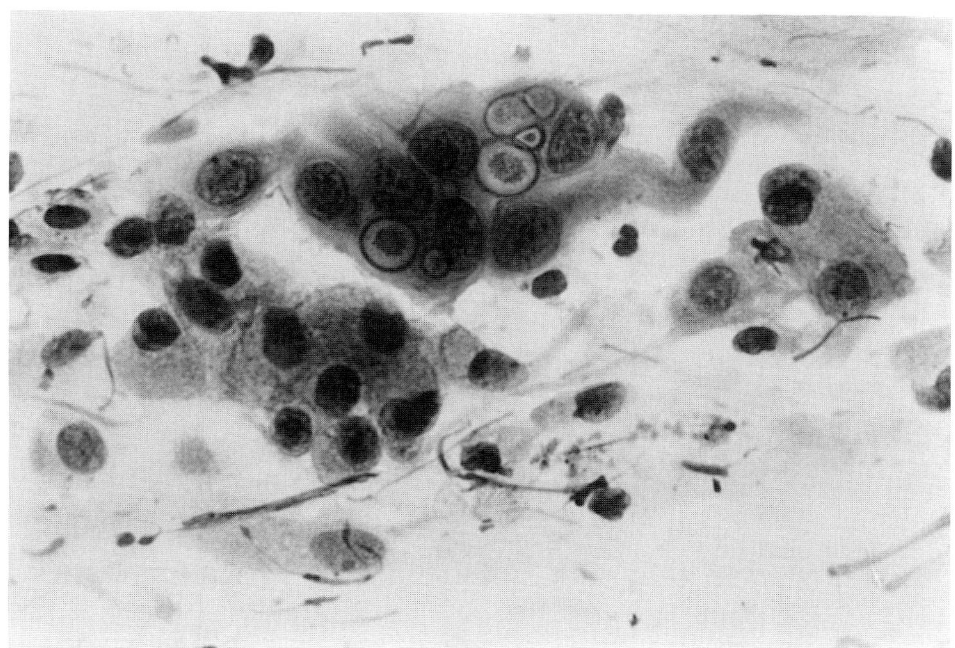

FIGURE 3.18.   Endocervical glandular cells with changes suggestive of Chlamydia. (40x) Multiple cytoplasmic vacuoles with distinct, sharp borders and containing centrally located amorphous, basophilic material are seen here. Using E.M. and antibody studies, Henry and colleagues (30) found that *Chlamydia* organisms are mostly present in thin-walled vacuoles that do not distend the cytoplasm nor displace the nuclei and contain finely granular inclusions.

mous cells or within neutrophils on Pap smears (8). Clinically, the patient may be asymptomatic or may present with a purulent discharge, urethritis, cervicitis, or an ascending infection. Although the organisms may be detected in the Pap smear, obtaining confirmatory cultures is necessary because of the significant social ramifications of the diagnosis (8). In vulvar lesions due to *C. granulomatis,* characteristic "Donovan bodies" are found within histiocytes. They appear as 0.6–2.0mm straight or dumbell-shaped rods with bipolar granules surrounded by clear capsules (18). Although these organisms are as easily noted in Pap-stained smears (using oil) as in Wright-Giemsa smears (18), confirming the diagnosis with special studies is always preferable.

The majority of **fungal** infections of the lower female genital tract are due to *Candida albicans.* These organisms have two forms—nonbranching pseudohyphae and budding yeasts (Fig.3.21). Occasionally, less common fungi are noted in Pap smears, including *Torulopsis glabrata* (very tiny budding yeasts), *Aspergillus* (thick, septate hyphae displaying 45° branching), *Geotrichum* (septate hyphae), and other fungi best classified by culture (Fig. 3.22).

The most common **parasitic** infection in these sites is *Trichomonas vaginalis* (8), which is easily recognizable in Pap smears. Nonetheless, Krieger and colleagues (47) found improved detection using culture, monoclonal antibodies, or wet mounts. Other rare parasites, such as *Enterobius vermicularis, Ascaris lumbricoides,Trichuris trichiuria, Entamoeba histolytica, Entamoeba gingivalis, Hymenolepsis nana, Pediculus humanus, Wuch-*

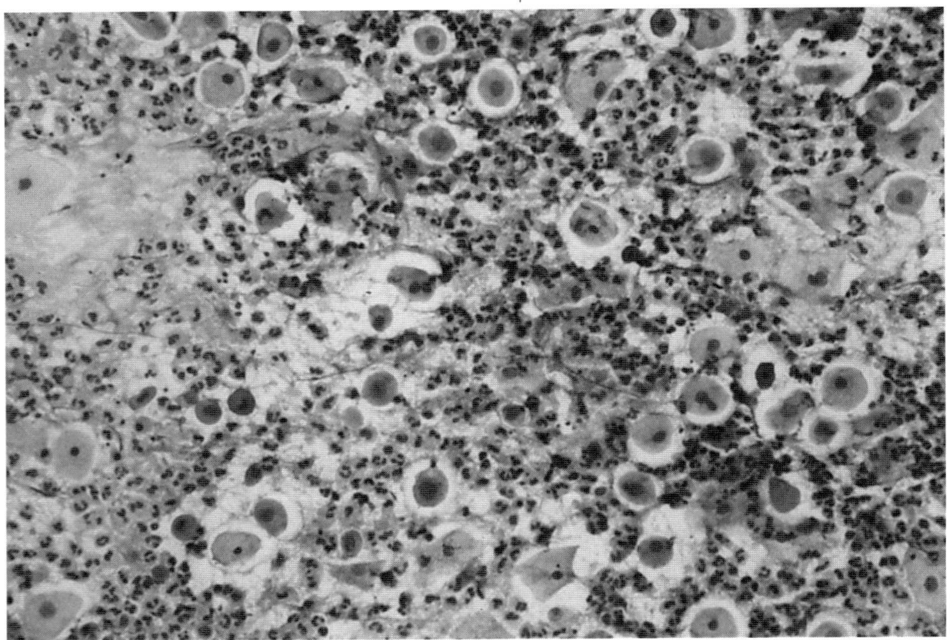

FIGURE 3.19. Atrophic vaginitis. Note the marked acute inflammation and the scattered parabasal cells, some of which have pyknotic, degenerating nuclei resembling parakeratotic cells, in this atrophic smear. (10x)

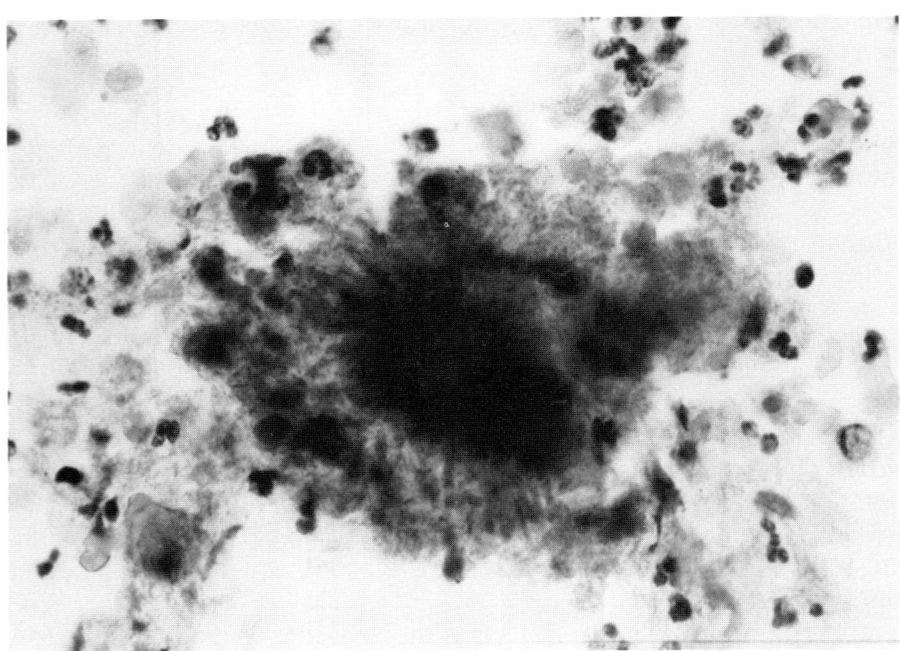

FIGURE 3.20. Actinomyces. This is a common finding in IUD users. Typically, the organisms form a "sulfur granule" with a dense core surrounded by peripherally radiating filaments. Calcific material may be present. Acute inflammation is in the background. (40x) (8)

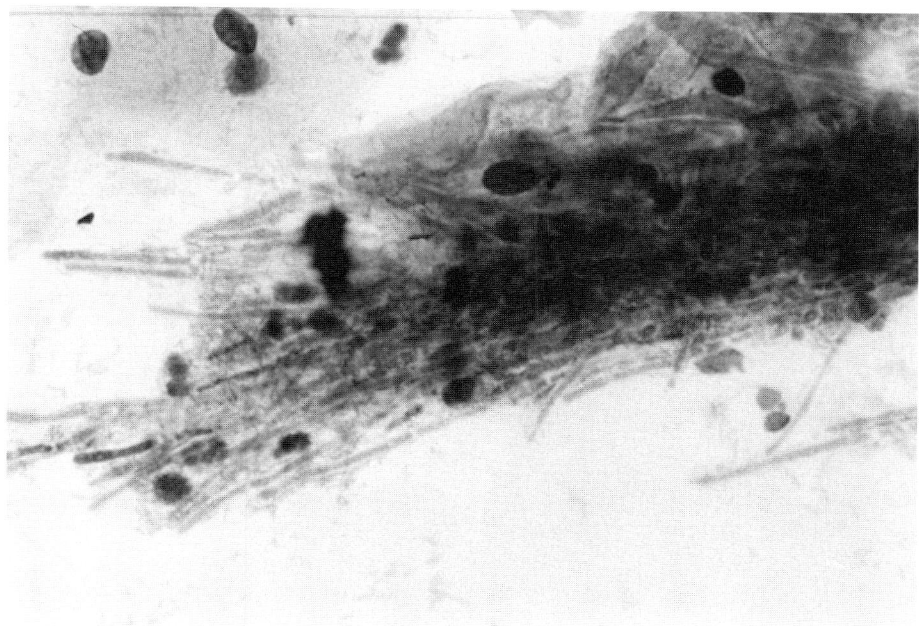

FIGURE 3.21. Candida. Numerous fungal elements of monilia are seen here. Note the parallel array of pseudohyphae and interspersed budding yeast forms. (40x).

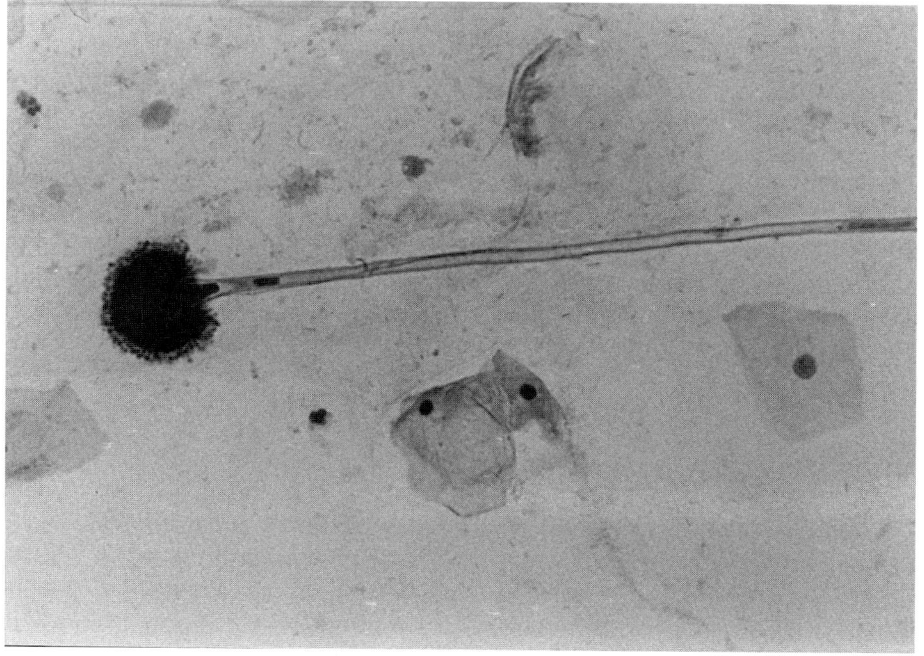

FIGURE 3.22. Isolated fruiting fungus found in a Pap smear, pathogen versus contaminant. In cases such as this, cultures are recommended. (20x)

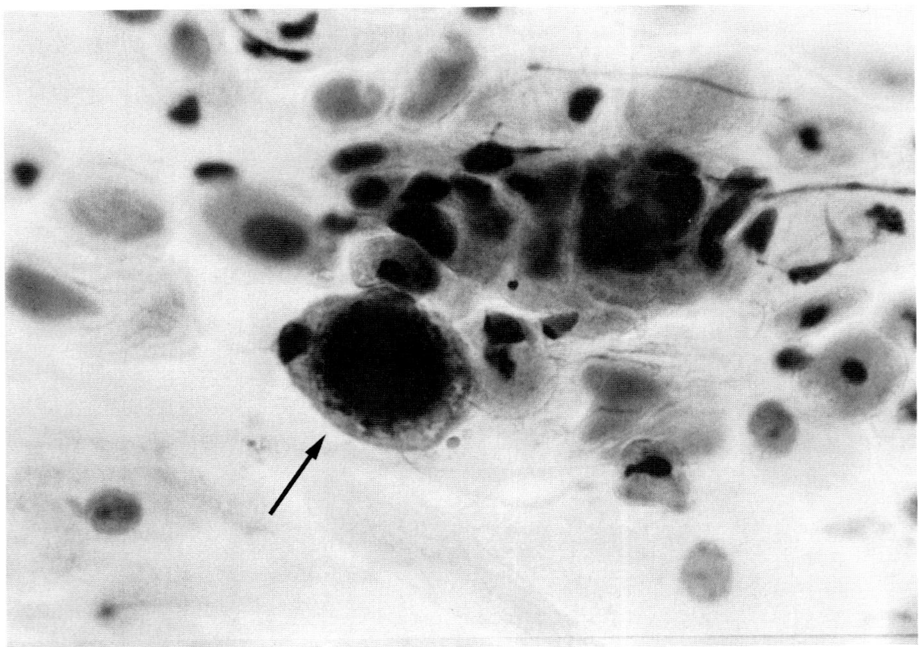

FIGURE 3.23.   Parasitic ova found in a Pap smear. Features such as lateral spines (*Schistosoma mansoni*) and clear polar knobs (*Trichuris trichiura*) are helpful in identifying the type of parasite. (40x)

ereria bancrofti, Balantidium coli, Schistosoma haematobium and *mansoni,* and *Taenia,* have been reported in the cytologic literature (8, 45, 51) (Fig. 3.23).

Viral involvement in this region is easily detected by Pap smear. Commonly, one sees the cytopathic changes associated with HPV, such as koilocytotic atypia (Fig. 3.15), and the squamous nuclear atypia diagnostic of squamous intraepithelial lesions (SIL, low-grade and high-grade). Herpes simplex 2 causes very characteristic cellular changes including "ground glass" nuclei, chromatin margination, nuclear molding, multinucleation, and red nuclear inclusions (Fig. 3.24). Less specific findings include cellular and nuclear enlargement or bizarre cells. Proper cytologic detection of herpes simplex virus (HSV) has significant clinical implications to both mother and fetus. Other viral entities that have been described cytologically include *CMV* (Fig. 3.10), Epstein Barr virus, measles (28), molluscum, polyomavirus, and varicella (45). According to TBS, the finding of infectious organisms (fungal, parasitic, or viral) should be reported as *"organisms morphologically consistent with," "cellular changes associated with,"* or *"cytopathic changes suggestive of,"* to emphasize the Pap smear's limitations (37).

THE VULVA

This region is primarily covered by a stratified squamous epithelium that is both keratinized and nonkeratinized. Smears taken from the vulva generally consist of anucleated squamous cells and benign, mostly superficial, squamous cells in a clean background (8, 43, 45). To obtain a good vulvar cytology sample, the site should first be moistened

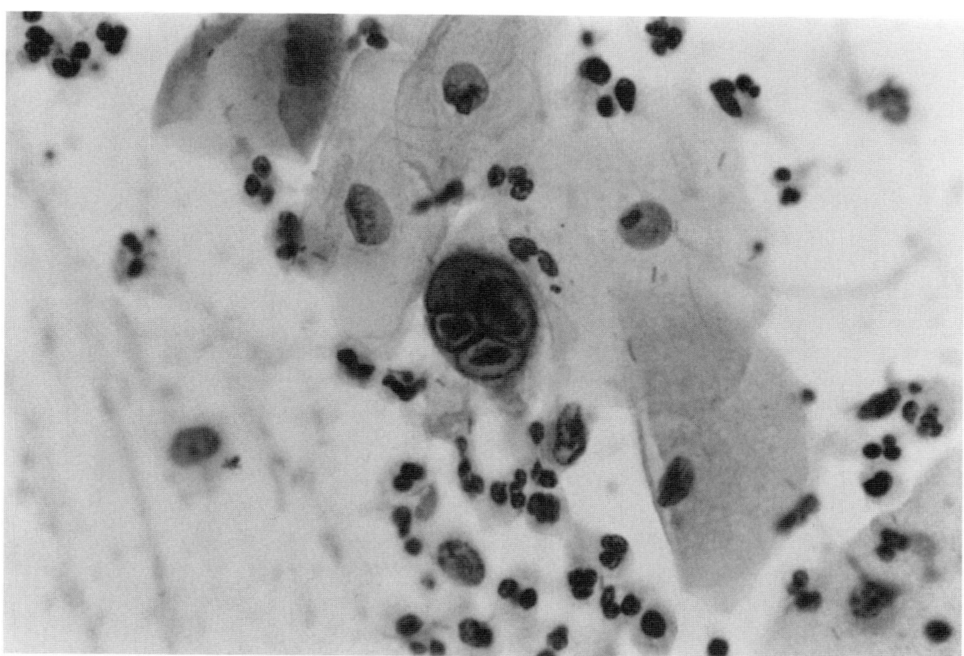

FIGURE 3.24.   Herpes. Cellular changes characteristic of HSV infection displayed here include multinucleation, nuclear molding, chromatin margination, and nuclear inclusions which are characteristically red. (40x)

with a saline-soaked towel, and then the excess soft keratin should be scraped off with a scalpel blade or the edge of a glass slide. After this initial scrape is discarded, the underlying lesion can be sampled properly (8, 17, 43).

Benign lesions of the vulva that have been diagnosed by cytologic means include papillary hidradenoma, fibroadenoma (ectopic breast), condyloma, endometriosis, vulvar dystrophy, granular cell tumor, Bartholin's cysts, and abscesses. The cytologic findings and salient diagnostic features are summarized in Table 3.1. In addition, benign vascular lesions occur in this location, but these have not yet been described in the cytology literature. We recently saw a case of a 20-year-old woman whose Pap smear showed an exuberant capillary network in a background of inflammatory cells and anucleated squamous cells (Fig. 3.25). Suggested diagnostic possibilities included angiokeratoma (13), pyogenic granuloma, and keratinous cyst with inflamed granulation tissue. No clinical follow-up is available to date. The various dermatologic conditions that may involve the vulva are best diagnosed histologically (see Chapter 1).

Cytologically detected **malignant vulvar tumors** (primary and secondary) include squamous cell carcinoma (invasive and in situ), comprising more than 85% of all malignant vulvar tumors (14); verrucous carcinoma; Paget's disease (Figs. 3.26 and 3.27); melanoma (Fig. 3.28); basal cell carcinoma; sarcomas, e.g., epithelioid sarcoma (32) and alveolar rhabdomyosarcoma; non-Hodgkin lymphoma (52); carcinomas of Bartholin's gland, e.g., adenocarcinoma and adenoid cystic carcinoma; and metastases. Key features of these lesions are summarized in Table 3.2.

TABLE 3.1.   Cytology of Benign Vulvar Lesions

Lesion	Gross Findings/ Clinical Presentation	Cytologic Findings	Differential Diagnosis
Papillary hidradenoma	Small, unifocal, ulcerated blue-raspberry-colored nodule. Usually asymptomatic; may be pruritic. Rare lesion. Occurs mostly in postpubertal women. (6)	Small glandular cells with fine, even chromatin and minimal anisonucleosis, occurring singly or in small clusters. (34)	Adenocarcinoma (6, 34), ectopic breast tissue, sweat gland or sebaceous carcinoma, melanoma, Paget's, and poorly differentiated squamous cell carcinoma.
Fibroadenoma in ectopic breast tissue	Firm, mobile mass with a white, trabeculated surface. May manifest clinically as a painful swelling. (66)	Uniform sheets and clusters of ductal cells with scant to moderate cytoplasm and round nuclei in a background of naked nuclei and stromal fragments. (66)	Hidradenoma
Condyloma	Warty, exophytic growth. Often multiple.	Koilocytotic atypica, dysplastic, larger squamous cells, and pearls.	Squamous cell carcinoma in situ, invasive squamous cell carcinoma, verrucous carcinoma.

Endometriosis	Solid or cystic mass which may bleed, cause pain, and swell cyclically. Rare in the vulva. (54, 78)	Uniform, small glandular cells, loosely arranged bipolar spindly stromal cells, vessels, and hemosiderin-laden macrophages. Biphasic cell population is essential to diagnosis. Epithelial cells have indistinct cell borders, are present in sheets or tubular structure, are evenly distributed, and have finely speckled chromatin and scanty cytoplasm. Mitoses may be seen in proliferative phase. (50, 57, 78)	Carcinosarcoma, malignant mixed Mullerian tumor.
Nonneoplastic epithelial disorders (lichen sclerosus, squamous hyperplasia)	Keratinized region.	Anucleated and parakeratotic squamous cells. Nonspecific findings. (43)	
Granular cell tumor		Loosely cohesive large cells with indistinct cell borders; small, round nuclei; and abundant, eosinophilic, granular cytoplasm. (57)	Skin adnexal tumor.
Bartholin's cyst and epidermal inclusion cyst	Cysts.	Benign epithelial cells and proteinaceous mucoid material. (57)	
Abscess	Fluctuant mass.	Numerous neutrophils, histiocytes, and proteinaceous material.	

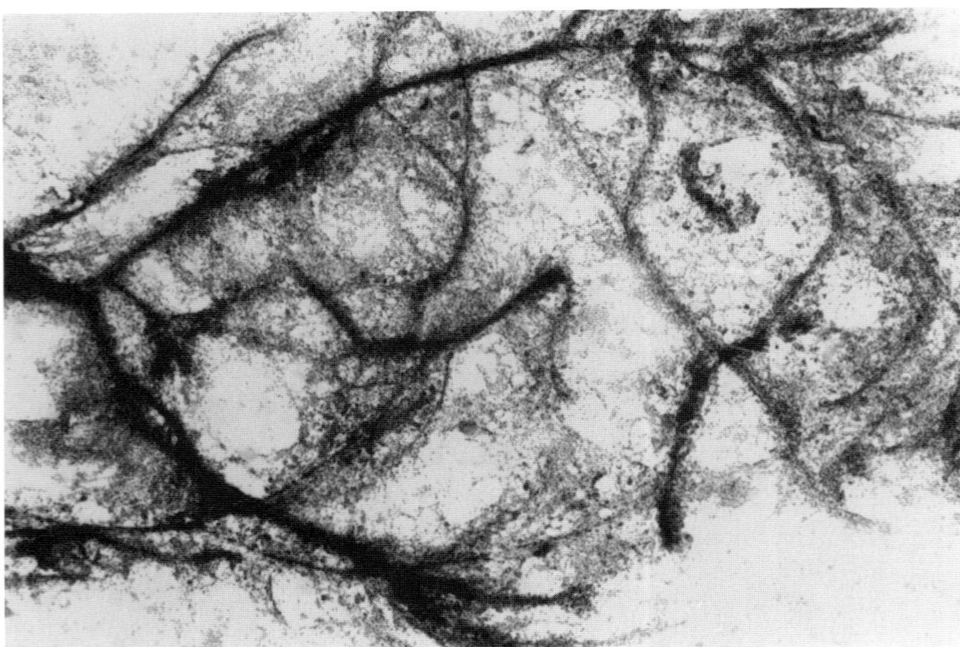

FIGURE 3.25.   Low-power view of delicate branching capillaries in a background of acute inflammatory cells and anucleated squamous cells. (2x)

THE VAGINA

The vagina is lined by a nonkeratinizing stratified squamous epithelium. The vaginal epithelial cells are hormonally sensitive and normally undergo cyclic changes in menstruating women. In squamous cells, the result of estrogen stimulation is an increase in the level of maturation toward superficial cells. Therefore, in conditions in which estrogen levels are elevated, e.g., when estrogen-producing ovarian tumors are present, full maturation of the squamous epithelium occurs. Conversely, in conditions in which estrogen is decreased or absent, e.g., in postmenopausal or postpartum women, a predominance of immature parabasal cells exists.

Evaluation of the degree of maturation of vaginal squamous cells is one means of assessing a patient's **hormonal status.** To obtain cells for this analysis, one should remove excess mucus secretion and then scrape the lateral vaginal wall (8). One must exercise care not to contaminate the specimen with metaplastic squamous cells from the transition zone because these small cells resemble immature parabasal cells, and misclassifying them would alter the results. Therefore, obtaining vaginal smears prior to manipulation of the cervix is recommended (8).

Several indices have been devised to define the hormonal status of the squamous epithelial cells. These include the karyopyknotic index, eosinophilic index, maturation index, maturation value, folded-cell index, and crowded-cell index (45). These indices, in conjunction with hormonal assays and/or endometrial biopsies, may be useful in determining the time of ovulation. The vaginal cytohormonal pattern may suggest a range of diagnoses or exclude some diagnostic possibilities (60). For example, vaginal smear cytology and sex chromatin determination are used to evaluate cases of primary

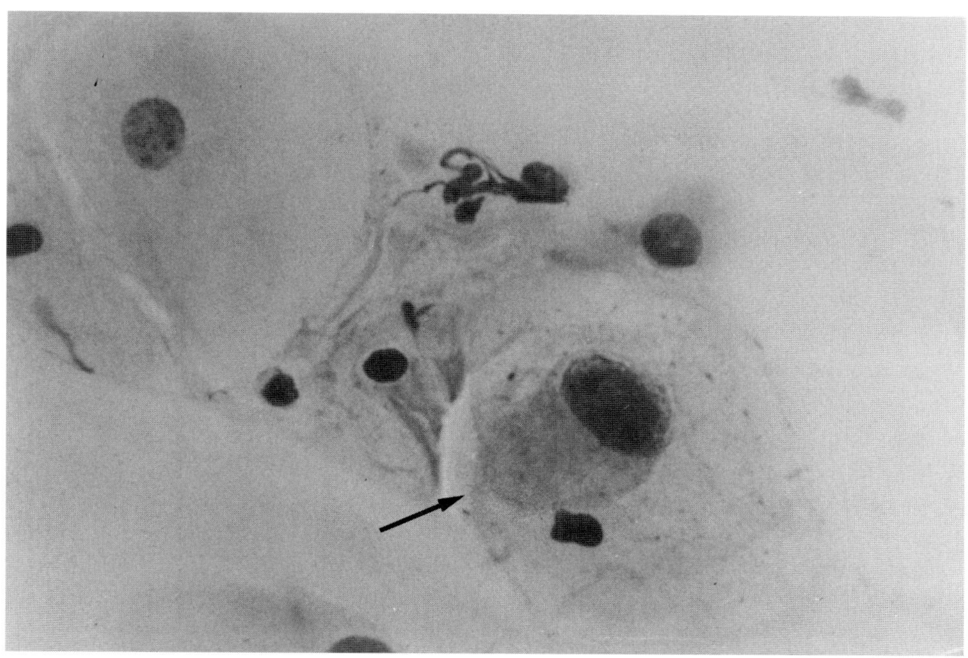

FIGURE 3.26. Vulvar Paget's disease: Cytology. A single, large, malignant Paget's cell is surrounded by benign squamous cells. Note the high N/C ratio, large nucleolus, clumped chromatin, and eccentric location of the nucleus. (44) This is a photo of a cervical/vaginal smear from a known case of vulvar Paget's. Another common feature, not seen here, is a cell-in-cell configuration ("cannibalism") (26). (40x)

amenorrhea. For instance, in cases of Turner's syndrome, both squamous cell maturation and the sex chromatin are absent, whereas in the syndrome of testicular feminization, squamous epithelial maturation is present, but the sex chromatin is absent (45). In accordance with the Bethesda system, a statement may be included in a cytology report indicating whether the hormonal cellular pattern of the vaginal smear is compatible with the patient's age and history (37).

Benign vaginal conditions amenable to cytologic diagnoses are uncommon. The cytologic findings in the more common benign lesions are listed in Table 3.3. Mullerian cysts, endometriosis, leiomyomas, benign tumors of Gartner's ducts, and other rare benign vaginal tumors are not usually diagnosed by cytology.

Rectovaginal fistulae, vesicovaginal fistulae, previous hysterectomy smears, presence of a neovagina, and malakoplakia are conditions that may have specific cytologic findings. Rectovaginal fistulae resulting from trauma, irradiation, neoplasm, or pelvic abscess may be detected on vaginal smears if fecal material and/or colonic glandular cells are present. In a cytologic study of rectovaginal fistulae, Angeles and Saigo (2) found cytology to be diagnostic in 65% of patients with the condition. Similarly, urothelial cells may be present in cases of vesicovaginal fistulae. Unlike the tall, mucus-producing colonic cells in rectovaginal fistulae, the smaller urothelial cells are not as easily identifiable in vaginal smears (45). In posthysterectomy vaginal smears, acute inflammatory cells and foreign body giant cells containing polarizable material have been reported (5). Rarely, columnar cells have also been noted; these are postulated to be

TABLE 3.2. Cytology of Malignant Vulvar Lesions

Lesion	Gross Findings/ Clinical Presentation	Cytologic Findings	Differential Diagnosis	Frequency
Squamous cell carcinoma	In situ: Slightly raised red, white, or pigmented lesion with well-defined border. Often pruritic. Invasive: Warty or ulcerated mass.	In situ: Atypical squamous cells, present singly and in "syncytia," with high N/C ratios, ± keratinization, parakeratosis, anucleated squames. Immature small cell or large cell varieties. Background is clean. Invasive: Spindle cells, macronucleoli, and necrosis may be seen. (43, 57)	In situ: Inflammatory lesion, warty lesion. Invasive: Ulcerated, herpetic lesion.	In situ: 25% of all malignant vulvar lesions. Invasive: 51% of all malignant vulvar lesions.
Verrucous carcinoma	Large, exophytic mass.	Nonspecific findings: parakeratosis, anucleated squames, squamous cell groups with minimal atypia. (43)	Condyloma, pseudoepitheliomatous hyperplasia.	
Paget's	Pruritis and burning. Lesions are sharply demarcated, erythematous, and sometimes weeping, indurated and excoriated. (26, 45)	Large cells, present singly and in small clusters, with large eccentric nuclei and nucleoli. Signet ring cells and cell-in-cell arrangements may be seen. Positive staining with mucicarmine, epithelial membrane antigen (EMA), and carcinoembryonic antigen (CEA). (26, 44, 45)	Large cell carcinoma, adenocarcinoma.	8% of all malignant vulvar tumors. Rarely diagnosed by cytology. (12)
Melanoma	Mass, possibly pigmented. May be pruritic or bleeding.	Large, possibly pleomorphic cells arranged singly or in loose aggregates. Round, eccentric nuclei, binucleation, large nucleoli, ± cytoplasmic melanin pigment. (9, 57)		Uncommon. 5% of all malignant vulvar tumors.
Basal cell carcinoma	Grossly identical to basal cell carcinoma of the skin.	Small, uniform, hyperchromatic cells with scanty cytoplasm. Nucleoli variable. Spindly cells and palisading may be noted.	Basaloid cloacogenic carcinoma.	2–3% of all malignant vulvar lesions.
Epithelioid sarcoma	Erythematous, edematous, ulcerated, well-circumscribed mass. Cut surface may be hemorrhagic and necrotic.	Polygonal cells with eosinophilic cytoplasm, which is centrally granular and peripherally vacuolated. Eccentric nuclei with chromatin clearing and one or more conspicuous nucleoli. Cells present singly and in small, loosely cohesive groups in a hemorrhagic and inflammatory background.	Inflammatory lesions.	1% of all malignant vulvar tumors. High recurrence rate. (32)

Alveolar rhabdomyosarcoma	Swollen, painful, solid, irregular mass. (35)	Spindle cells may be present. Positive staining with vimentin and cytokeratin. (32) Uniform population of malignant cells with clear or scanty cytoplasm, round to oval nuclei with granular chromatin and nucleoli, frequent mitoses, and occasional multinucleation. No cross striations seen. Cells present singly, in sheets, or in a reticular pattern. Positive staining with desmin, vimentin, and myoglobin. (35)		Rare. Leiomyosarcoma is more common. (35)
Embryonal rhabdomyosarcoma		Small, single cells with dense, eosinophilic cytoplasm, eccentric nuclei, and cross striations.		
Non-Hodgkin's lymphoma	Well-demarcated, painless nodule. (52)	Monomorphic population of dispersed lymphoid cells with open chromatin, sparse cytoplasm, and nucleoli adherent to the nuclear membranes. Single cell necrosis is present. Positive staining with leukocyte common antigen (LCA) and negative staining with EMA. (52)	Epithelial tumors.	Seven cases reported in the literature. Vulvar involvement in 4%. (52)
Adenocarcinoma of Bartholin's gland	Painful mass exuding mucoid material. (36)	Malignant glanular cells arrranged in acini and clusters and displaying oval or crescentic nuclei, nucleoli, increased chromatin, and abundant basophilic cytoplasm. Microcalcifications, tumor diathesis, and psammoma bodies may be present. (36)	May be clinically mistaken for cyst or abscess.	Primary carcinomas of Bartholin's gland account for 2–7% of all vulvar cancers. (36)
Adenoid cystic carcinoma of Bartholin's gland	Painful mass, which may be elevated. (36)	Small, monotonous cells with oval to round, eccentric nuclei, finely increased chromatin, and abundant cytoplasm. Tubules and/or pseudorosettes containing hyaline material may be present.	Infected cyst, syringoma, microcystic adnexal carcinoma, mixed tumors, adenoma.	Adenoid cystic carcinomas constitute 10% of Bartholin's gland carcinomas and 1% of all female genital tract neoplasms.

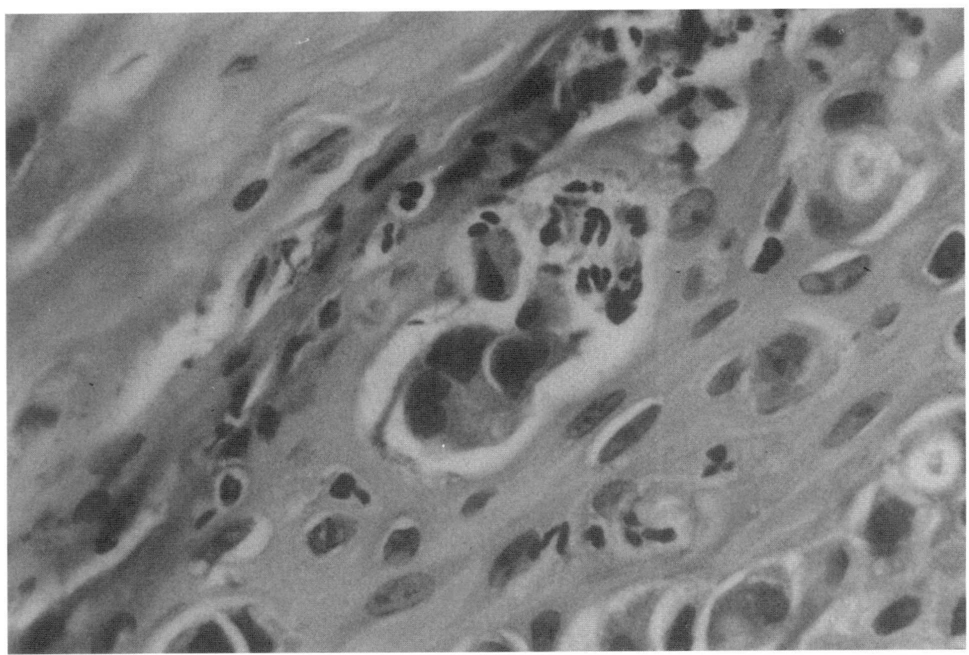

FIGURE 3.27. Vulvar Paget's disease: Histology. Vulvar biopsy showing intraepithelial clusters of large, malignant Paget's cells surrounded by a clear zone. (40x)

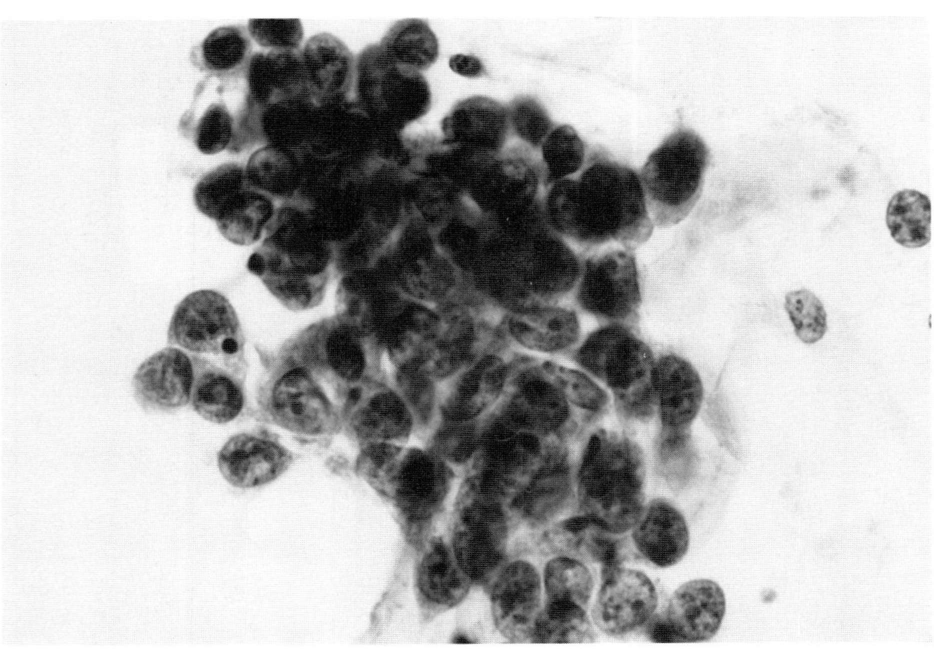

FIGURE 3.28. Recurrent malignant melanoma. The malignant cells are present singly and in clusters. Note the high N/C ratio, granular chromatin, large nucleoli, and occasional eccentric location of the nuclei. Other features, which are not present in this photograph, include cytoplasmic pigmentation, binucleation, and spindle cells. (40x) (9, 57)

TABLE 3.3.   Benign Vaginal Lesions

Lesion	Gross Findings/ Clinical Presentation	Cytologic Findings	Comments
Vaginal Inclusion Cyst	Usually located in posterior wall of the distal third of vagina. (29)	Keratinous debris. (8)	Usually occurs as a result of trauma or surgery. (29) Cytologic material may be obtained by FNA biopsy.
Adenosis	Occurs in upper third of vagina and adjacent cervix (45). Presents as a small cystic lesion or as solid, reddened epithelium. (29)	Columnar epithelial cells resembling normal endocervical cells, ± squamous metaplastic cells.	In obtaining the sample, care must be taken to avoid contamination with material from the endocervix.
Fibroepithelial polyp	Most often found in older women. Appears as a firm, irregular lesion measuring 1–2 cm in diameter. (29)	Normal squamous cells. (8)	Uncommon lesion.
Endometriosis	Usually one or more red or blue-red 2–5 mm cystic lesions in posterior vaginal fornix. (29)	See Table 3.1.	

derived from benign mucinous cells or goblet cell metaplasia in atrophic vaginal epithelium (7). Neovaginal cytology is used to monitor for disease recurrence in patients who have undergone radical surgery and/or irradiation for the treatment of gynecologic malignancies. The typical findings in benign neovaginal smears include anucleated squamous cells admixed with parabasal, intermediate, and superficial squamous cells. Cases of malakoplakia involving the vagina and cervix are rare, and the cytologic features have been described in the literature (56, 69, 8). Clinically, patients with this condition often have a vaginal discharge. In vaginal smears, the characteristic intracytoplasmic Michaelis-Gutmann bodies may be seen within histiocytes. These appear as concentrically laminated basophilic inclusions that stain positive for iron and calcium (8).

One of the most common benign vaginal lesions diagnosed by cytologic methods is vaginal adenosis. In this condition, glandular epithelium, most commonly of endocervical type, is present in the vagina or outer rim of the uterine cervix, where squamous epithelium is normally found. Vaginal adenosis may be associated with early exposure to diethylstilbestrol (DES) in utero, but it also occurs in patients who have no known exposure history. When sampling for adenosis, a circumvaginal scraping technique or, alternatively, a four quadrant (anterior, posterior, and lateral walls) downward directional scrape is recommended (8, 45). Typical smear findings include columnar cells (usually resembling endocervical cells, or, less commonly, endometrioid-type cells) with or without squamous metaplastic cells. In one study of 575 DES-exposed patients, only 34% of vaginal scrapes and 54% of portio scrapes yielded these cell types in patients with known adenosis (68). Adenosis has been noted to coexist with clear cell carcinoma in 95% of the clear cell carcinoma cases studied (8). Conversely, in a report of approximately 2000 DES-exposed women who were screened over an 8-year period, only four women subsequently developed clear cell adenocarcinoma while under observation (46). Melnick and colleagues (55) estimated the risk of vaginal adenocarcinoma to be 1 case per 1,000 DES-exposed women through age 34. Of even greater concern is the risk of developing squamous cell carcinoma, due to the presence of a larger transformation zone in DES-exposed patients (45).

Dysplastic squamous epithelial changes and carcinoma-in-situ of the vagina have been termed "squamous intraepithelial neoplasia" (SIL), as in the cervix. The cytologic appearance of these lesions is indistinguishable from their cervical counterparts. In our experience, many of the low-grade vaginal intraepithelial lesions are often more subtle than those of cervical origin. Koss (45) mentions that, in contrast to the cervix, where the cytologic appearance fairly accurately predicts the degree of histologic abnormality, considerable overlap exists in the cytologic features of all grades of squamous intraepithelial lesions and invasive squamous cell carcinoma of the vagina.

Primary malignant neoplasms of the vagina are infrequent, and the most common type is squamous cell carcinoma, which accounts for 75–90% of all primary vaginal cancers (29). The proof of the presence of HPV in vaginal squamous neoplasms is not as extensive as it is for cervical and vulvar squamous cell carcinomas and precursor lesions, yet the vaginal disorders show the same patterns as cervical disease and share identical cytologic, histologic, and biologic backgrounds (1, 45). In approximately 50% of cases of invasive vaginal squamous cell carcinomas, a synchronous or metachronous squamous cell carcinoma of the cervix is also present (45).

Adenocarcinoma accounts for only 10–12% of all vaginal cancers (29). Primary adenocarcinomas, previously rare, became more common because of their association with adenosis. Most cases of primary clear cell adeocarcinomas of the vagina (so-named because of the transparent appearance of the cytoplasm of the malignant cells in histologic sections in many of these tumors) are associated with DES exposure. Now that most DES-exposed women are over 40 years of age, these tumors are again rare (29). Non-DES-related adenocarcinomas of the vagina are rare. The cytologic features of vaginal adenocarcinomas are listed in Table 3.4. In 60% of cases of vaginal adenocarcinomas associated with adenosis, the cervix is not involved; therefore, obtaining vaginal pool specimens or direct vaginal wall scrape smears in women at risk for adenosis and adenocarcinoma is critical (45).

Very rare malignant tumors occurring in the vagina include sarcomas (21, 38, 63), lymphomas, small cell neuroendocrine carcinomas (42), and malignant melanomas. Melanomas account for 0.5–2.6% of all primary vaginal cancers (11). **Metastatic disease** comprises 84% of all vaginal neoplasms (8). Most carcinomas metastatic to the vagina, which include cervical, endometrial (21), colorectal (29), ovarian (27, 57) breast (39, 64), transitional cell (53), and renal cell carcinomas, display cytologic features similar to those of the primary tumor.

THE CERVIX

A Pap smear of the uterine cervix should contain a representative population of both the ectocervical squamous cells and endocervical columnar cells. In addition, squamous

TABLE 3.4. Malignant Vaginal Lesions

Lesion	Gross Findings/ Clinical Presentation	Cytologic Findings	Comments
SIL I–III of vaginal source	Predominantly affects upper vagina. (3) In most cases, lesions are multifocal. (29) On colposcopic exam, lesions appear similar to cervical SIL lesions. Most patients with CIS are asymptomatic and have no visible or palpable lesion. (31)	Cytology is indistinguishable from counterpart lesions in cervix. Koilocytes may be present in low grade lesions. CIS may be composed of large, keratinizing cells or small cells.	Vaginal pool smears and/or direct scrape smears of the vaginal wall may be used. Note: The cytologic appearances of vaginal low grade lesions, CIS, and invasive squamous cell carcinoma show significant overlap. (45)
Invasive squamous cell carcinoma	Mean age is 63. (63) Vaginal bleeding and discharge are the most common presenting symptoms. (29) No distinctive gross appearance; may be exophytic and fungating, nodular, flat, or ulcerating. (29) Most frequent location is in upper third of vagina. (29)	Cytologically indistinguishable from counterpart lesion in cervix (see Table 3.6); however, necrosis is less common in vaginal tumors. Most tumors are keratin-producing. (45)	
Verrucous carcinoma	Slowly growing, exophytic, locally invasive type of squamous cell carcinoma. (8)	Hyperkeratotic or parakeratotic cells with little pleomorphism. (8)	Uncommon variant of squamous cell carcinoma
Primary adenocarcinoma	Mean age is 51. (63) Most patients present with vaginal bleeding or abnormal cytology. Most arise in association with adenosis; most patients with DES-related clear cell adenocarcinoma were between 18 and 24 years of age at the time of diagnosis. Most frequent location is anterior vaginal wall; posterior and lateral aspects are less frequent sites. Clear cell adenocarcinomas most frequently arise in upper third of vagina. Early lesions frequently present as a submucosal nodule. Later, tumors may ulcerate or grow as polypoid, fungating lesions. (29)	Polygonal or columnar cells present singly and in clusters, with delicate, transparent, or sometimes vacuolated cytoplasm which may contain neutrophils. Nuclei are finely granular and may contain large nucleoli. (45)	Adenocarcinomas associated with adenosis affect girls and very young women, many of whom are initially asymptomatic. (45) Vaginal pool smears, direct scrape smears, or cervical scrape smears (if the cervix is involved) are sources of diagnostic material. (45)

metaplastic cells derived from the transition zone may be seen. Specimen adequacy largely depends on retrieval of sufficient numbers of these cell types. Although some squamous lesions are detected in smears lacking endocervical and squamous metaplastic cells, many studies have shown a significantly higher detection rate of high-grade lesions in smears containing these cells (37). The endocervical cells may be smeared together with the squamous cells over the entire slide and still be recognized easily and examined without difficulty. Smearing the endocervical cells separately at the edges of the slide is unnecessary; this process results in delayed fixation and often contributes to unnecessary air drying artifact, which hinders interpretation. Other factors that determine the adequacy of the specimen include the following: 1) completeness of patient and specimen identification, 2) pertinent clinical information, and 3) technical interpretability (37).

To optimize the detection of cervical lesions, various sampling devices have been used. In one study, the cytobrush yielded greater numbers of endocervical cells than the Q-tip applicator or Cervex brush (22). The swab produces the lowest numbers of endocervical cells and the greatest cellular distortion (22). Luzzatto and colleagues (49) noted that diagnostic cells were found more often in the cytobrush smears (endocervical sample) than in wooden spatula smears (ectocervical). In this large study, the cytobrush detected 79% of low-grade (CIN 1 and CIN 2) squamous lesions, whereas the spatula detected only 64% of these lesions. Interestingly, 37% of the high-grade (CIN 3) lesions were detectable in the cytobrush smear alone, whereas only 1% of these high-grade lesions were detected exclusively in the spatula smear. Of the invasive squamous cell

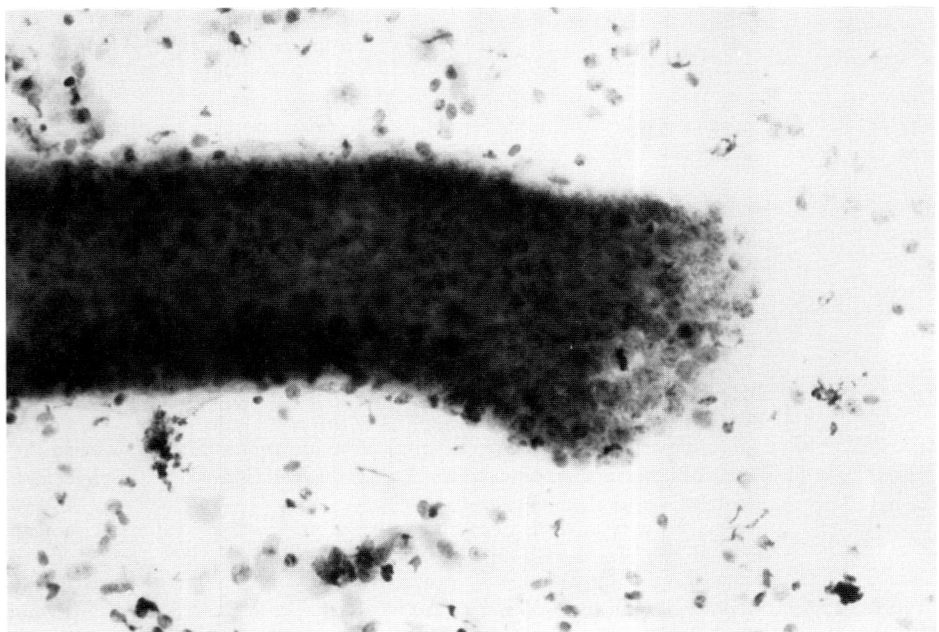

FIGURE 3.29.   Lower uterine segment cytology. Cells from the lower uterine segment are often present in cytobrush smears. Cytologic features include sheets and glandular sleeves of tightly cohesive and crowded endometrial cells with speckled chromatin and occasional mitotic figures (proliferative). In contrast to AIS, the cells are smaller and the chromatin more evenly speckled. (20x)

carcinomas, 93% were found with both instruments, and 7% of these invasive lesions were detected exclusively in the cytobrush smears. In 76% of the adenocarcinomas, both samples were positive, and in 23% of the adenocarcinomas, only the cytobrush smear was diagnostic.

With the continuing use of the cytobrush, pathologists must now recognize a broader range of normal cell types, including cells derived from the lower uterine segment (Fig. 3.29), brush artifact of normal endocervical cells (Fig. 3.30), and tubal metaplasia (Fig. 3.31) from higher and deeper glands (41, 85). Because of increased cellularity and hyperchromasia, these entities may be misinterpreted as high-grade lesions (glandular and squamous).

Various **benign** entities involve the cervix and may be diagnosed using cytologic information. In addition to the reactive, reparative, and inflammatory-related changes previously discussed, other benign epithelial and nonepithelial lesions that occur in this area include tubal metaplasia, microglandular hyperplasia (Fig. 3.32), Arias-Stella reaction, cervical polyps, and endometriosis. These are summarized in Table 3.5.

Epithelial cell abnormalities of cervical lesions can be subdivided into those of squamous cell origin and those of endocervical glandular cell origin. Reactive/reparative/infectious-related cell changes are considered benign changes and are excluded from these categories. The term "atypical squamous cells of undetermined significance"

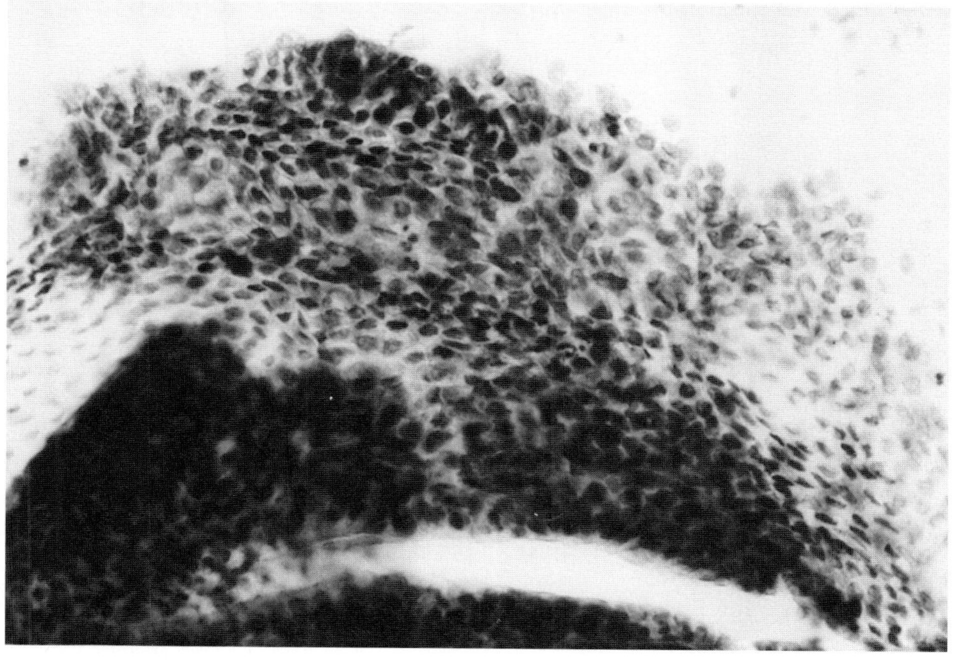

FIGURE 3.30.   Brush artifact of benign endocervical cells. The cytobrush often extracts large sheets of endocervical cells, which, when smeared, roll up and display pulled-out at edges. Thicker areas where the cells are doubled upon each other may be misinterpreted as showing crowding, whereas pulled areas may be misinterpreted as feathering. Examination of the center of the sheet away from these areas of artifactual changes reveals the benign nature of the sheet, with evenly spaced, normally sized cells arranged in a honeycomb pattern. (20x)

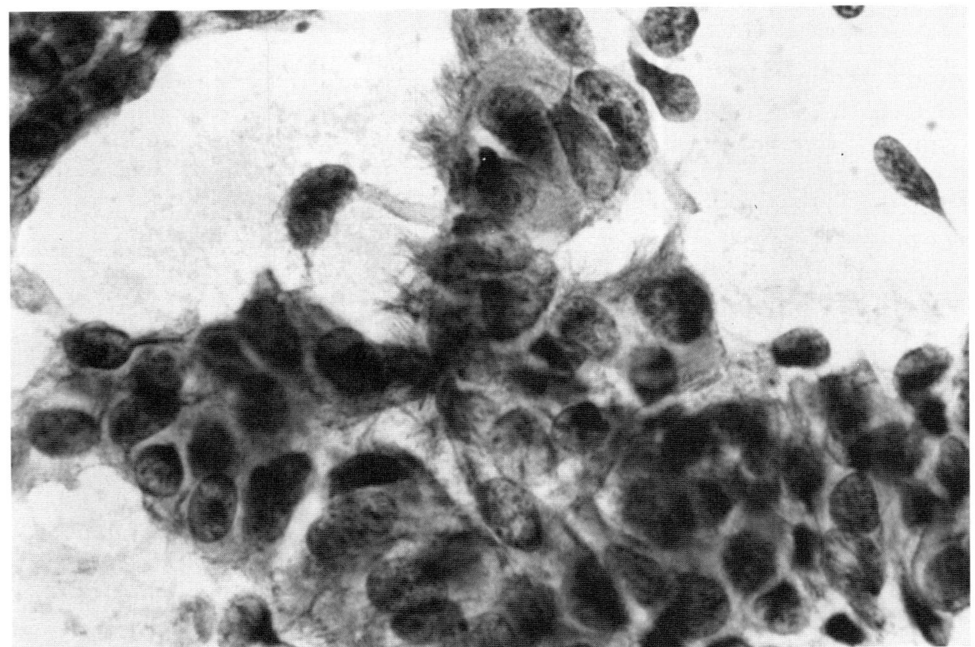

FIGURE 3.31. Tubal metaplasia. The cells have a flat, two-dimensional appearance. Nuclear hyperchromasia and enlargement are frequent findings. The apical surfaces show characteristic terminal bars and cilia. Peg cells are difficult to detect. (40x)

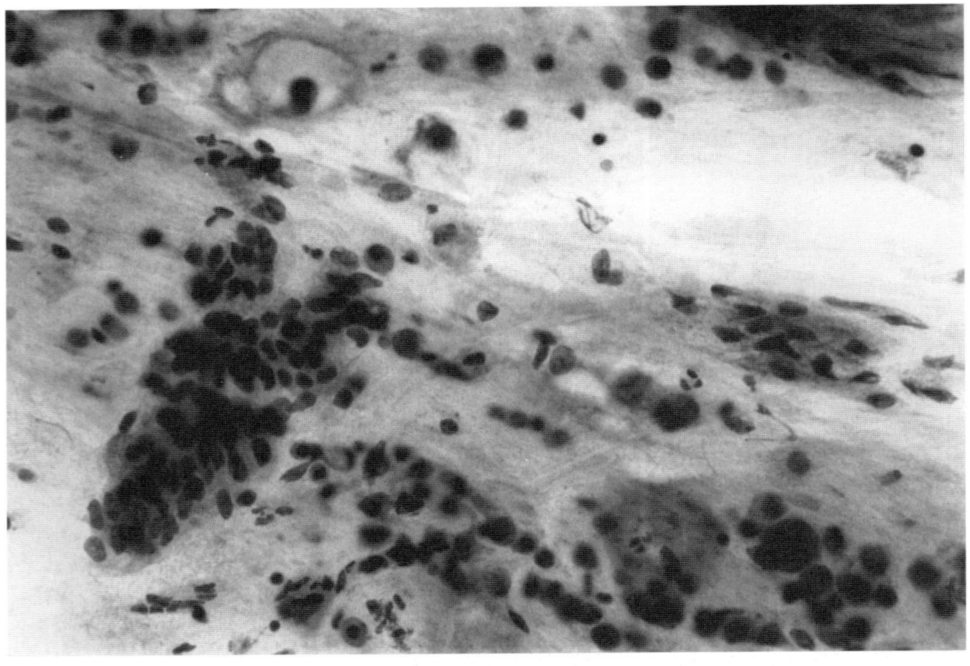

FIGURE 3.32. Microglandular hyperplasia. Cytologic findings are variable, and range from groups of tiny, benign glandular cells—as shown here in the cervical mucus—to atypical glandular cells. (20x)

TABLE 3.5. Cytology of Benign Cervical Lesions

Lesion	Gross Findings/ Clinical Presentation	Cytologic Findings	Differential Diagnosis
Tubal metaplasia	More frequent in upper endocervix and deep endo-cervical glands. Normally present in $\frac{1}{3}$ to $\frac{2}{3}$ of population. (41)	Evenly spaced glandular cells arranged in flat groups. Oval, enlarged, polarized nuclei are characteristic. Terminal bars and cilia are diagnostic. Peg cells not easily detected. Low cellularity. Absence of feathering and rosettes. Rare or no mitoses. (59)	Glandular dysplasia and AIS, glandular involvement by SIL. (41)
Microglandular hyperplasia	May be associated with oral contraceptive use or pregnancy. (15)	Variable findings. Small, reactive-appearing cells with less cytoplasm and enlarged, eccentric nuclei. Mitoses and nucleoli are infrequent. Cytoplasm may be clear. Cellular arrangements include small glandular clusters, sheets, strips, papillae, and rosettes. (15)	Glandular neoplasia, squamous neoplasia, parakeratosis.
Arias-Stella reaction	Intrauterine or extrauterine pregnancy.	Enlarged glandular cells with large, eccentric, hyperchromatic, round nuclei. Cytoplasm often appears vacuolated.	Adenocarcinoma.
Benign cells from lower uterine segment	Normal anatomy	Small, uniformly but closely spaced glandular cells with scanty cytoplasm arranged in 3-dimensional groups, sheets, and glandular sleeves. Mitoses may be seen in proliferative phase.	AIS
Cervical polyps	Polypoid mass; may be inflamed or ulcerated.	Reparative changes or reactive endocervical cells may be seen. 3-dimensional papillary structures covered by cuboidal or columnar epithelium. Squamous metaplasia is common.	Atypical glandular cells of undetermined significance, atypical repair.
Endometriosis	See Table 3.1.		

(ASCUS) is used when significant cellular alterations not diagnostic of a squamous intraepithelial lesion (SIL) exist. These changes include nuclear enlargement (2–3× normal size), mild nuclear membrane irregularities, nuclear molding, altered chromatin pattern, and binucleation or multinucleation. The term "ASCUS" is often applied when the pathologist is confronted with the finding of rare or few atypical cells exhibiting only one or two of these features and the findings are insufficient to allow determination of the nature of the lesion. On the other hand, in other ASCUS cases, the atypia may be diffuse but so subtle (e.g., enlarged, bland nuclei) that, again, a definitive diagnosis is not possible (Fig. 3.33). Atypical squamous metaplasia and atypical parakeratosis (Fig. 3.34) are also reported as ASCUS because of the frequent association of these findings with HISIL on biopsy. In cases diagnosed as "atypical repair" (Fig. 3.35), cellular sheets share many features in common with a reparative process but display a degree of atypia, architectural abnormality, or mitotic rate above the level seen in typical reactive/reparative processes. In such cases, the pathologist may elect to include a statement in the report such as "a neoplasm cannot be ruled out" to alert the clinician that worrisome features are present (16).

Determining optimal management for a patient with an ASCUS diagnosis is controversial. For this reason, in many institutions, the pathologist will qualify the atypia in an attempt to assist the clinician in treatment choice (e.g., by stating "favor a reactive process" versus "favor HPV-related changes"). A repeat smear taken 3–6 months later will often yield more information. However, in some cases, the repeat diagnosis remains equivocal, resulting in a patient with a persistent ASCUS diagnosis. Pearlstone and colleagues (62) studied a group of patients with persistent atypia (ASCUS) and noted that

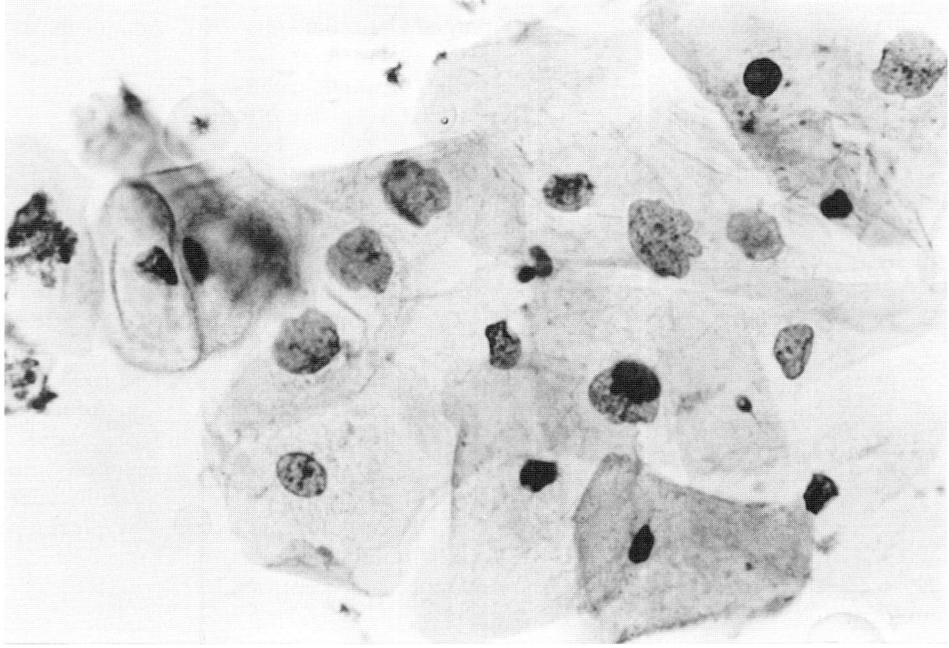

FIGURE 3.33. ASCUS. Subtle nuclear changes including mild nuclear enlargement and lobulated nuclear membranes were present in this case, which was reported as "ASCUS with cellular changes suggestive of low-grade SIL." (40x)

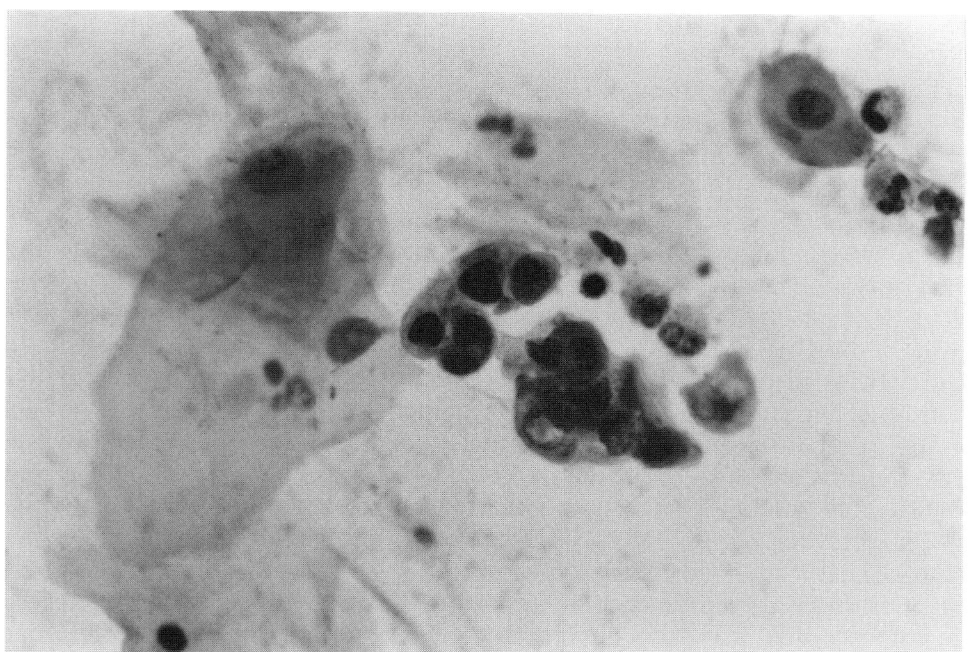

FIGURE 3.34. ASCUS: Atypical parakeratosis. A group of tiny, keratinized parakeratotic cells with atypical features including enlarged hyperchromatic nuclei and nuclear angulation are present. Atypical parakeratosis is included in the ASCUS category. (40x)

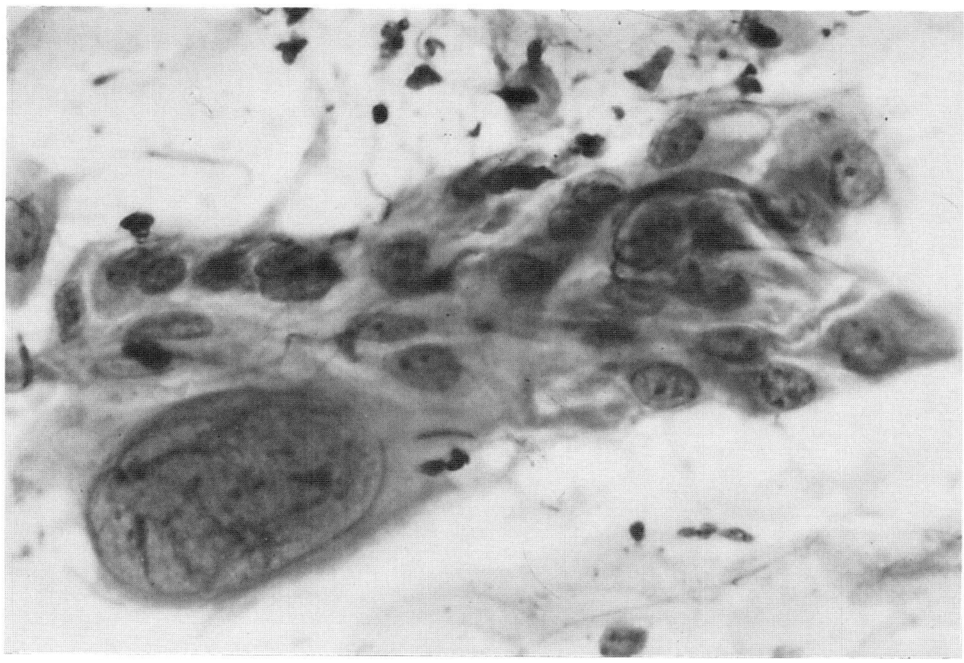

FIGURE 3.35. ASCUS: Atypical repair. Nuclear enlargement (without proportionally enlarged cytoplasm), three-dimensional cellular configurations, and a high mitotic rate are worrisome features in this case, which was interpreted as showing atypical repair. (40x)

18% of the patients had dysplasia on colposcopically guided biopsies and 25% had evidence of HPV. These findings are consistent with similar studies on patients with repeat ASCUS reports. Goff and colleagues found that ASCUS findings on Pap smears are associated with SIL in 19–30% of cases, whereas cytologically diagnostic dysplastic findings are associated with SIL in up to 90% of cases (24). The rate of ASCUS reports may vary between laboratories, and a high-risk population may raise this rate. In view of this, The National Cancer Institute Guidelines for Management of Abnormal Cervical Cytology state that acceptable rates of ASCUS may be two to three times that of SIL (48).

Most SILs arise at the squamocolumnar junction, and they more often involve the anterior lip of the cervix (8). The current nomenclature of "low-grade SIL" and "high-grade SIL" has reduced the confusion associated with previous classification systems (class system, dysplasia, CIN). The term "low-grade SIL" encompasses CIN 1 (Fig. 3.36) and condyloma (koilocytosis, koilocytotic atypia) (Figs. 3.15 and 3.37), which have a greater tendency to regress. These lesions behave similarly and are frequently associated with low-risk HPV types (primarily types 6 and 11) (37). Management of patients with this diagnosis is controversial, and ranges from following with a repeat cytologic study and/or colposcopy to laser, LEEP, or cryotherapy procedures. The Bethesda system combines the previous CIN 2 and 3 into **high-grade SIL** (Figs. 3.38 and 3.39) based on the more aggressive behavior of these lesions. These are frequently associated with high-risk HPV types (including 16 and 18), which are also noted in invasive lesions (37). Management of these lesions usually includes colposcopy and biopsy, followed by more

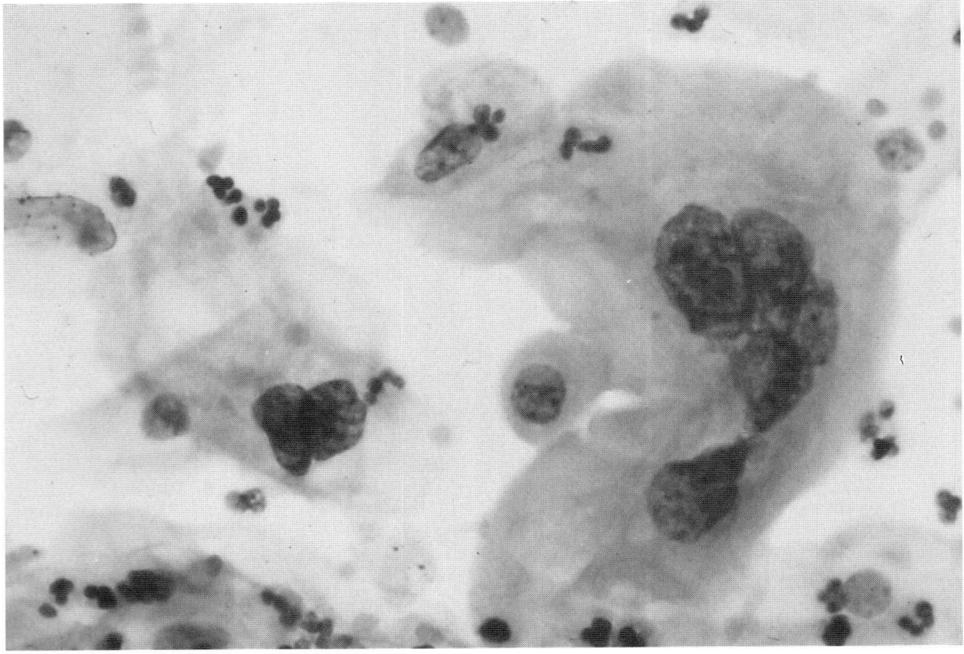

FIGURE 3.36. Low-grade SIL. Two cells displaying features of low-grade SIL are present. Features include binucleation and multinucleation; nuclear molding; coarse, unevenly distributed chromatin; and cytomegaly. In binucleated cells, the nuclei often touch at one end, mold together, or are parallel to each other. (40x)

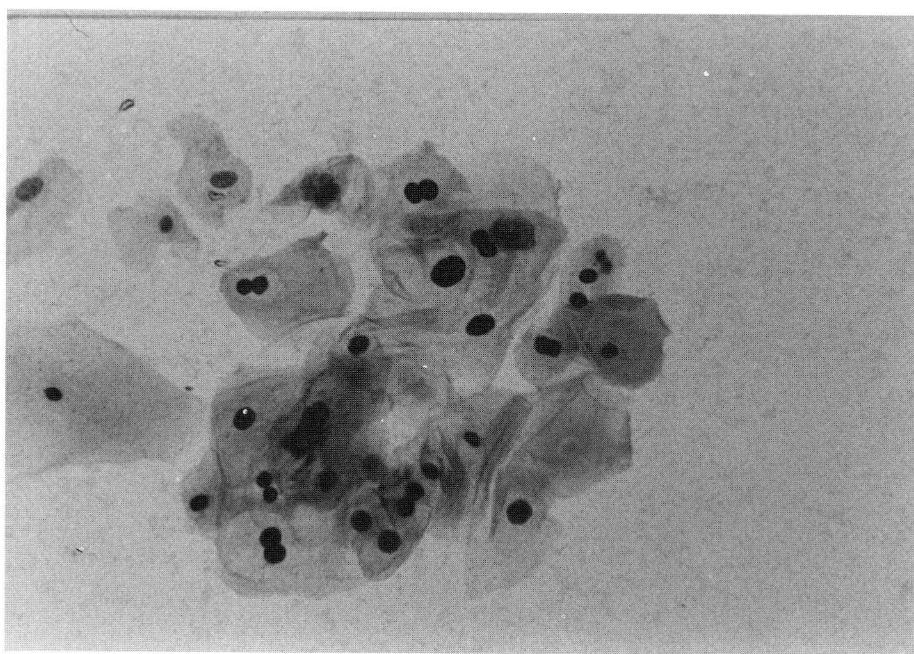

FIGURE 3.37. Low-grade SIL. In addition to the classic koilocytotic changes shown in Figure 3.15, a population of binucleated superficial squamous cells with darkly staining small nuclei (with or without nuclear molding) may be present in condylomatous lesions and should not be overlooked. At least a half dozen binucleated squamous cells are present in this field alone. Some cells may have perinuclear clearings but lack diagnostic koilocytotic features. (20x).

definitive treatment. The diagnoses of carcinoma-in-situ (CIS) and CIS with possible microinvasion are not included in TBS, but may supplement the diagnosis (37). Less-differentiated cells found in syncytial aggregates are features of a CIS; however, if nucleoli and granular chromatin are also noted, **microinvasion** should be considered (8).

Invasive squamous cell carcinoma of the cervix can been subdivided into keratinizing, nonkeratinizing, and small cell types. Typically, the keratinizing variety has bizarre, sometimes elongated squamous cells with darkly staining, irregular nuclei and bright orange, keratinized cytoplasm (Fig. 3.40)(8). In contrast, the nonkeratinizing type has smaller, rounder squamous cells with increased N/C (nuclear size/cytoplasm) ratios, irregularly clumped chromatin, and cyanophilic cytoplasm (Fig. 41) (8). The small cell variant, as its name implies, consists of smaller malignant cells having high N/C ratios and hyperchromatic nuclei. According to TBS, subclassification into these types is unnecessary and is left to the discretion of the individual laboratory (37).

Endocervical cell atypia is included in the category "atypical glandular cells of undetermined significance" (AGUS). The reported incidence of endocervical atypia is approximately 0.5%, and the affected mean age (44 years) is higher than that of squamous lesions (30–39 years) (24). Cervical adenocarcinoma now constitutes 10–20% of all invasive cervical cancers (59), but rates from 5–34% have been reported (4, 19). Patients with cervical adenocarcinoma may present with bleeding, vaginal discharge,

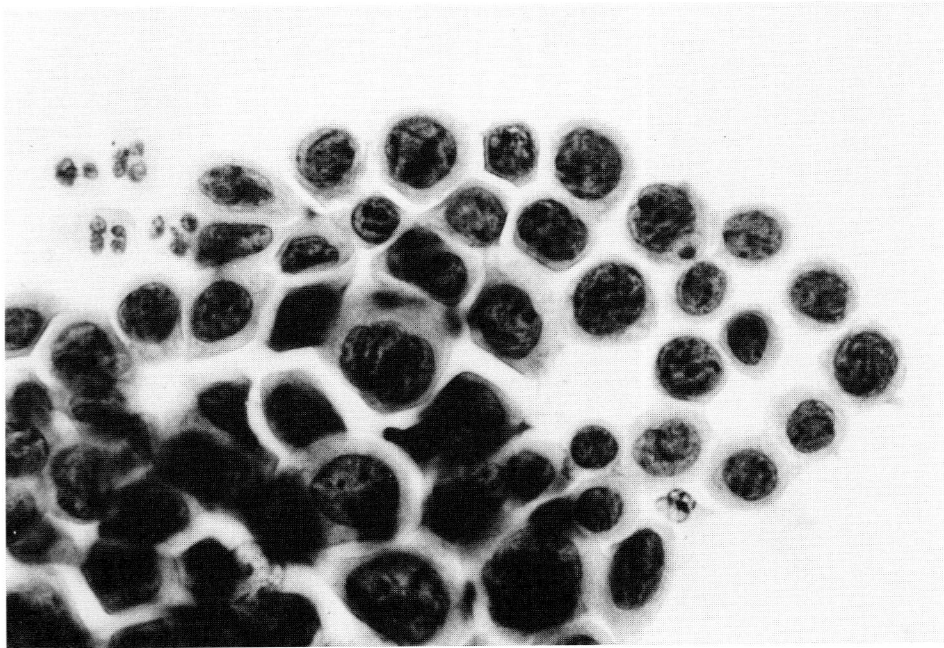

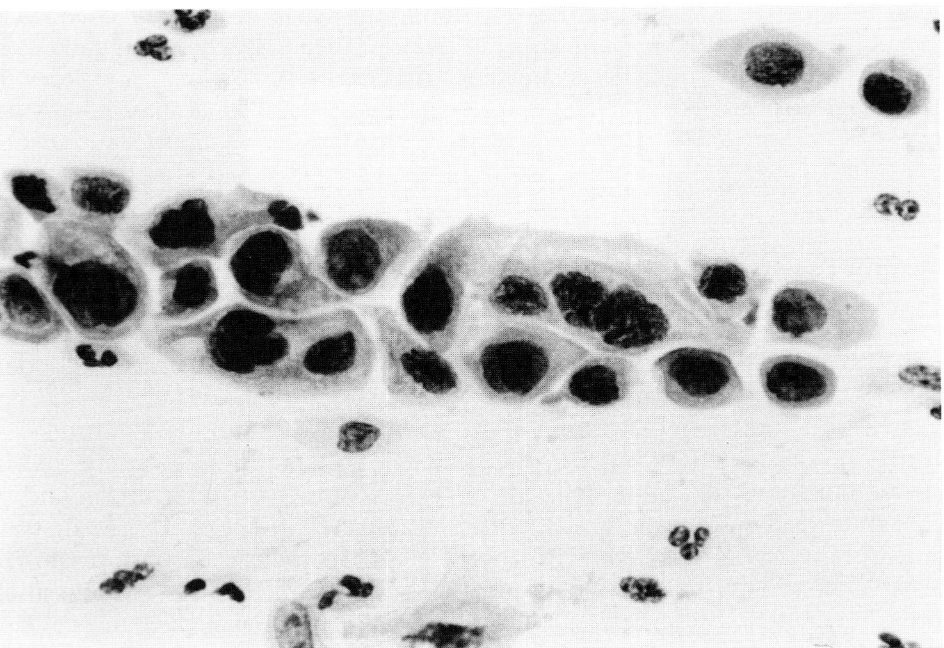

FIGURE 3.38. AND 3.39. High-grade SIL. In these high-power views of CIN 3, or high-grade SIL, small, markedly atypical cells with very high N/C ratios, nuclear membrane irregularities, and clumped chromatin are present. To appreciate the small size of these cells, compare their size to the neutrophils in the background. (40x)

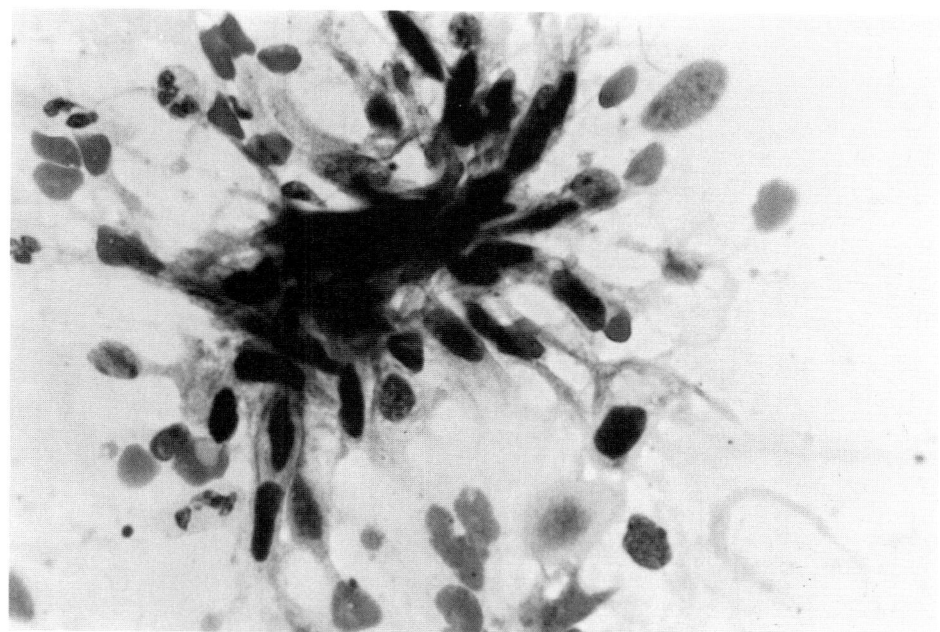

FIGURE 3.40. Keratinizing squamous cell carcinoma. Spindly squamous cells with darkly staining enlarged nuclei are present in a bloody background in this case. (40x) In addition to these cells, larger, bizarre, bright orange (keratinized) squamous cells with marked nuclear hyperchromasia and irregularities are usually present. (40x)

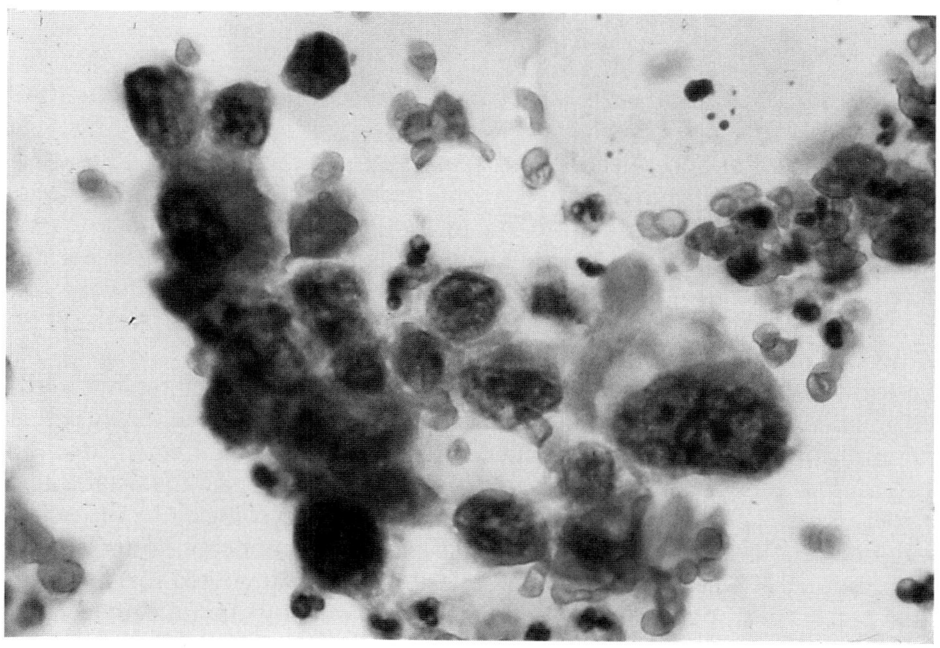

FIGURE 3.41. Nonkeratinizing squamous cell carcinoma. Small, malignant squamous cells with cyanophilic cytoplasm, enlarged nuclei, marked nuclear membrane irregularities, and occasional nucleoli are present in a bloody background. (40x) In this case, the biopsy revealed moderately differentiated invasive squamous cell carcinoma.

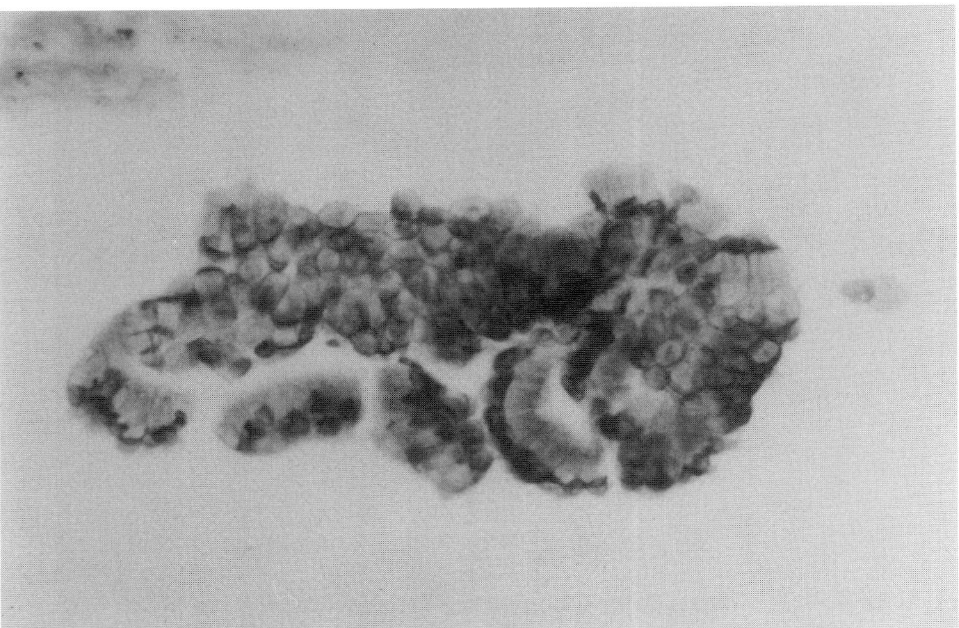

FIGURE 3.42. Benign endocervical cells. The cells are arranged in two-dimensional sheets and strips with basally aligned nuclei. When viewed on end, a honeycomb pattern is evident. In many endocervical lesions, this equal spacing of cells is lost as the cells become crowded and overlapped. (20x)

or a visible lesion. Glandular lesions may coexist with squamous lesions in 30–50% of cases (24, 58, 59).

The spectrum of endocervical lesions spans from reactive (Figs. 3.42 and 3.43) to in situ (Figs. 3.44–3.50) and invasive adenocarcinoma (Table 3.6). The lesions in-between fall into the AGUS category and include atypia secondary to polyps, atypia from glandular involvement of SIL, and low-grade endocervical dysplasia. Because early endocervical lesions do not have any specific clinical symptoms or colposcopic findings, the importance of routine cytologic recognition cannot be overemphasized. The features differentiating these entities are summarized in Table 3.6.

Cervical adenocarcinoma can be categorized into the following types: endocervical (including adenoma malignum and villoglandular), endometrioid, clear cell, serous, mesonephric, intestinal, signet-ring, adenosquamous, glassy cell carcinoma, adenoid basal carcinoma, adenoid cystic carcinoma, mixed, small cell, and metastatic adenocarcinoma (91). Several of these variants have been described cytologically, including minimal deviation adenocarcinoma, villoglandular papillary adenocarcinoma, and adenoid cystic carcinoma. The key features of these lesions are summarized in Table 3.7.

Other cervical lesions that have been detected by cytology include metastatic breast carcinoma (Figs. 3.51 and 3.52) (20), metastatic melanoma (Fig. 3.28) (9), primary lymphoma (Fig. 3.53) (10), metastatic adenocarcinoma from the gallbladder, metastatic gastric signet ring cell carcinoma (54), metastatic ovarian carcinoma (Fig. 3.54) (27), preleukemic granulocytic sarcoma (75), fallopian tube carcinoma (Fig. 3.55) (33), and metastatic mesothelioma (Fig. 3.56).

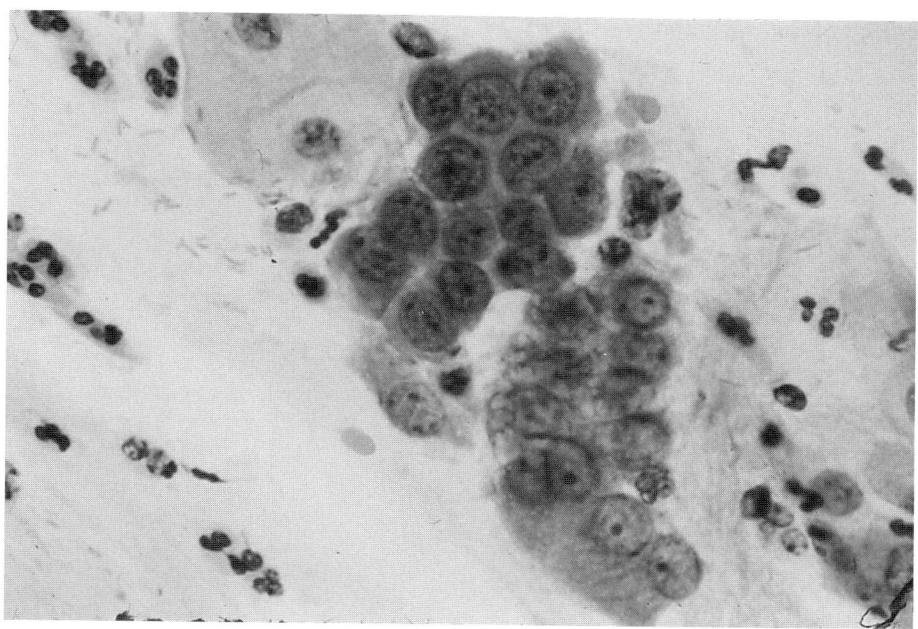

FIGURE 3.43. Reactive endocervical cells. Reactive features displayed here include mild nuclear enlargement, an open chromatin pattern, and nucleoli. The cells are still equally spaced, and the nuclei are basally situated. (40x) Another feature of reactive endocervical cells is multinucleation (Fig. 3.8).

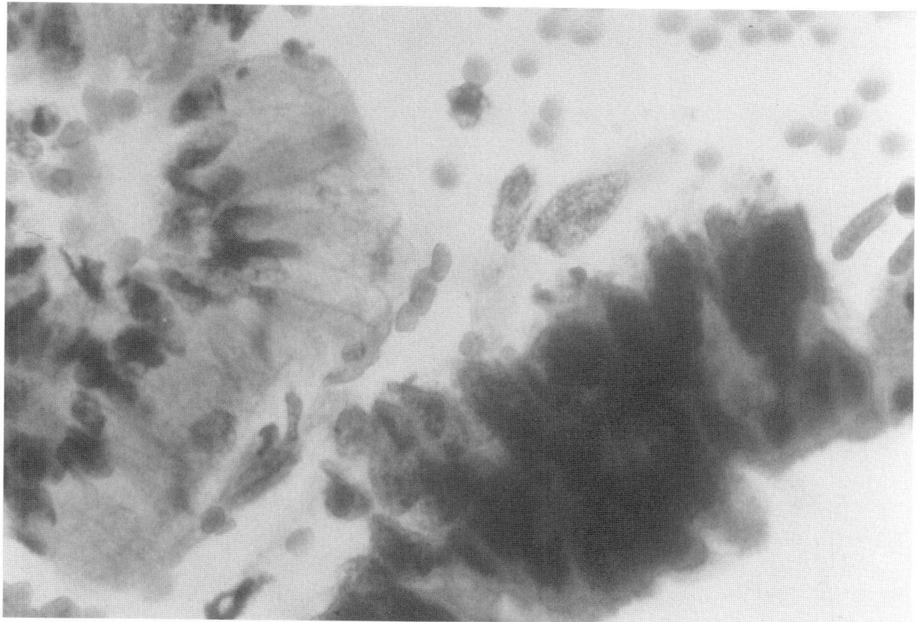

FIGURE 3.44. Adenocarcinoma-in-situ: AIS. A strip of AIS cells is adjacent to a strip of benign endocervical cells. Note the marked nuclear pseudostratification (nuclei located basally as well as apically), elongation (cigar shape), and coarse chromatin in the neoplastic cells. (40x)

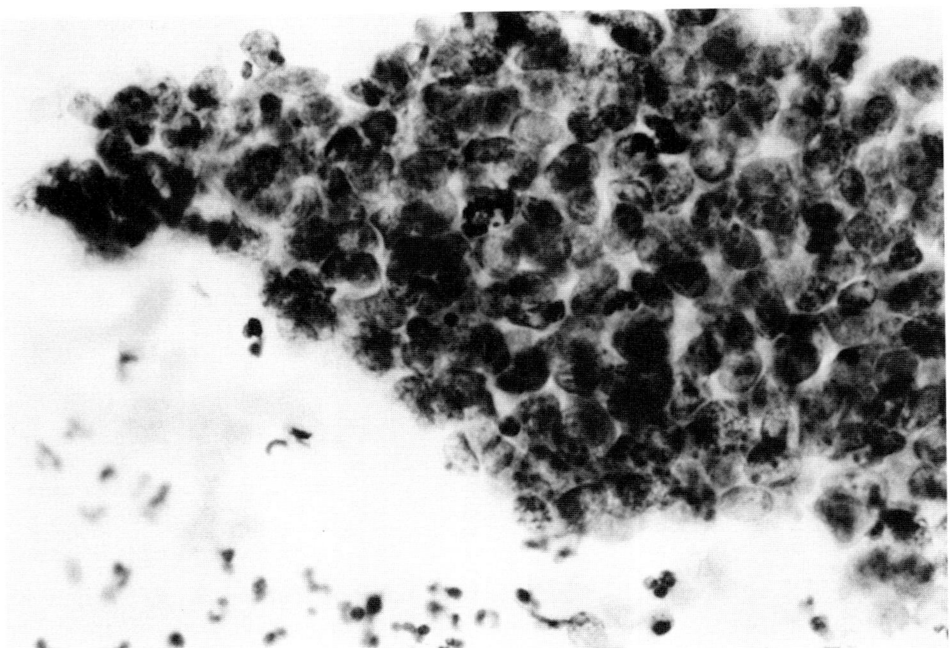

FIGURE 3.45. AIS. A cluster of AIS cells showing marked nuclear overlap, loss of polarity, mitoses, and intense chromatin stippling. (40x).

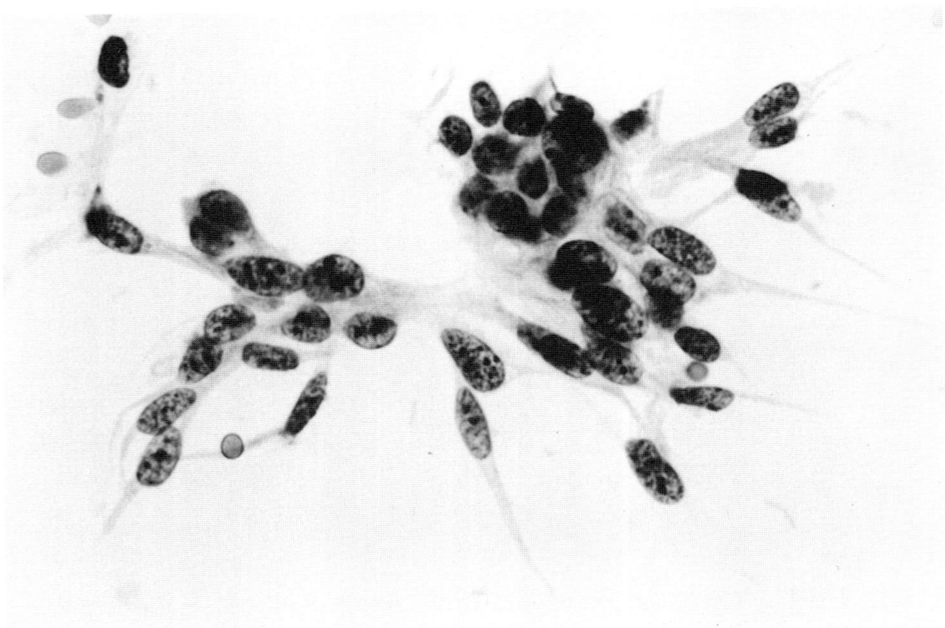

FIGURE 3.46. AIS. This cluster of AIS cells demonstrates "feathering" (stretching out of cytoplasm at the edges of the clusters), which is one of the more diagnostic features of this lesion. Note the coarse chromatin pattern and oval-to-cigar shaped nuclei. (40x)

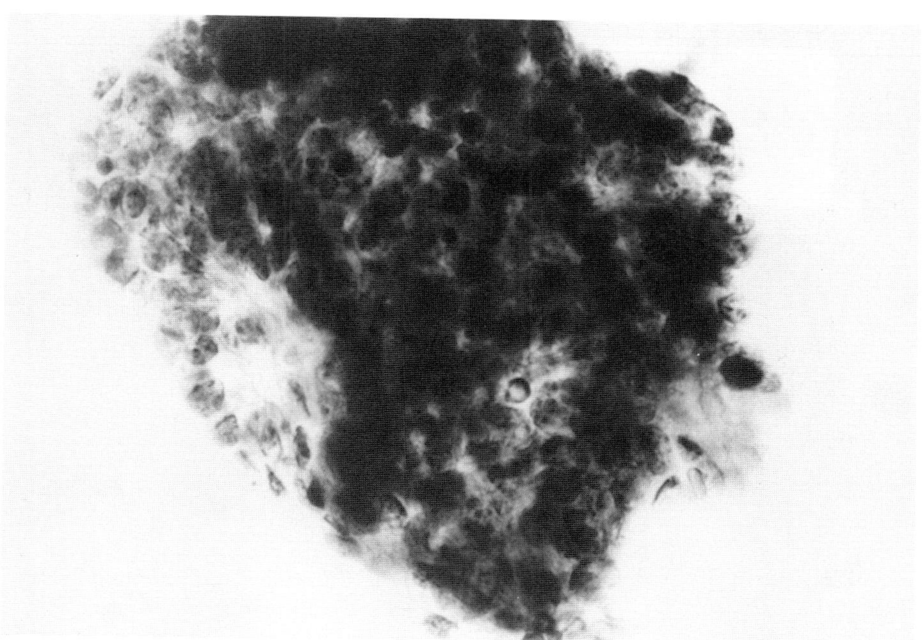

FIGURE 3.47. AIS. Note the rosette formation and marked nuclear overlap and crowding in this group of AIS cells. (40x)

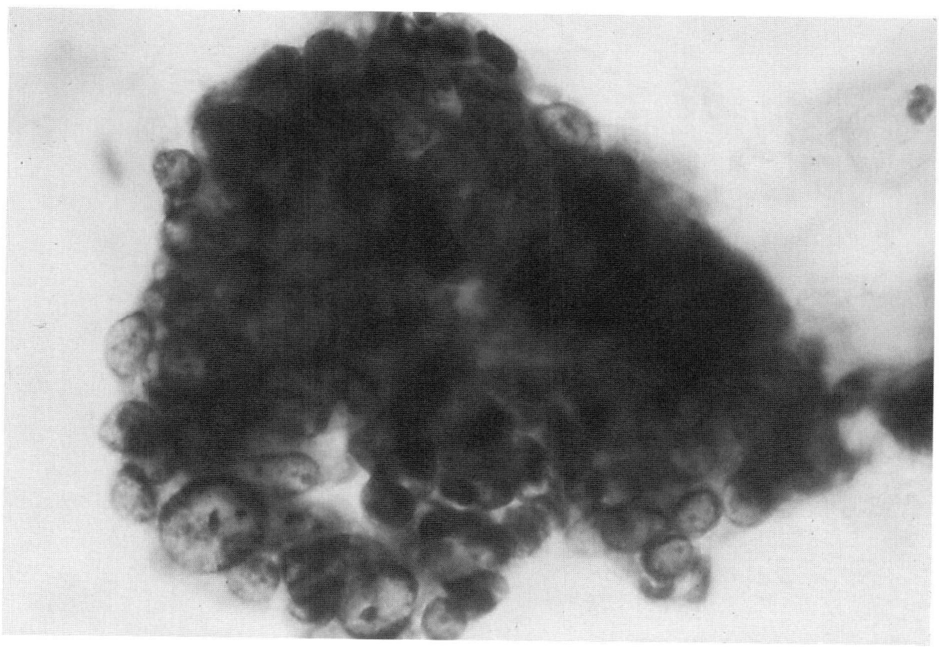

FIGURE 3.48. AIS. One type of AIS has smaller nuclei displaying a very open chromatin pattern and resembling a group of grapes, as shown here. In contrast to the hyperchromatic, cigar-shaped variety, these cells with small, round, pale nuclei may be easily overlooked. Note the crowding, variation in nuclear size, and occasional nucleoli. (40x)

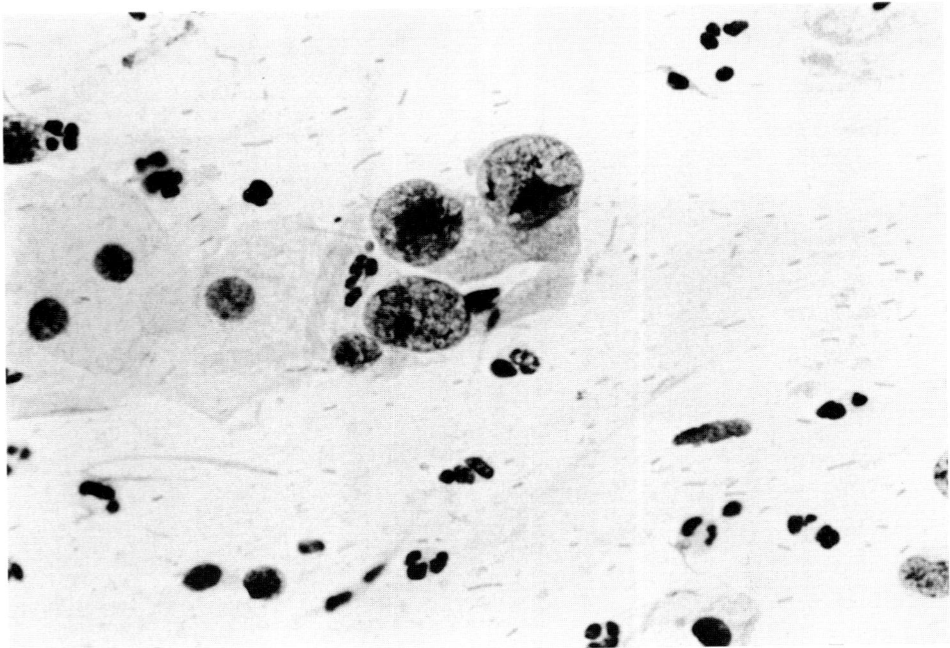

FIGURE 3.49. AIS. Single AIS cells with enlarged nuclei and coarse chromatin pattern are present in the center of this photo. (40x)

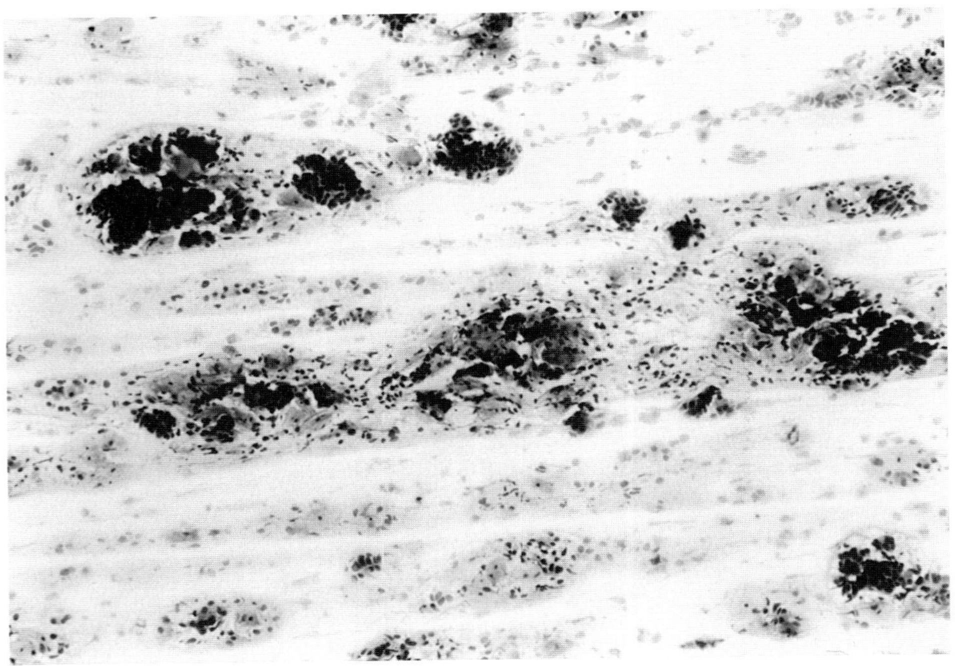

FIGURE 3.50. AIS. Note the darkly staining groups of AIS cells in contrast to the paler benign endocervical cells in this low-power view. Many of these clusters show branching, a feature best appreciated at low power. (4x)

TABLE 3.6. Lesions of the Endocervix

	Reactive (19, 24, 58)	AGUS (19, 24, 58, 83, 84)	Low Grade Glandular Dysplasia (19, 58, 83, 84)	High Grade Glandular Dysplasia (19, 59, 83, 84)	Invasive Adenocarcinoma (19, 59, 83, 84)	SIL Involving Endocervical Glands (72)
Cell borders	Well-defined		Ill-defined	Feathered edges	Variable; may be feathered	Smooth cell borders
N/C ratios	Normal	Increased	Mild increase	Increased	Marked	Increased
Nuclear overlap (crowding)	Absent–minimal; honeycomb sheets	Minimal	Moderate	Marked	Marked	Central loss of polarity with spindling
Nuclear shape	Round to oval; no nuclear irregularities	Variable	Oval or minimally elongated; some nuclear irregularities	Oval to elongated	Pleomorphic	Round to oval
Chromatin	Fine	Mildly increased	Mildly increased	Coarse or open	Coarse, irregular, or open	Increased; hyperchromatic
Nucleoli	Prominent	Variable	Inconspicuous	Inconspicuous	Prominent	None
Rosettes	Rare	Rare	Occasional	Common	Very common	None
Cell strip stratification	Rare		Few	Very common (loss of polarity)	Moderate	None
Background	Inflammatory		Clean	Clean	"Dirty"; tumor diathesis	SIL may be present
Single cells	Rare	Minimal	None	Moderate	Common	Common
Mitoses	Rare		Occasional	Common	Common	Increased
Cellularity	Low		Less	Marked	Marked	None
Papillations (cell clusters)	None	None	None	Occasional	Many	

TABLE 3.7. Variants of Adenocarcinoma

Lesion	Gross Findings/ Clinical Presentation	Cytologic Findings	Differential Diagnosis
Adenoma malignum	Profuse vaginal discharge, menometrorrhagia, and menorrhagia. Indurated, beefy red cervix which may be hemorrhagic and friable. Accounts for 1–3% of all cervical adenocarcinoma. May be associated with Peutz-Jeghers Syndrome. Prognosis may be poor. (25)	Subtle changes. Vacuolated cells with bland, enlarged nuclei ($2\times$ normal size), fine chromatin pattern, small nucleoli, and occasional nuclear grooves. Cells usually arranged in honeycombed sheets which may be branched and multilayered. Mucin and cytoplasmic tails have been reported. Atypical endocervical cells with thickened. irregular nuclear membranes and nucleoli may be noted. (25)	Microglandular hyperplasia, clear cell carcinoma, tubal metaplasia. Histologically, differential diagnosis includes hyperplastic mesonephric remnants and adenomatous hyperplasia.
Adenoid cystic carcinoma (cylindromatous)	Postmenopausal bleeding and cervical nodule or polypoid mass. May be associated with squamous dysplasia, invasive squamous cell carcinoma, adenocarcinoma, or small cell carcinoma.	Small, uniform cells with scanty cytoplasm and slightly granular, hyperchromatic chromatin. Cells characteristically arranged in small, round, compact acini forming papillary groupings. Acini may contain a core of hyaline material or may appear empty. Nucleoli are inconspicuous. (67)	Endometrial cells, endometrial adenocarcinoma, brush artifact, adenoid basal carcinoma. (67)

	Rare tumor, constituting 1–3% of all cervical adenocarcinoma. Poor prognosis. (67)		
Villoglandular adenocarcinoma	Friable, papillary or polypoid, exophytic mass arising in endocervical canal and causing abnormal bleeding. Most patients under 40 years of age. Favorable prognosis. (4)	Cellular smears composed of large sheets, tight clusters, and papillary configurations of tumor cells with small, dark, oval, crowded and overlapping nuclei. Chromatin is even, and nucleoli are inconspicuous. Tumor cells at the periphery of cell groups appear flattened or palisading. Mitoses are present. (4)	AIS, CIS involving endocervical glands, endometrial cells, reactive endocervical cells. Histologically, differential diagnosis includes chronic cervicitis, Mullerian papilloma, and adenofibroma. (4)
Well-differentiated adenocarcinoma with abundant mucus secretion	Induration and swelling, with rubber ball-like resilience, profuse watery discharge, and, less commonly, bleeding. Colposcopically, abundant mucus and very large, irregular glandular openings. Net-like pattern observed following acetic acid application.	Abundant mucus and slight nuclear atypia.	

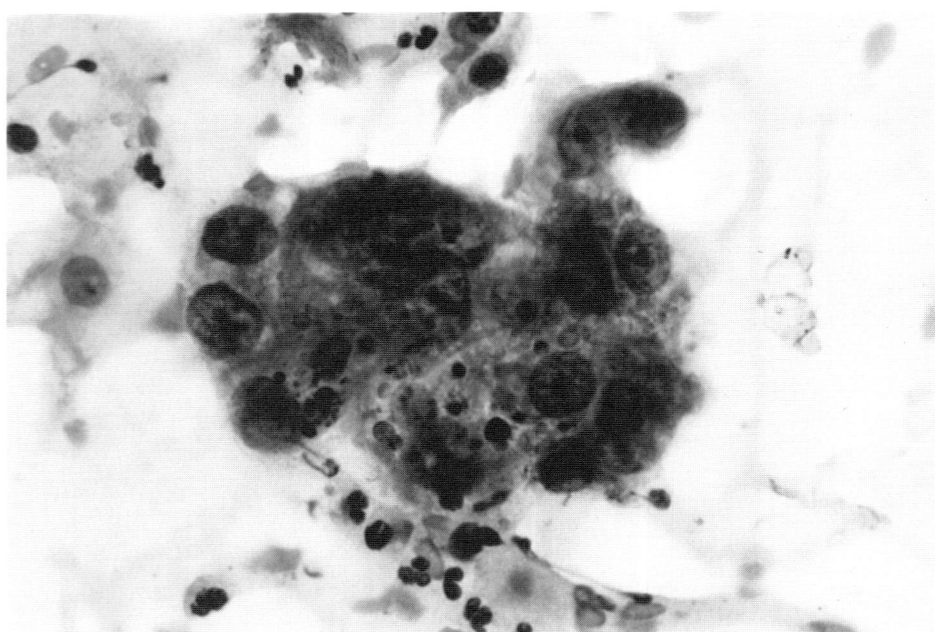

FIGURE 3.51. Metastatic breast carcinoma. A cluster of metastatic mammary carcinoma cells from a patient with a known history of breast carcinoma. Note the enlarged nuclei with prominent nucleoli. More often, breast carcinoma cells are not so obviously atypical, making detection more difficult. (40x)

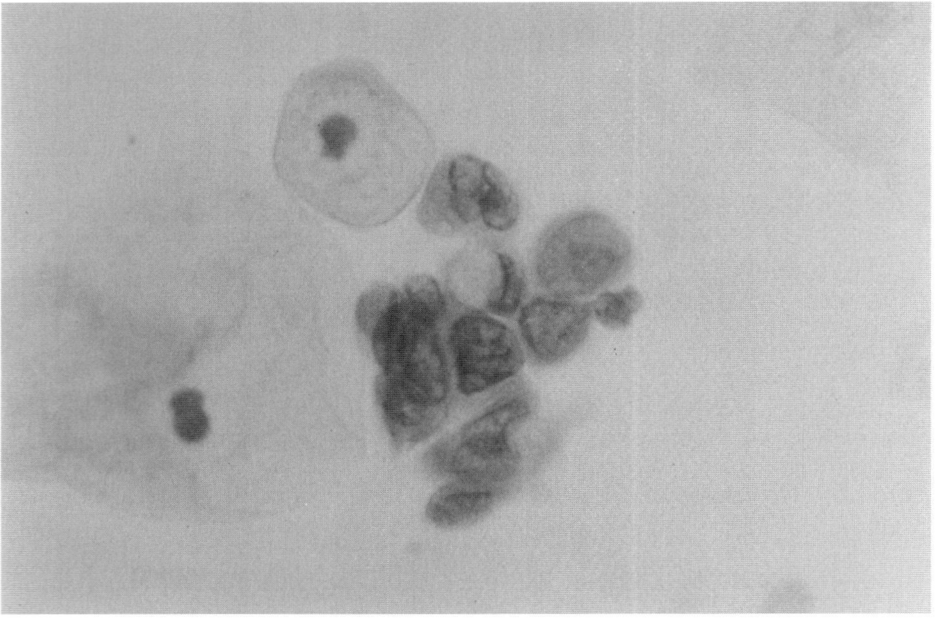

FIGURE 3.52. Metastatic breast carcinoma. In this case of metastatic mammary carcinoma, the atypia is more subtle. Note the signet cell in the center. (40x) (20)

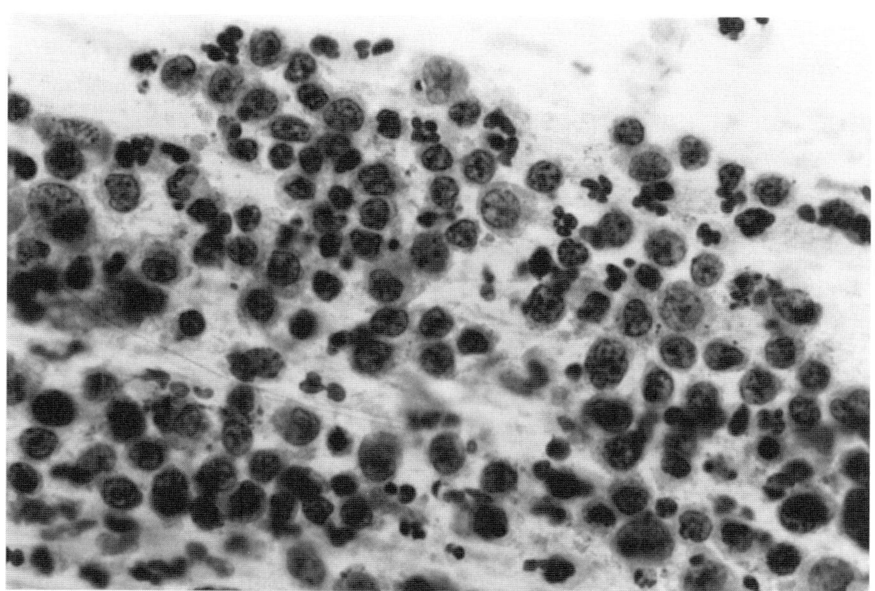

FIGURE 3.53. Primary malignant lymphoma of the uterine cervix. The dispersed population of atypical lymphocytes displays marked nuclear membrane irregularities (lobulations and snouts) and an altered chromatin pattern. (40X) The lack of cohesion is typical of a lymphoid population. Clinically, bleeding per vagina and diffuse enlargement of the cervix are common. Cytology is positive in only 40–50% of the cases. (10)

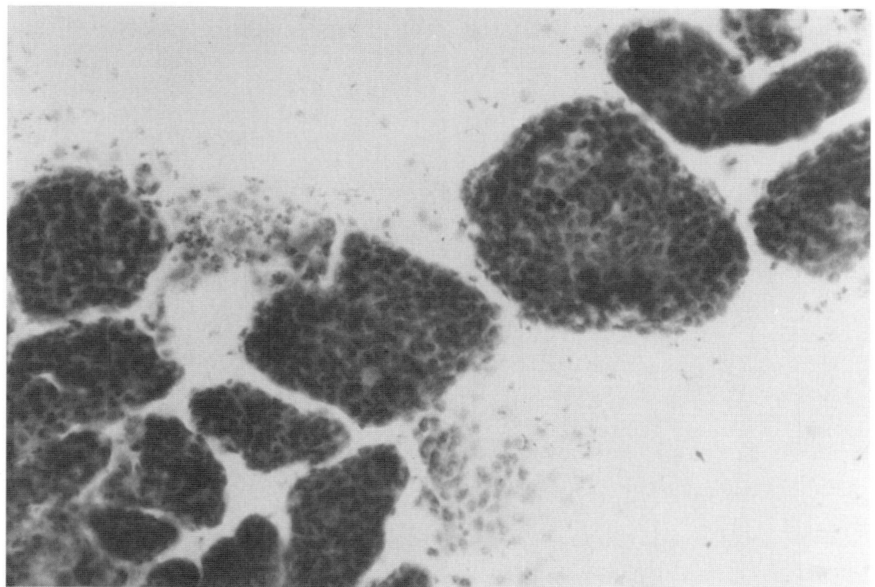

FIGURE 3.54. Metastatic ovarian carcinoma. In this example, multiple papillary clusters of neoplastic cells are present in a clean background. Sometimes, psammoma bodies are present within the papillary groupings. The finding of metastatic ovarian carcinoma in the lower genital tract is rare. (10x) (27)

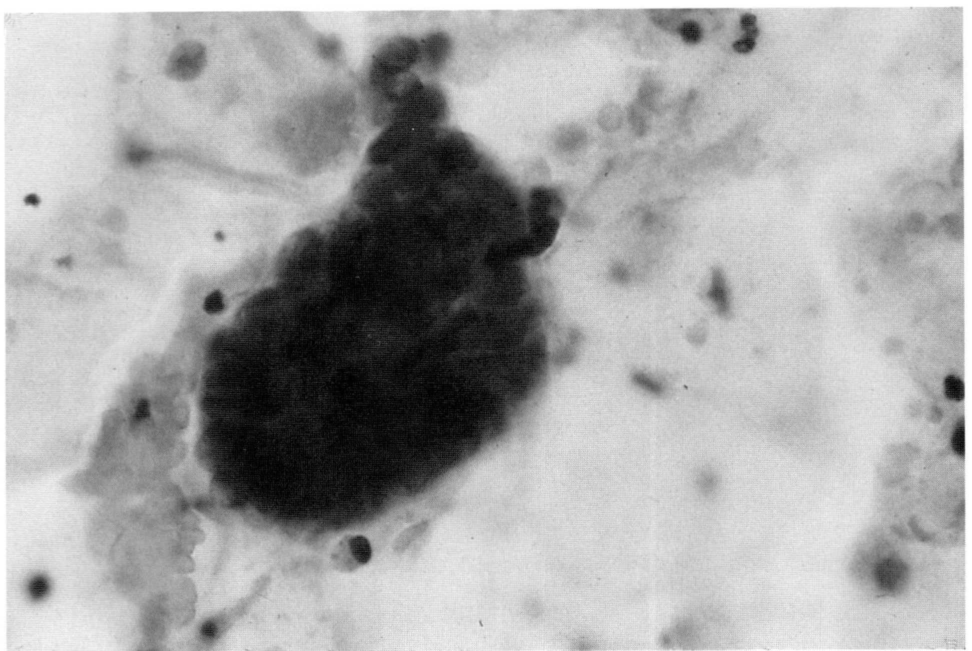

FIGURE 3.55.   Metastatic fallopian tube carcinoma. This is a case of early fallopian tube carcinoma detected in a routine Pap smear. In this cluster, the malignant cells at the periphery appear columnar. Only a few cell clusters were present, and most appeared endometrioid in nature. (40x) The rate of cytologic detection of this rare lesion varies from 0–60%. Endometrial aspirates are diagnostic more often than cervical, endocervical, and vaginal smears. (33)

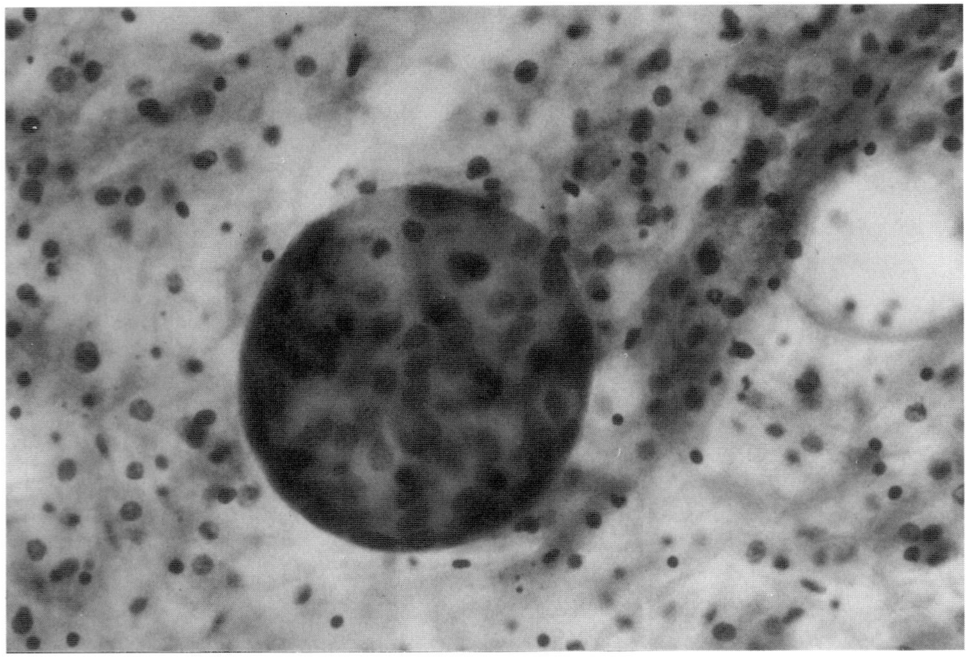

REFERENCES

1. Angeles MA, Saigo PE. Cytologic findings in rectovaginal fistulae. Acta Cytol 1994;38(3): 373–376.
2. Ballo MS, Silverberg SG, Sidawy MK. Cytologic features of well-differentiated villoglandular adenocarcinoma of the cervix. Acta Cytol 1996;40(3):536–540.
3. Bardales RH, Valente PT, Stanley MW. Cytology of suture granulomas in post-hysterectomy vaginal smears. Diagn Cytopathol 1995;13(4):336–338.
4. Basta A, Madej JG Jr. Hydradenoma of the vulva. Incidence and clinical observations. Eur J Gynaecol Oncol 1990;11(3):185–189.
5. Bewtra C. Columnar cells in posthysterectomy vaginal smears. Diagn Cytopathol 1992; 8(4):342–345.
6. Bibbo M. Comprehensive Cytopathology. Philadelphia: WB Saunders, 1991.
7. Bokun R, Perkovic M, Bakotin J, et al. Cytology and histopathology of metastatic malignant melanoma involving a polyp on the uterine cervix. A case report. Acta Cytol 1985;29(4):612–615.
8. Bou Saba C, Houkayem J, Afif N, et al. Primary lymphoma of the uterine cervix. A case report and literature review. J Med Liban 1992;40(4):207–210.
9. Cohen GJ. Vulvar Paget's disease. Cytologic and immunohistologic diagnosis of a case. Acta Cytol 1988;32(5):727–730.
10. Cohen PR, Young AW, Tovell HMM. Angiokeratoma of the vulva: diagnosis and review of the literature. Obstet & Gynec Survey 1989;44(5):339–346.
11. Daniele E, Nuara R, Morello V, et al. Microglandular hyperplasia of the uterine cervix. Histo-cytopathological evaluation, differential diagnosis and review of the literature. Pathol 1993;85(1100):607–635.
12. Davey DD, Naryshkin S, Nielsen ML, et al. Atypical squamous cells of undetermined significance: interlaboratory comparison and quality assurance moniters. Diagn Cytopath 1994;11(4):390–396.
13. de Boer A, de Boer F, Van der Merwe JV. Cytologic identification of Donovan bodies in granuloma inguinale. Acta Cytol 1984;28(2):126–128.
14. Dennerstein GJ. Cytology of the vulva. J Reprod Med 1988;33(8):703–704.
15. DiTomasso JP, Ramzy I, Mody DR. Glandular lesions of the cervix. Validity of cytologic criteria used to differentiate reactive changes, glandular intraepithelial lesions and adenocarcinoma. Acta Cytol 1996;40(6):1127–1135.
16. Fiorella RM, Beckwith LG, Miller LK, et al. Metastatic signet ring carcinoma of the breast as a source of positive cervicovaginal cytology. A case report. Acta Cytol 1993;37(6): 948–952.
17. Germain M, Heaton R, Erickson D, et al. A comparison of the three most common Papanicolaou smear collection techniques. Obstet Gynecol 1994;84(2):168–173.

FIGURE 3.56 Metastatic mesothelioma. This is a case of a woman with a known history of adenocarcinoma whose Pap smear showed scattered papillary balls such as the one in this photomicrograph. Little or no cytologic atypia is present, but the pattern in the smear is that of a metastatic lesion. The possibility of a metastatic adenocarcinoma was suggested. A clinical workup revealed a second primary—mesothelioma. In retrospect, the cellular balls were noted to display flattened cells around the periphery, a finding more characteristic of mesothelioma. (40x). No other reports of metastatic mesothelioma presenting in this way appear in the medical literature.

18. Giacomini G, Schnadig VJ . The cervical Papanicolaou smear: bacterial infection and the Bethesda System [letter]. Acta Cytol 1992;36(1):109–110.
19. Goff BA, Atanasoff P, Brown E, et al. Endocervical glandular atypia in Papanicolaou smears. Obstet Gynecol 1992;79(1):101-104.
20. Granter SR, Lee KR. Cytologic findings in minimal deviation adenocarcinoma (Adenoma Malignum) of the cervix. A report of seven cases. Am J Clin Pathol 1996;105(3):327–333.
21. Guarner J, Cohen C. Vulvar Paget's disease. Acta Cytol 1988;32(5):727–730.
22. Guidozzi F, Sonnendecker EW, Wright C. Ovarian cancer with metastatic deposits in the cervix, vagina, or vulva preceding primary cytoreductive surgery. Gynecol Oncol 1993;49(2):25–28.
23. Heimann A, Scanlon R, Gentile J, et al. Measles cervicitis. Acta Cytol 1992;36(5):727–730.
24. Henry MR, de Mesy Jensen KL, Skoglund CD, et al. *Chlamydia trachomatis* in routine cervical smears: a microscopic and ultrascopic analysis. Acta Cytol 1993;37(3):343–352.
25. Hernandez-Linares W, Puthawala A, Nolan JF, et al. Carcinoma in situ of the vagina: past and present management. Obstet Gynecol 1980;56(3):356–360.
26. Hernandez-Ortiz MJ, Valenzuela-Ruiz P, Gonzalez-Estecha A, et al. Fine needle aspiration cytology of primary epithelioid sarcoma of the vulva: a case report. Acta Cytol 1995;39(1):100–103.
27. Hirai Y, Chen JT, Hamada T, et al. Clinical and cytologic aspects of primary fallopian tube carcinoma. A report of ten cases. Acta Cytol 1987;31(6):834–840.
28. Hustin J, Donnay M, Hamels J. Identification of papillary hidradenoma of the vulva by imprint cytology (letter). Acta Cytol 1980;24(5):466–467.
29. Imachi M, Tsukamoto N, Kamura T, et al. Alveolar rhabdomyosarcoma of the vulva: report of two cases. Acta Cytol 1991;35(3):345–349.
30. Imachi M, Tsukamoto N, Shigematsu T, et al. Cytologic diagnosis of primary adenocarcinoma of Bartholin's gland: a case report. Acta Cytol 1992;36(2):167–170.
31. International Academy of Cytology. The Bethesda system for reporting cervical/vaginal cytologic diagnoses. Acta Cytol 1993;37(2):115–124.
32. Johnson CA, Lorenzetti LA, Liese BS, et al. Clinical significance of hyperkeratosis on otherwise normal Papanicolaou smears. Fam Pract 1991;33(4):354–358
33. Jonasson JG, Wang HH, Antonioli DA, et al. Tubal metaplasia of the uterine cervix: A prevalence study in patients with gynecologic pathologic findings. Internat J of Gynecol Pathol 1992;89–95.
34. Joseph RE, Enghardt MH, Doering DL, et al. Small cell neuroendocrine carcinoma of the vagina. Cancer 1992;70(4):784–789.
35. Kashimura M, Matsuura Y, Kawagoe T, et al. Cytology of vulvar squamous neoplasia. Acta Cytol 1993;37(6):871–875.
36. Kashimura Y, Kashimura M, Horie A. Cytologic, histologic, DNA ploidy and electron microscopic analyses of a case of vulvar Paget's disease. Anal Quant Cytol Histol 1989;11(6):413–418.
37. Kern SB. Significance of anucleated squames in Papanicolaou-stained cervicovaginal smears. Acta Cytol 1991;35(1):89–93.
38. Koike N, Higuchi T, Sakai Y. Goblet-like cells in atrophic vaginal smears and their histologic correlation. Acta Cytol 1990;34(6):785–788.
39. Koss LG. Diagnostic cytology and its histopathologic bases. 4th ed. Philadelphia: JB Lippincott, 1992.
40. Krieger JN, Tam MR, Stevens CE, et al. Diagnosis of trichomoniasis. Comparison of conventional wet-mount examination with cytologic studies, cultures, and monoclonal antibody staining of direct specimens. JAMA 1988;259(8):1223–1227.
41. Luzzatto R, Boon ME. Contribution of the endocervical cytobrush sample to the diagnosis of cervical lesions. Acta Cytol 1996;40(6):1143–1147.

42. Mahmud N, Kusuda N, Ichinose S, et al. Needle aspiration biopsy of vulvar endometriosis. Acta Cytol 1992;36(4):514–516.
43. Mali BN, Joshi JV. Vaginal parasitosis. An unusual finding in routine cervical smears. Acta Cytol 1987;31(6):866–868.
44. Marcos C, Martinez L, Esquivias JJ, et al. Primary non-Hodgkin lymphoma of the vulva. Acta Obstet Gynecol Scand 1992;71(4):298–300.
45. McGill F, Adachi A, Karimi N, et al. Abnormal cervical cytology leading to the diagnosis of gastric cancer. Gynecol Oncol 1990;36(1):101–105.
46. Mihaescu A, Gloor E, Chobaz C. Malacoplakia of the vagina. Cytological, histological and ultrastructural study of a case. Arch Anat Cytol Pathol 1991;39(3):109–115.
47. Nadji M, Defortuna S, Sevin BU, et al. Fine-needle aspiration cytology of palpable lesions of the lower female genital tract. Int J Gynecol Pathol 1994;13(1):54–61.
48. Nasu I, Meurer W, Fu YS. Endocervical glandular atypia and adenocarcinoma: a correlation of cytology and histology. Int J Gynecol Pathol 1993;12(3):208–218.
49. Novotny DB, Maygarden SJ, Johnson DE, et al. Tubal metaplasia: a frequent potential pitfall in the cytologic diagnosis of endocervical glandular dysplasia on cervical smears. Acta Cytol 1992;36(1):1–10.
50. Pearlstone AC, Grigsby PW, Mutch DG. High rates of atypical cervical cytology: occurrence and clinical significance. Obstet Gynecol 1992;80(2):191–195.
51. Platz-Christensen JJ, Larsson P, Sundstrom E, et al. Detection of bacterial vaginosis in wet mount, Papanicolaou stained vaginal smears and in Gram stained smears. Acta Obstet Gynecol Scand 1995;74:67–70.
52. Prasad KRK, Kumari GS, Aruna CA, et al. Fibroadenoma of ectopic breast tissue in the vulva. A case report. Acta Cytol 1995;39:791–792.
53. Ravinsky E, Safneck JR, Chantziantonioun. Cytologic features of primary adenoid cystic carcinoma of the uterine cervix: a case report. Acta Cytol 1996;40(6):1304–1308.
54. Schust DJ, Moore DH, Baird DB, et al. Primary adenocarcinoma of the gallbladder presenting as primary gynecologic malignancy: a report of two cases. Obstet Gynecol 1994;83(5pt2):831–834.
55. Selvaggi SM. Cytologic features of squamous cell carcinoma in situ involving endocervical glands in endocervical cytobrush specimens. Acta Cytol 1994;38(5):687–692.
56. Selvaggi SM, Haefner HK, Lelle RJ, et al. Neovaginal cytology after total pelvic exenteration for gynecological malignancies. Diagn Cytopathol 1995;13(1):22–25.
57. Spahr J, Behm FG, Schneider V. Preleukemic granulocytic sarcoma of cervix and vagina: initial manifestations by cytology. Acta Cytol 1982;26(1):55–60.
58. Spiegel CA. Bacterial vaginosis. Clin Microbiol Rev 1991;4(4):485–502.
59. Tabbara SO, Copvell JL, Abbitt PL. Diagnosis of endometriosis by fine-needle aspiration cytology. Diag Cytopath 1991;7(6):606–610.
60. Ueki M, Ueda M, Okamura S, et al. Clinicopathological features of well-differentiated cervical adenocarcinoma with abundant mucus secretion. J of Medicine 1995;26(1/2): 17–30.
61. Van Aspert-van Erp AJM, van't Hof-Grootenboer AB, Brugal G, et al. Endocervical columnar cell intraepithelial neoplasia: discriminating cytomorphologic criteria. Acta Cytol 1995;39(6):1199–1214.
62. Van Aspert-van Erp AJM, van't Hof-Grootenboer AB, Brugal G, et al. Endocervical columnar cell intraepithelial neoplasia: grades of expression of cytomorphologic criteria. Acta Cytol 1995;39(6):1216–1232.
63. Van Le L, Novotny D, Dotters DJ. Distinguishing tubal metaplasia from endocervical dysplasia on cervical Papanicolaou smears. Obstet Gynecol 1991;78(2):974–975.
64. Vogelsang PJ, Nguyen GK, Honore' LH. Exfoliative cytology of adenoma malignum (minimal deviation adenocarcinoma) of the uterine cervix. Diagn Cytopath 1995;13(2): 146–150.
65. Vuong PN, Neveux Y, Schoonaert MF, et al. Adenoid cystic (cylindromatous) carcinoma associated with squamous cell carcinoma of the cervix uteri. Acta Cytol 1996;40(2):289–294.

66. Yahr LJ, Lee KR. Cytologic findings in microglandular hyperplasia of the cervix. Diagnos Cytopathol 1991;7(3):248–251.
67. Yamagiwa S, Niwa K, Yokoyama Y, et al. Primary adenoid cystic carcinoma of Bartholin's gland. A case report. Acta Cytol 1994;38(1):79–82.
68. Young RH, Scully RE. Invasive adenocarcinoma and related tumors of the uterine cervix. Seminars in Diag Pathol 1990;7(3):205–227.
69. Young RH, Scully RE. Villoglandular papillary adenocarcinoma of the uterine cervix: a clinicopathologic analysis of 13 cases. Cancer 1989;63:1773–1779.

BENIGN DISEASES OF THE VULVA

Debra S. Heller, MD

■

Normal Anatomy and Histology of the Vulva
Congenital Anomalies
Sexually Transmitted Diseases (STDs)
Other Infections and Inflammations
Benign Disorders of Pigmentation
Nonneoplastic Epithelial Disorders
Cystic Lesions of the Vulva
Papillary Lesions of the Vulva
Other Tumor-like Lesions of the Vulva
Benign Neoplasms

Vulvar symptomatology will frequently cause a patient to seek medical attention. The clinical approach to the patient with a vulvar complaint was discussed in Chapter 1. The approach to the patient with a vulvar condition may need to be multidisciplinary, and gynecological, dermatological, and pathological input may be necessary. One must remember that in addition to conditions specific to the vulvar area, a wide variety of dermatologic disorders can affect the vulva as well as the rest of the body. These conditions are covered in depth in dermatology texts.

The liberal use of biopsy is particularly important in assessing and treating vulvar disease because visual inspection alone cannot always be relied upon to lead to the correct diagnosis.

NORMAL ANATOMY AND HISTOLOGY OF THE VULVA

The anatomy of the vulvar region is illustrated in Figure 4.1. The vulva consists of the mons pubis, labia majora, labia minora, clitoris, perineum, and vestibule. The outer labia majora is covered by keratinized squamous epithelium containing apocrine and eccrine sweat glands, sebaceous glands, and hair follicles (Fig. 4.2). The inner labia majora is nonhairbearing and generally lacks sweat glands although sebaceous glands

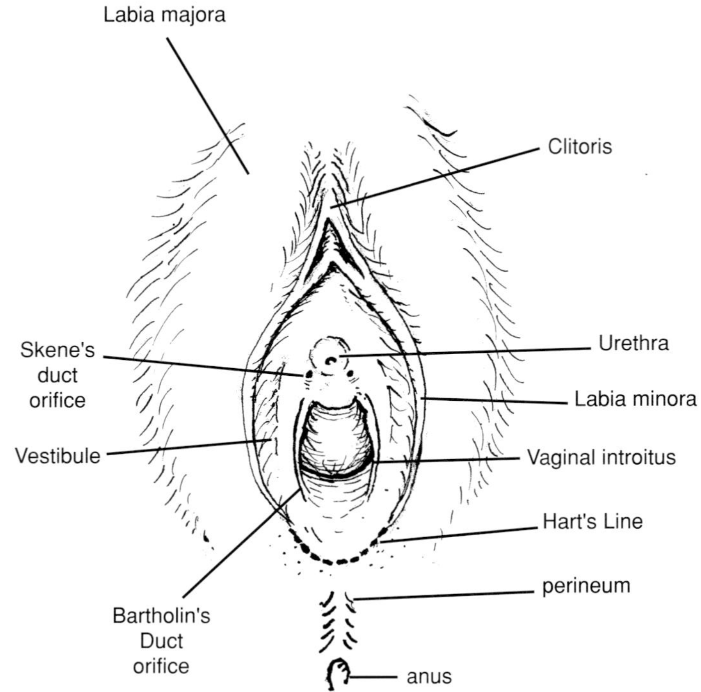

FIGURE 4.1. Anatomy of the vulvar region.

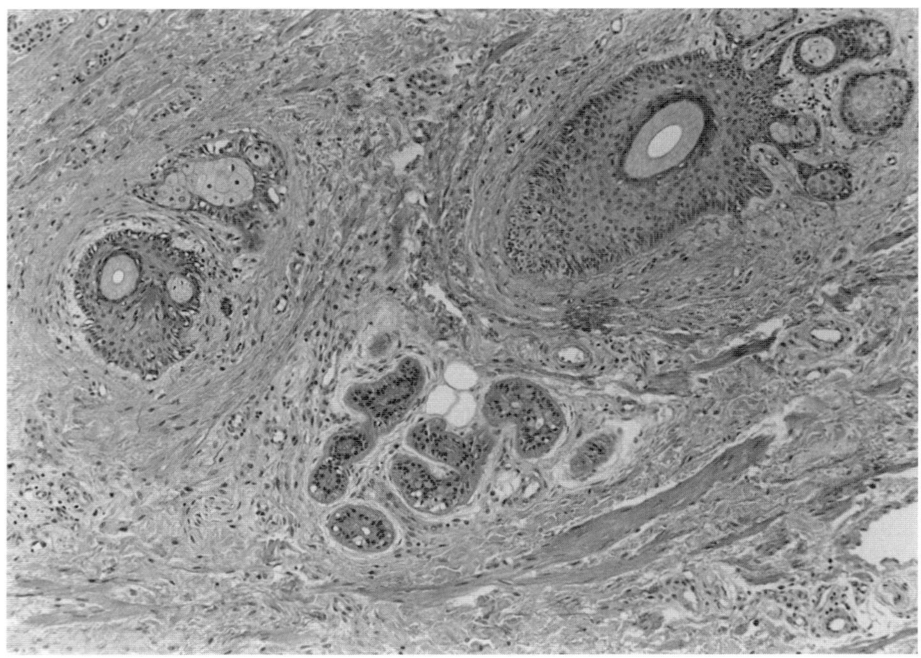

FIGURE 4.2. Labia majora. Hair follicles, sweat, and sebaceous glands are seen in the dermis.

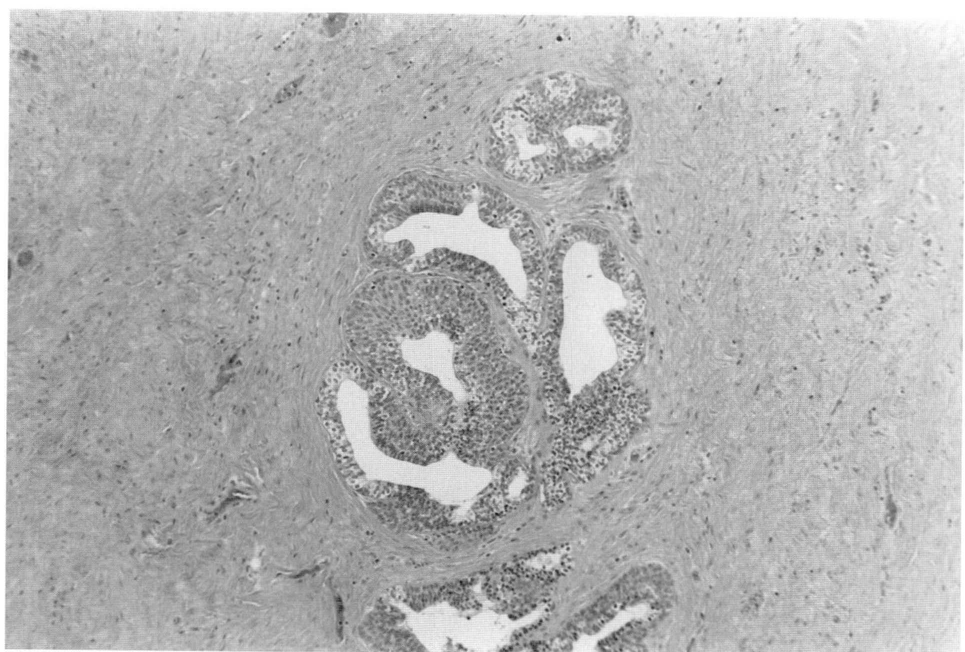

FIGURE 4.3.   Skene's duct lined by transitional epithelium.

are present. The labia minora are nonhairbearing, and glands are usually absent. The labia minora have a lateral, thin, keratinizing layer, which is absent medially. Sebaceous glands end external to Hart's line, which delineates the vestibule from the rest of the vulva. These sebaceous glands may be seen grossly as small yellow spots, known as Fordyce spots. The vestibule is the area internal to Hart's line and external to the hymen, and it is nonkeratinized. There are no sebaceous glands and generally no sweat glands in the vestibule. The vagina, urethra, Skene's and Bartholin's ducts, and minor vestibular glands empty into the vestibule. The Skene's ducts open onto either side of the urethra posterolaterally, and are lined by transitional epithelium (Fig 4.3). The Skene's glands are composed of pseudostratified mucinous columnar epithelium. The minor vestibular glands open directly into the vestibule, and are lined by mucinous columnar epithelium. The Bartholin's (major vestibular) ducts open into the vestibule at the 4 o'clock and 8 o'clock positions. Bartholin's glands are composed of acini, lined by mucinous epithelium (Fig.4.4). The ducts are lined by transitional epithelium, or a combination of mucinous and transitional epithelium. The vestibule is lined by nonkeratinized squamous epithelium. The urethra is lined by transitional epithelium (1–3).

CONGENITAL ANOMALIES

A discussion of the wide range of conditions resulting in ambiguous genitalia is beyond the scope of this book. Most cases of ambiguous genitalia in a 46XX infant are due to female pseudohermaphroditism, with increased intrauterine androgen exposure to a 46XX individual with ovaries (Table 4.1). Other anomalies, including imperforate hymen, and labial duplication, are rare.

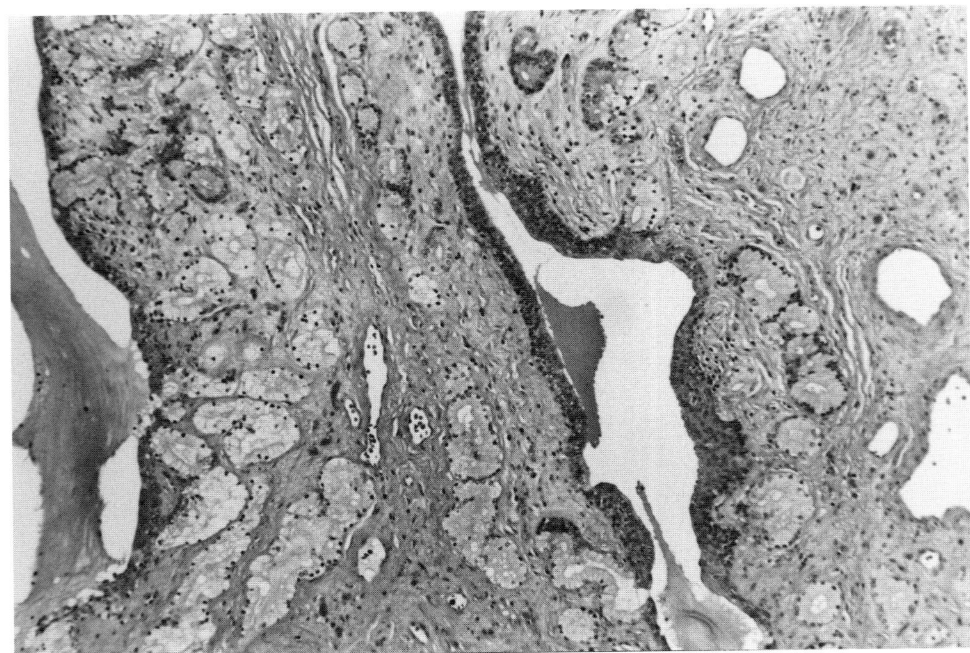

FIGURE 4.4. Bartholin's gland and duct. The mucinous epithelium-lined acini of the Bartholin's glands surround the duct, lined by transitional epithelium.

TABLE 4.1. Conditions That May Result In Ambiguous Genitalia in an Infant with a 46XX Karyotype

Female pseudohermaphroditism
    Congenital adrenal hyperplasia (adrenogenital syndrome)
    Virilizing maternal tumor
    Maternal intake of progestins/androgens
True Hermaphroditism with a 46XX Karyotype

Adapted from material in Robboy SJ, Bernhardt PF, Parmley T. Embryology of the female genital tract and disorders of abnormal sexual development. In Kurman RJ, ed. Blaustein's Pathology of the Female Genital Tract. 4th ed. New York: Springer-Verlag, 1994:3–29.

SEXUALLY TRANSMITTED DISEASES (STDs)

Many of the ulcerative vulvar lesions are secondary to sexually transmitted diseases (Table 4.2). Identifying STDs and treating them adequately is important, and a thorough treatment regimen should include counseling and partner therapy. If one STD is present, multiple STDs may be present; thus, a full screening should be performed.

CONDYLOMA ACCUMINATUM

Vulvar condyloma may be single or multiple. The presenting complaint is generally one of painless papillary growths although pruritus may occur. Most vulvar condyloma

TABLE 4.2.   Vulva Lesions That May Manifest as Ulcers (2, 10)

Syphilis
Herpes
Granuloma Inguinale
Chancroid
Lymphogranuloma Venereum
Sarcoid
Tuberculosis
Fungal infection
Bacterial infection
Hailey-Hailey disease
Darier disease
Behcet's syndrome
Pyoderma gangrenosum
Hidradenitis suppurativa
Pemphigus vulgaris
Pemphigoid
Erythema multiforme (Stevens-Johnson syndrome)
Reiter's syndrome
Fixed drug eruption
Contact dermatitis
Factitial/Trauma
Crohn's disease
Varicella
Cytomegalovirus
Epstein-Barr virus
Herpes zoster
AIDS
Insect bites
Pediculosis pubis
Scabies
Histiocytosis X
Malignancy

are associated with low oncogenic potential HPV types 6 and 11 (4). A high percentage of patients with vulvar HPV infection also have cervical HPV infection. HPV infection is common in male partners of women with HPV (5).

Grossly, condylomas are "warty" in appearance, and they may be single or multiple (Fig. 4.5). Histologically, lesions may show papillomatosis, acanthosis, koilocytosis, dyskeratosis, hyperkeratosis, or parakeratosis (Figs. 4.6 and 4.7); however, the histologic findings may not be pronounced, depending on the age and location of the lesion (Fig. 4.8). An increase in the granular cell layer may be noted in hairbearing areas. In cases in which the diagnosis is unclear, it should be documented that the lesion is suggestive but not diagnostic of condyloma, and in-situ hybridization for human *Papillomavirus* can be performed if the clinician requests it. Therapeutic options include trichloroacetic

FIGURE 4.5. Multiple condylomas of the vulva. Reprinted by permission of Chapman & Hall.

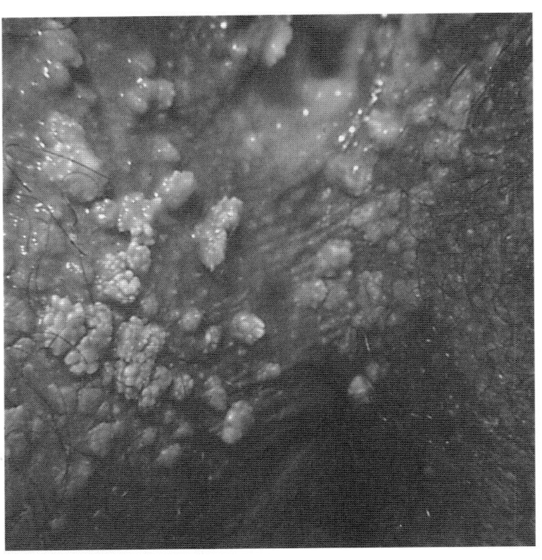

FIGURE 4.6. Condyloma. Typical papillary configuration of vulvar condyloma.

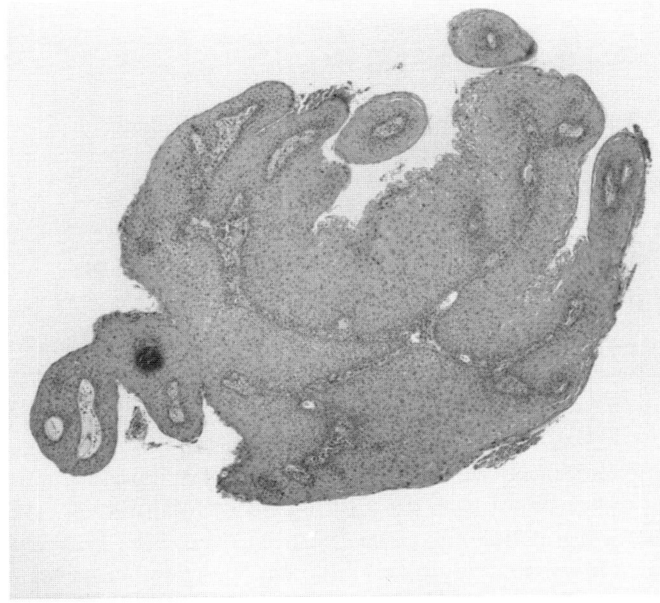

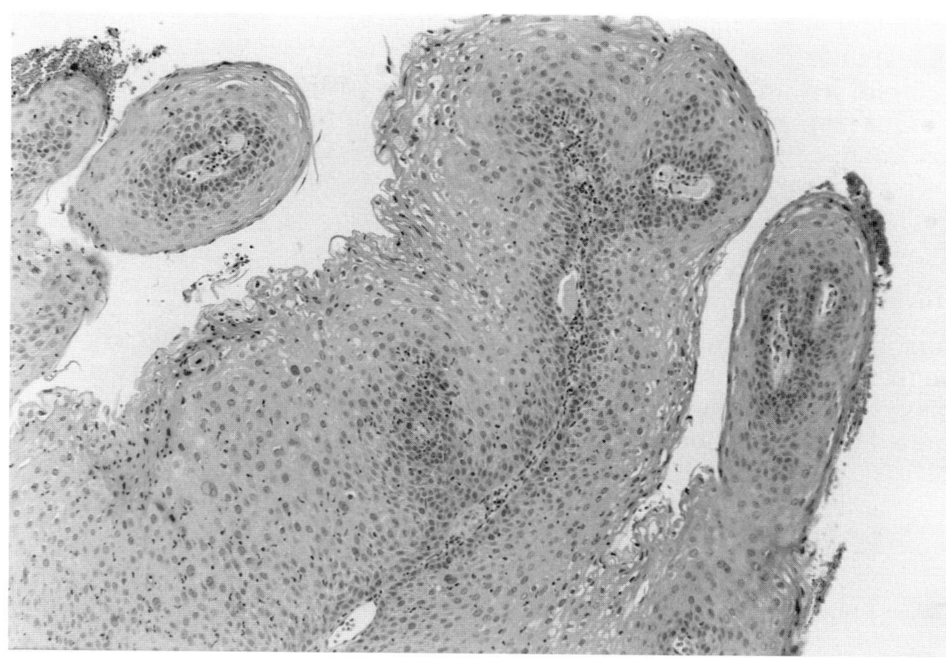

FIGURE 4.7.   Condyloma. The lesion shows koilocytosis.

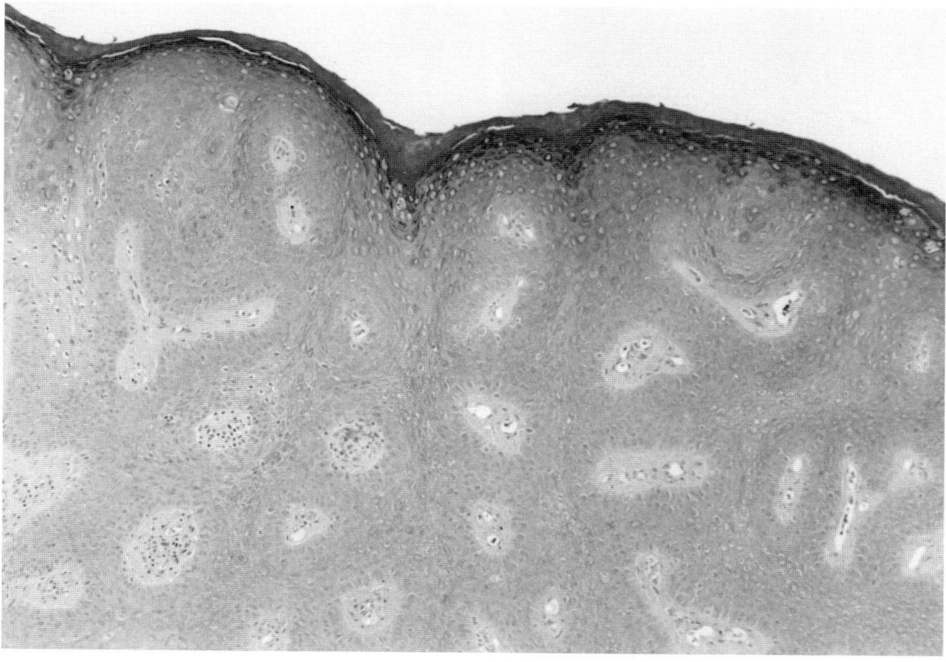

FIGURE 4.8.   Rule out condyloma. Lesions such as this, with hyperkeratosis, acanthosis, and an increased granular cell layer, are suggestive but not diagnostic of condylomas. Tangential sectioning often adds to the diagnostic difficulty. In-situ hybridization for HPV can be performed in these cases.

acid or podophyllin application, laser therapy, loop electrosurgical excision procedure (LEEP), and interferon injections (6).

Recurrent lesions are frequent. Condylomas are particularly difficult to control in the immunosuppressed patient. If lesions are resistant to therapy, biopsies to rule out neoplasia may be performed. Biopsies should not be taken shortly after podophyllin therapy because the resin induces changes that may be mistaken for vulvar intraepithelial neoplasia (VIN).

HERPES

The number of women with antibodies to herpes simplex virus type 2 (HSV-2) exceeds the number with a clinical history of infection. Primary infection with genital herpes is usually severe, with multiple vesicular or ulcerating lesions (Fig. 4.9A,B). The severe pain caused when urine touches these ulcers often prompts the patient to seek medical

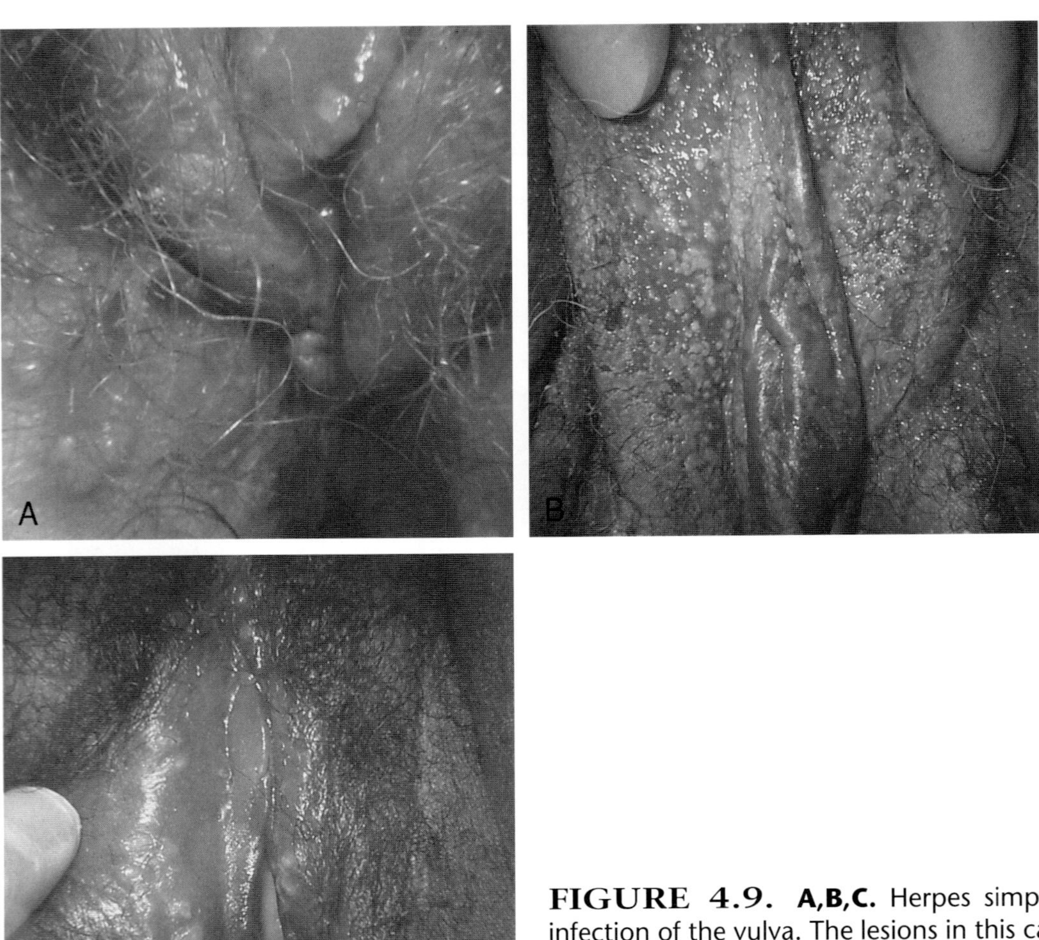

FIGURE 4.9. A,B,C. Herpes simplex infection of the vulva. The lesions in this case of primary herpes infection are initially vesicular **(A)** and then ulcerative **(B).** Recurrent episodes **(C)** are less severe. Reprinted with permission from Chapman & Hall, New York.

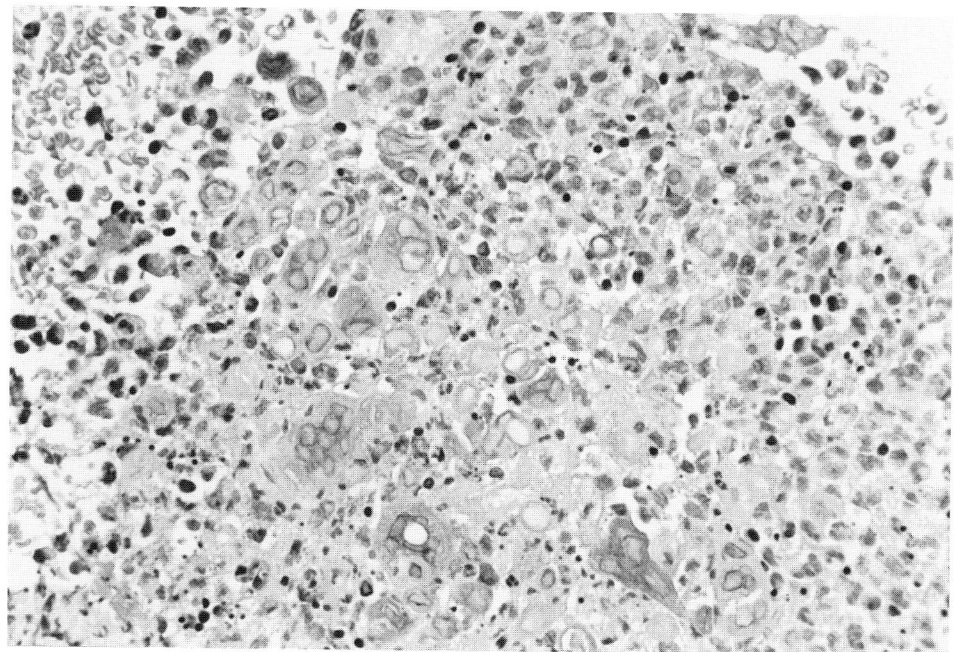

FIGURE 4.10.   Herpes simplex of the vulva. Multinucleation and ground-glass nuclei are seen.

attention and may even lead to urinary retention. Recurrent episodes are often mild and of shorter duration (Fig. 4.9C). Occasionally, the lesion is examined by biopsy, and the characteristic multinucleation and ground-glass intranuclear inclusions may be seen (Fig. 4.10). Immunohistochemistry may be helpful in nondiagnostic biopsies. The virus is harbored in the dorsal root ganglia, and asymptomatic viral shedding may occur (7). While most genital herpes is secondary to HSV-2, HSV-1 (cold sores) may be isolated as well. Therapy for genital herpes is with drugs such as acyclovir.

MOLLUSCUM CONTAGIOSUM

Molluscum contagiosum is caused by a DNA virus of the Poxvirus family, and this condition occurs on the pubis and inner thighs, as well as in nongenital areas. It is transmitted by close contact with an infected individual. Grossly, the condition is manifested by papules, usually multiple and frequently containing a central umbilication (Fig 4.11). Histologically, characteristic intracytoplasmic viral inclusions are seen (Fig 4.12). Molluscum contagiosum is often asymptomatic although it may cause pruritus. Diagnosis and treatment are effected by scraping the lesions or by extruding the material with a comedone extractor; however, the condition may resolve spontaneously. Liquid nitrogen therapy has also been performed (8).

CHANCROID

Chancroid is a sexually transmitted disease caused by Hemophilus ducreyi, a gram-negative bacillus. The initial papular lesions become ulcerative (Fig 4.13). In distinction

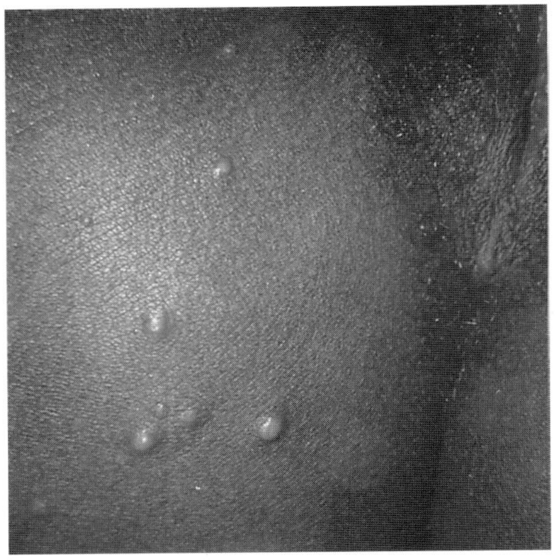

FIGURE 4.11. Molluscum contagiosum. The lesions are papules with central umbilication. Reprinted with permission from Chapman & Hall, New York.

from other ulcerative sexually transmitted diseases, chancroid is usually painful. Regional adenopathy with bubo formation can occur, and these may become chronic draining sinuses. Histology when examined by biopsy is generally one of a nonspecific inflammation although Freinkel (9) describes three zones of inflammation, a superficial zone of degenerating leukocytes, a middle zone with vascular changes, and a deep zone with a plasma cell and lymphocytic infiltrate. The diagnosis is made by culture. Organisms may be seen on a Gram's stain, but this is neither sensitive nor specific. Treatment is with antibiotics (8–17).

SYPHILIS

Syphilis, caused by *Treponema pallidum,* progresses in three stages. The first stage is manifested by a genital chancre, a painless ulceration with well-demarcated edges (Fig. 4.14). Diagnosis can be made using dark-field microscopy and confirmed through the use of serology. Biopsies are rarely performed on chancres; however, histology is characterized by a periarterial plasma cell infiltrate (Fig. 4.15). The spirochetes may be identifiable with Warthin-Starry or Dieterle stains. Secondary syphilis is systemic in nature and may be manifested on the vulva as condyloma lata, multiple pale plaque-like lesions (Fig. 4.16). Serological testing is the most accurate diagnostic modality at this point. The lesions of condyloma lata show similar perivascular plasma cell infiltrates with adjacent epithelial hyperplasia, and silver stains may identify the organisms. Tertiary syphilis involves the central nervous and cardiac systems. Treatment for syphilis is the use of antibiotics (8–10).

LYMPHOGRANULOMA VENEREUM (LGV)

LGV is caused by specific serotypes of *Chlamydia trachomatis* (L1, L2, L3) and is sexually transmitted. LGV usually presents in three stages, a primary painless genital papule or ulceration, regional adenopathy that may lead to draining sinuses, and finally, scarring and edema (Fig. 4.17). Diagnosis is usually made by serological testing (complement

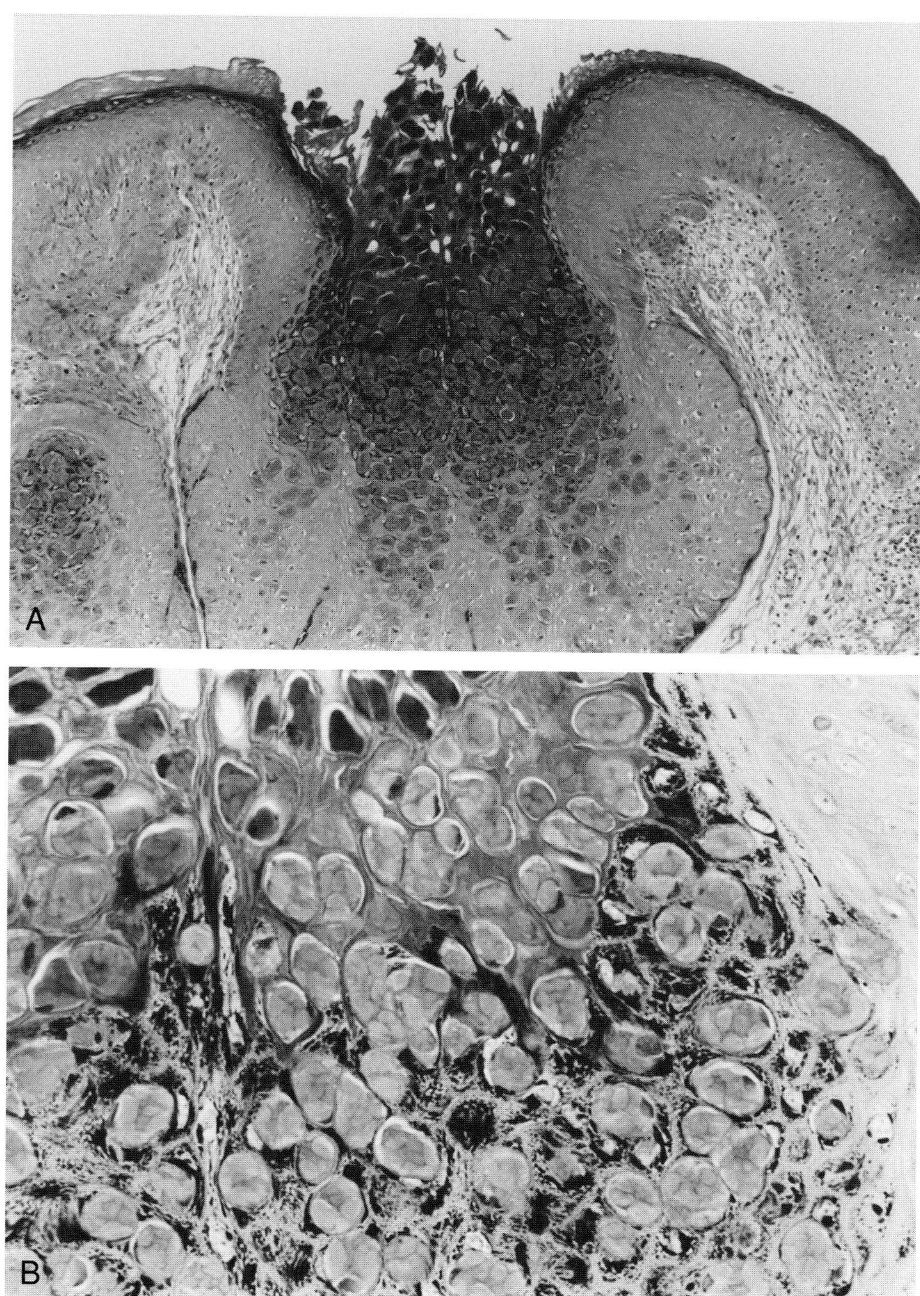

FIGURE 4.12.   Mollucum contagiosum. **A.** The central umbilication seen grossly corresponds to this crater-like configuration. **B.** Intracytoplasmic viral inclusions may be seen.

FIGURE 4.13. Chancroid. The initial presenting lesion is usually a painful ulcer. Reprinted with permission from Chapman & Hall, New York.

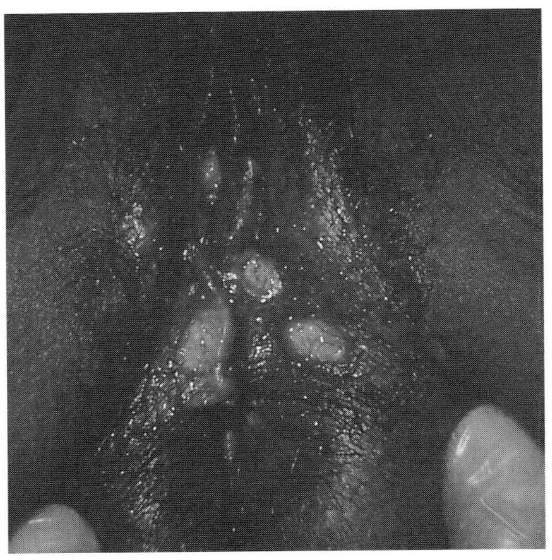

FIGURE 4.14. Syphilis. The chancre of stage 1 syphilis is usually painless and well-demarcated. Reprinted with permission from Chapman & Hall, New York.

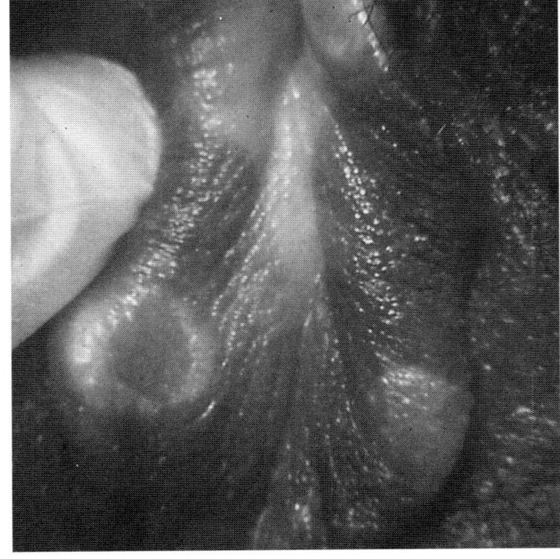

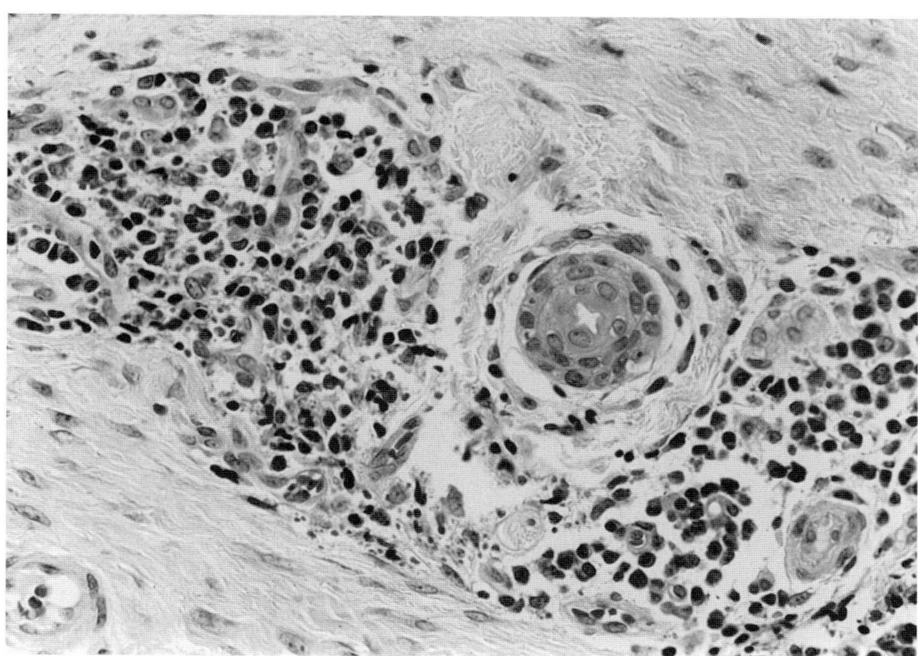

FIGURE 4.15.   Syphilis. A biopsy of a chancre will show a perivascular plasma cell infiltrate.

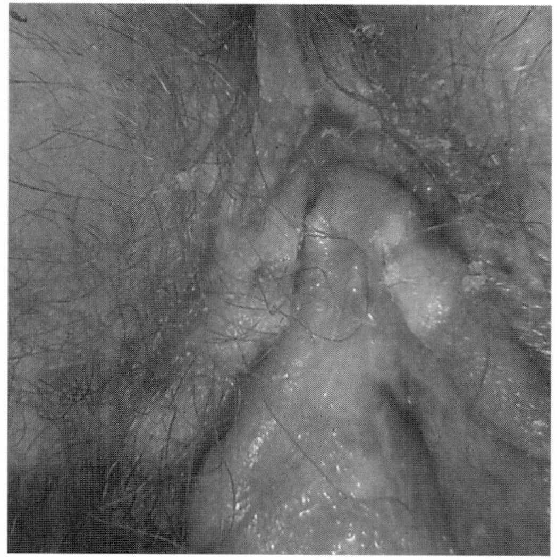

FIGURE 4.16.   Condyloma Lata-Secondary syphilis presents on the vulva as the papules of condyloma lata. Reprinted with permission from Chapman & Hall, New York.

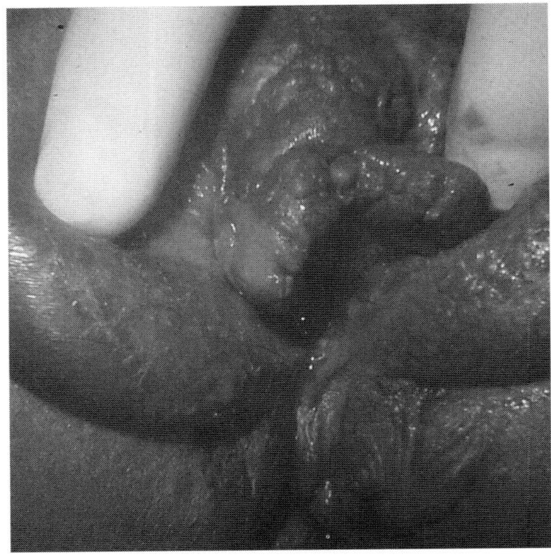

FIGURE 4.17. Lymphogranuloma venereum. LGV showing vulvar ulceration and edema. Reprinted with permission from Chapman & Hall, New York.

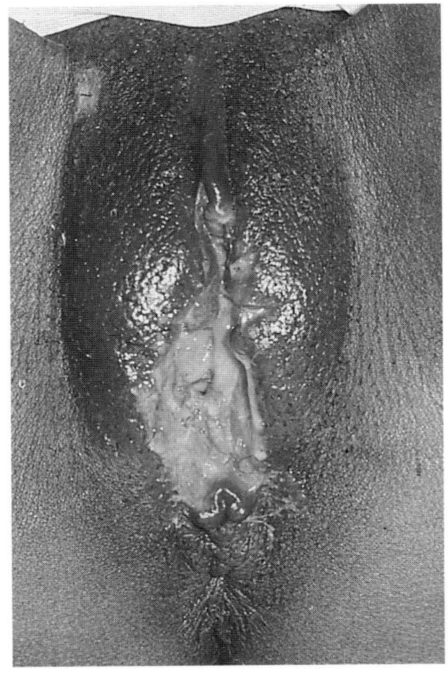

FIGURE 4.18. Granuloma Inguinale. This case of granuloma inguinale presented with ulceration. Reprinted with permission from Chapman & Hall, New York.

fixation) or can be made by direct immunofluorescence or other adjunctive laboratory techniques on obtained lesional smears. The histology— one of chronic granulomatous inflammation with lymphocytes and plasma cells—is nonspecific. Therapy is with antibiotics (8–11).

GRANULOMA INGUINALE

Granuloma inguinale is a sexually transmitted disease caused by *Calymmatobacterium granulomatis,* a gram-negative bacillus. Early vulvar manifestations include painless pap-

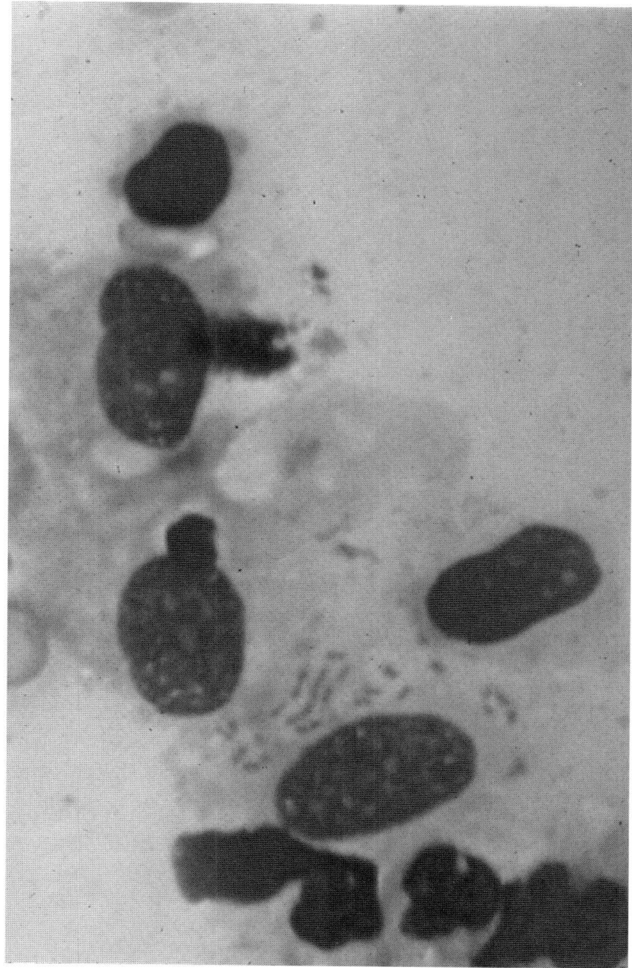

FIGURE 4.19. Granuloma inguinale. Donovan bodies (encapsulated organisms in histiocytes) may be seen on lesional imprints stained with Giemsa stain. Reprinted with permission from Chapman & Hall, New York.

ules and ulcers (Fig. 4.18). Later in the disease course, vulvar edema and fibrosis occurs. Lesional smears or imprints may be fixed in methanol and stained with Giemsa stain to identify Donovan bodies (encapsulated organisms within histiocytes) (Fig 4.19). Histology is one of a nonspecific granulomatous inflammation, although Donovan bodies may be identified with Giemsa, Wright's, or Warthin-Starry stains. Antibiotics are the treatment of choice (8–11).

OTHER INFECTIONS AND INFLAMMATIONS
VESTIBULITIS

Many symptomatological patterns to vulvar pain and burning exist, which are all classified under the umbrella term "vulvodynia." A good review of vulvodynia has been provided by McKay (12). A particularly frustrating condition for both patients and physicians is vestibulitis, a type of vulvodynia. This condition is often of long duration and frequently interferes with sexual intercourse. Physical findings consist of point vestibu-

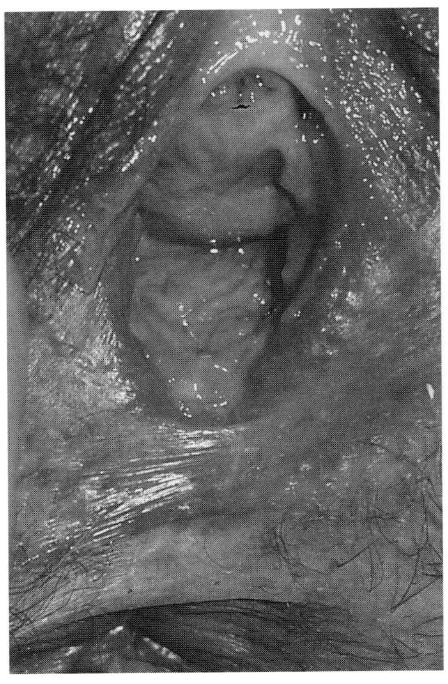

FIGURE 4.20.   Vulvar vestibulitis. There is erythema of the vestibule. Reprinted with permission from Chapman & Hall, New York.

lar tenderness, elicited on examination by palpation with a cotton swab (see Chapter 1), and variable erythema of the vestibular area (Fig. 4.20). Biopsies are not generally helpful. There may be no histological findings, or nonspecific chronic inflammation, usually in the lamina propria of the mucosa and secondarily in the tissue around minor vestibular ducts and glands (Fig. 4.21). Vestibulitis is not commonly associated with the usual vulvar types of human *Papillomavirus* (13, 14).

MALAKOPLAKIA

Rarely, malakoplakia may affect the vulva. Histologically, the finding of Michaelis-Guttman bodies within a monomorphous histiocytic infiltrate is diagnostic (Fig. 4.22). E. coli has been identified in some cases (15).

BEHÇET'S SYNDROME

This condition is characterized by oral and genital ulcers (Fig 4.23) and variable ocular lesions. Histologically, necrotizing arteritis is seen. Topical steroids are the first line of treatment for vulvar lesions (1, 16).

PEMPHIGUS AND PEMPHIGOID

Although any dermatologic condition can affect the vulva, it rarely is affected by bullous diseases (Fig. 4.24, Table 4.3). Biopsy will help distinguish the subepidermal bullae of pemphigoid from the intraepidermal bullae of pemphigus vulgaris (Fig. 4.25). With pemphigus, intercellular IgG deposition within the squamous epithelium exists, whereas with pemphigoid, the IgG deposition is located at the dermal-epidermal junc-

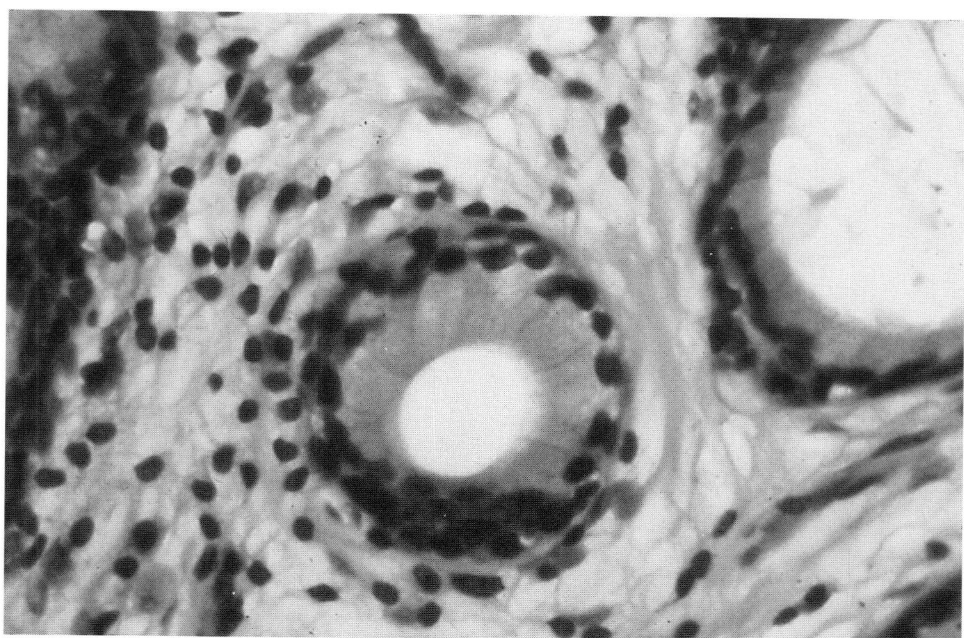

FIGURE 4.21.   Vulvar vestibulitis. Biopsies are not generally helpful. Here, a nonspecific chronic inflammatory infiltrate is seen adjacent to a minor vestibular gland. Reprinted with permission from Chapman & Hall, New York.

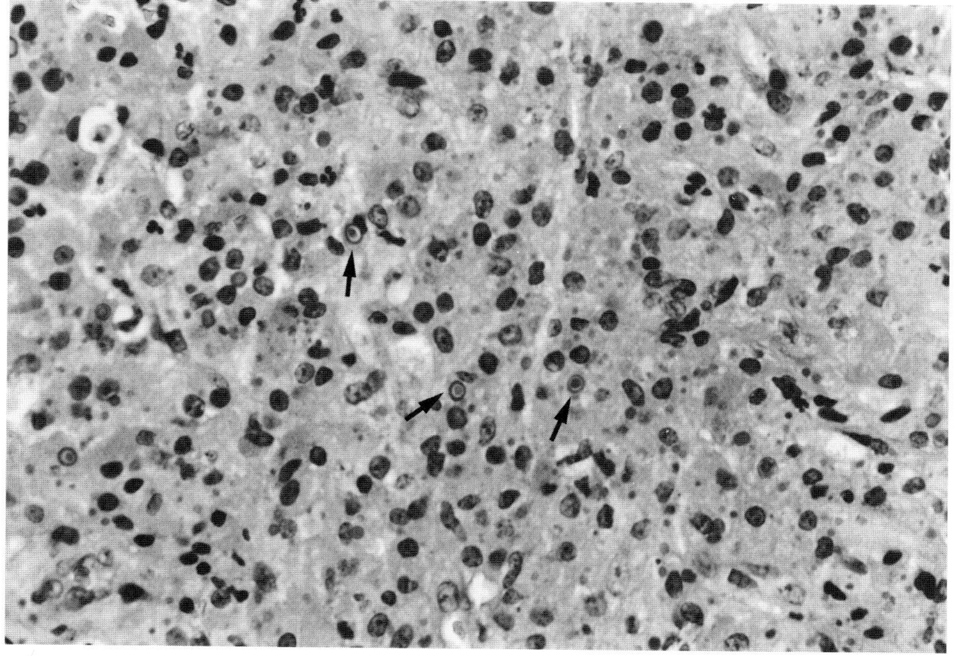

FIGURE 4.22.   Malakoplakia. The lesion consists of a histiocytic infiltrate. The diagnostic Michaelis-Guttman bodies may be seen (arrow).

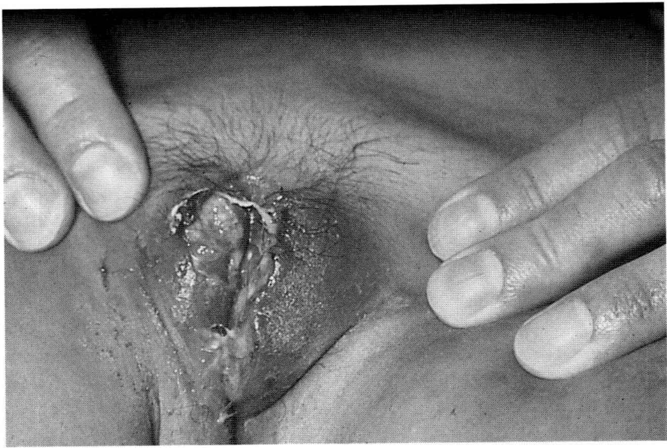

FIGURE 4.23. Behçet's disease. Vulvar ulceration can be seen with many conditions. Oral and opthalmologic manifestations should be looked for. Reprinted with permission from Chapman & Hall, New York.

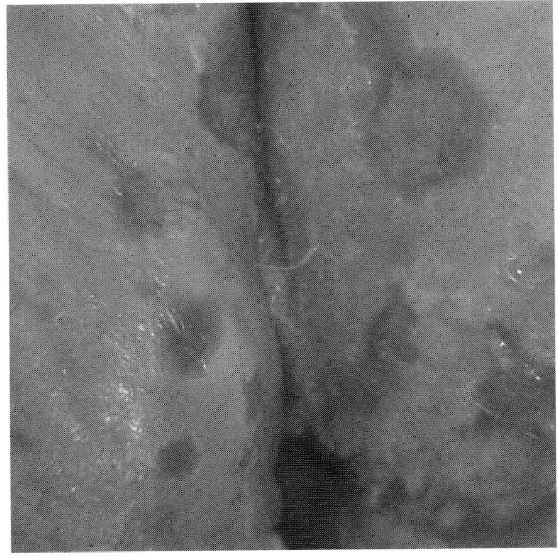

FIGURE 4.24. Pemphigus vulgaris. Multiple ruptured bullae are seen. Reprinted with permission from Chapman & Hall, New York.

tion. Distinction is important, as pemphigus vulgaris can be life-threatening; pemphigoid is not (1, 17, 18).

FOX-FORDYCE DISEASE

This pruritic condition may affect the vulva as well as the axillae. The disease consists of dilatation of apocrine glands, which are plugged by keratinaceous material that spills into the adjacent dermis. Grossly, multiple papules are noted. Treatment with local antipruritics and with oral contraceptives, which may suppress apocrine secretion, has been used (1, 2).

HIDRADENITIS SUPPURATIVA

This is a chronic inflammation of apocrine glands and may present on both the vulva and axilla (Fig 4.26). Multiple communicating abscesses are characteristic. Destruction

TABLE 4.3.   Lesions of the Vulva That May
Manifest as Bullae (1, 2, 18)

Herpes simplex
Herpes zoster
Varicella
Pemphigus
Pemphigoid
Hailey-Hailey disease
Darier disease
Dermatitis herpetiformis
Localized acantholytic disease of the vulva
Herpes gestationis
Erythema multiforme (Stevens-Johnson syndrome)
Warty dyskeratoma
Linear IgA disease
Polymorphic eruption of pregnancy
Fixed drug eruption

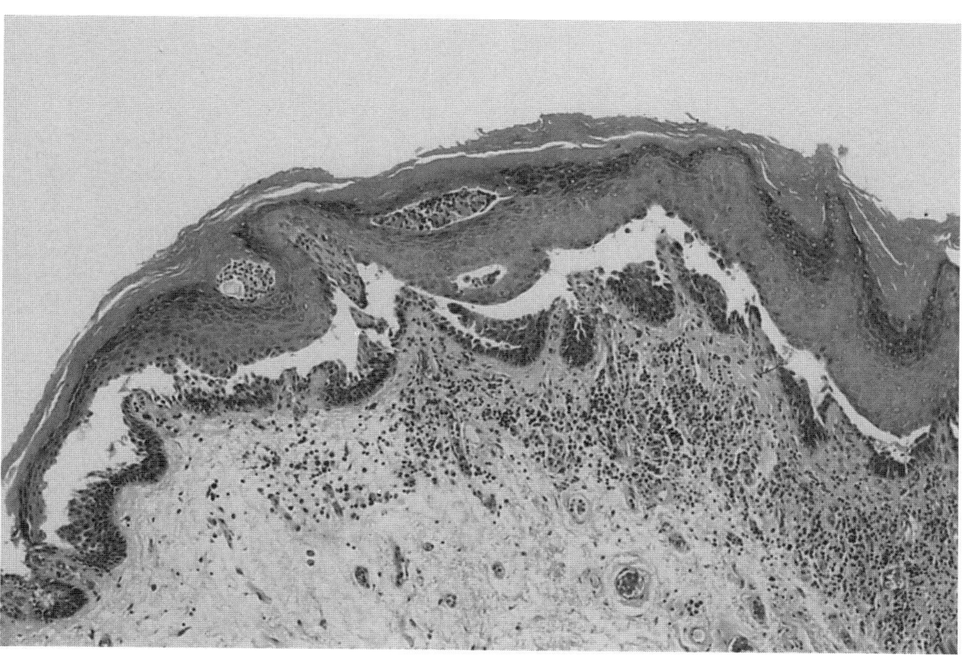

FIGURE 4.25.   Pemphigus vulgaris-intraepithelial bulla formation is seen.

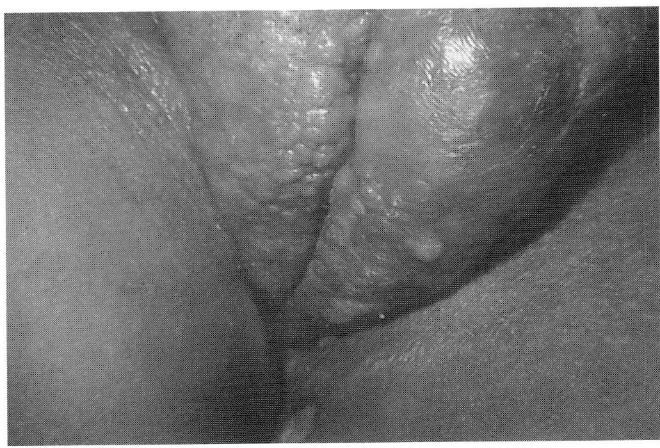

FIGURE 4.26. Hidradenitis suppurativa. Multiple draining abscesses are seen. Reprinted with permission from Chapman & Hall, New York.

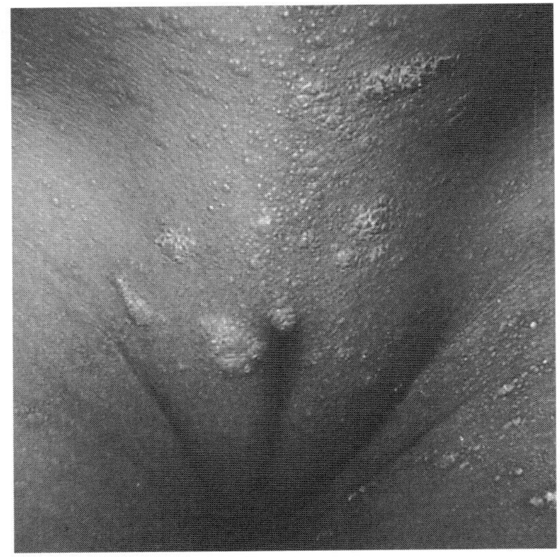

FIGURE 4.27. Lichen planus. Lichen planus may be seen on the vulva. Reprinted with permission from Chapman & Hall, New York.

of dermal appendages and eventual scarring occurs. A variety of medical therapies have been employed, as has surgical excision of the affected area (1, 2).

LICHEN PLANUS

Lichen planus (Fig. 4.27), a well-known dermatologic condition, can appear in the vestibule and vagina as a macular eruption or may be desquamative. Histologically, the lesion is characterized by acanthosis, basal cell degeneration (spongiosis), and a band-like dermal lymphoid infiltrate (Fig. 4.28). A variety of topical and oral medications have been used for therapy of this condition (19).

PSORIASIS

The typical silver, scaled erythematous lesions of psoriasis can be seen on the vulva, particularly in the genitocrural folds and external labia majora (Fig. 4.29). The usual

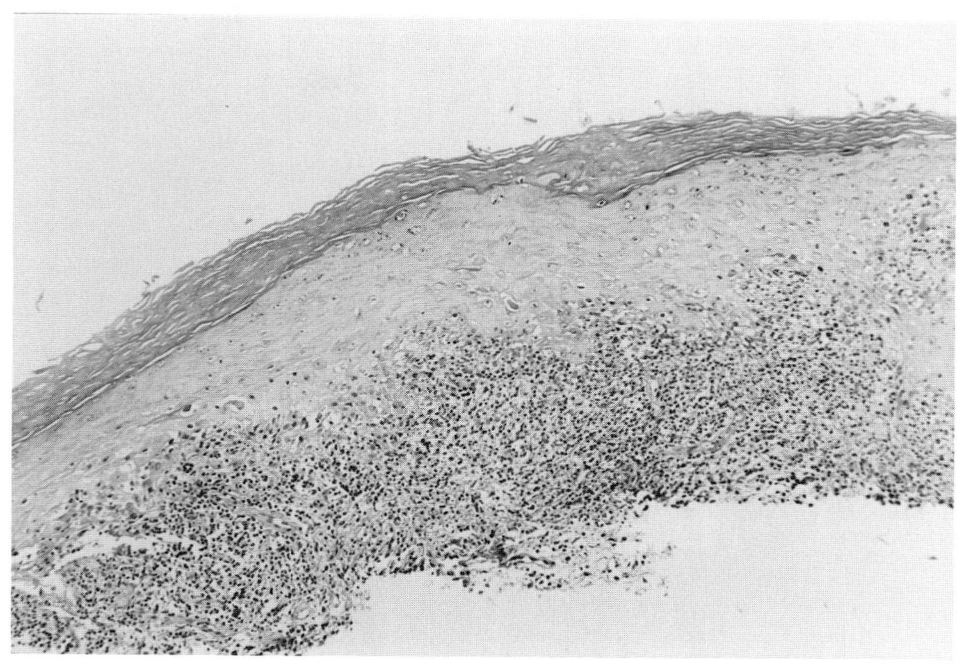

FIGURE 4.28.   Lichen planus. Spongiosis and a characteristic band-like chronic inflammatory infiltrate are seen.

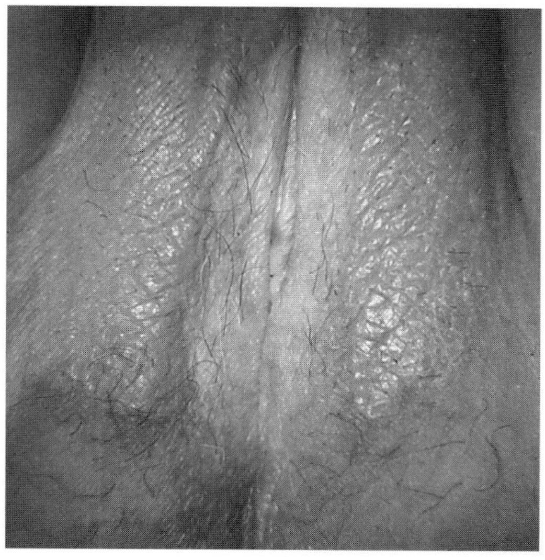

FIGURE 4.29. Psoriasis of the vulva. Note the characteristic shiny and scaley appearance. Reprinted with permission from Chapman & Hall, New York.

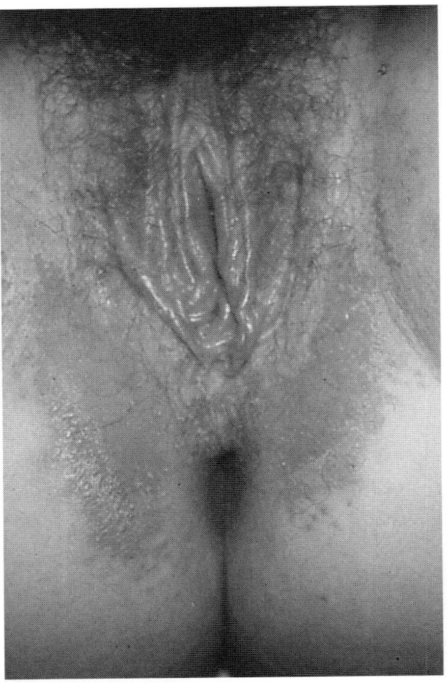

FIGURE 4.30. Cutaneous candidiasis. Cutaneous candidiasis appears as a well-demarcated red lesion. Reprinted with permission from Chapman & Hall, New York.

histological picture of hyperkeratosis, parakeratosis, acanthosis, and Munro microabscesses can also be seen (1, 2). The histology may resemble cutaneous *Candida*, which can be distinguished by stains for fungal organisms.

CANDIDA

Although rarely examined by biopsy, vulvar skin with candidiasis may occasionally be submitted as a specimen in cases of resistance to therapy or when the diagnosis is uncertain. Grossly, vulvar candiasis appears as a well-delineated red lesion with scaling on the labia majora and inner thighs, with frequent satellite lesions (Fig. 4.30). These lesions are usually scraped rather than examined by biopsy (see Chapter 1 for technique). Histologically, the epithelium contains polymorphonuclear leukocytes (Fig. 4.31), and candidal pseudohyphae may be seen penetrating the superficial epidermal layers with fungal stains (Fig. 4.32). If the polymorphonuclear leukocytes aggregate into microabscesses, the differential diagnosis includes psoriasis. Vulvar candidiasis is treated initially with topical antifungal agents. The presence of diabetes mellitus should always be considered (1, 20).

TINEA CRURIS AND VERSICOLOR

Infection with tinea cruris resembles cutaneous candida in the vulvar region (Fig. 4.33). Tinea versicolor presents as hypopigmented scaly areas. Tinea is usually scraped rather than examined by biopsy, and if tinea is present in a tissue biopsy, fungi may be identified in the keratin layer with PAS stain on biopsies (1). Topical antifungal agents are used for therapy.

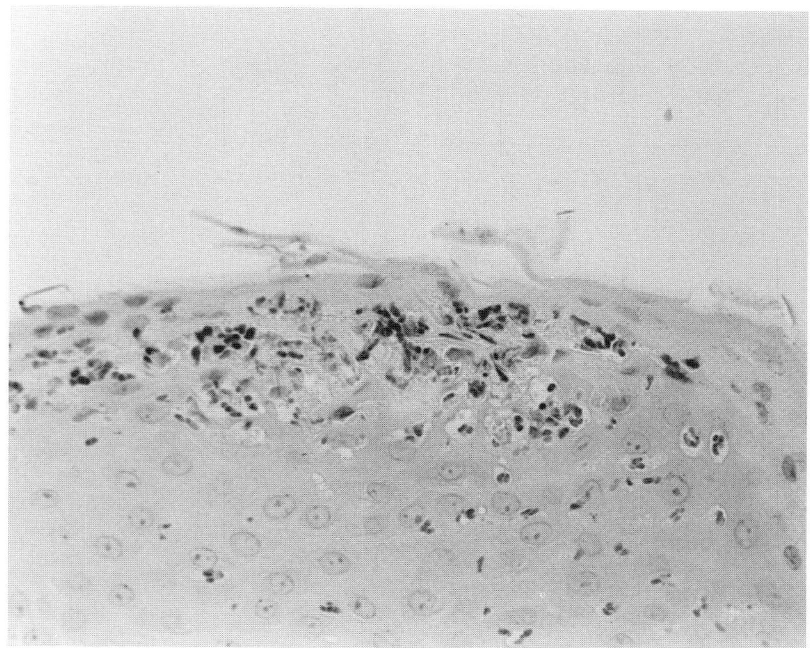

FIGURE 4.31. Cutaneous candida. Collections of leukocytes are seen in the epidermis.

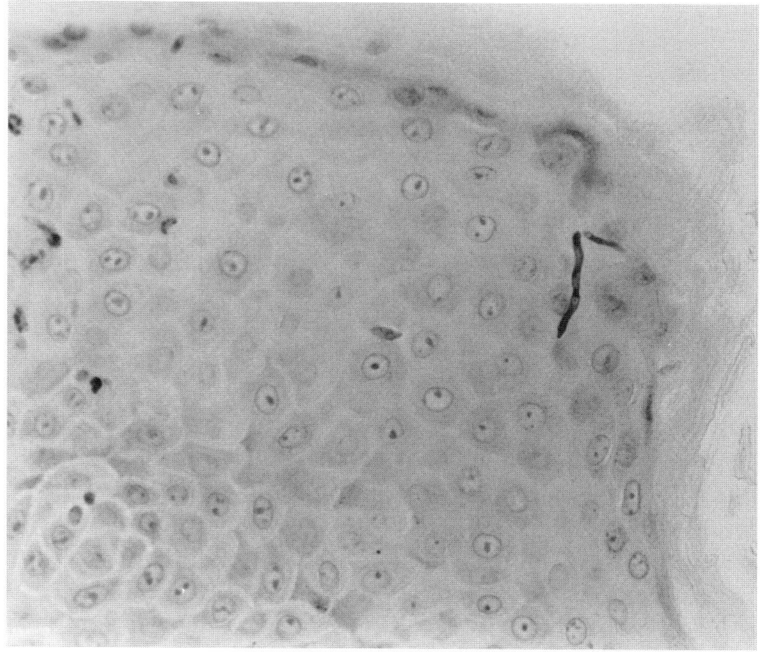

FIGURE 4.32. Cutaneous candida. On PAS or GMS stain, the fungal hyphae may be seen invading the superficial layers of the epithelium.

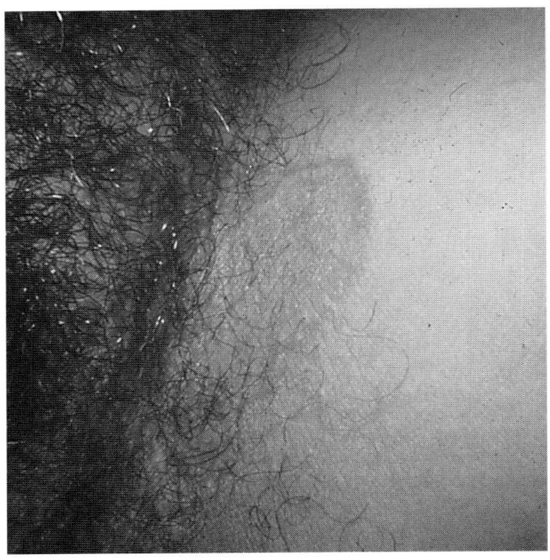

FIGURE 4.33. Tinea cruris. The lesion resembles cutaneous candida. Reprinted with permission from Chapman & Hall, New York.

PEDICULOSIS PUBIS AND SCABIES

Pediculosis pubis is secondary to the crab louse and is confined to the pubis. Scabies, due to the itch mite, is a systemic cutaneous condition. Scrapings examined under the microscope may reveal the offending organisms. Therapy is topical, with disinfection of clothes and linens, and often treatment of close contacts (8).

CROHN'S DISEASE

Vulvar ulcers secondary to Crohn's disease are unique in appearance, resembling a knife cut (1). Extensive perineal and perianal involvement leads to draining sinuses and recto-vaginal fistulas (Fig. 4.34).

BENIGN DISORDERS OF PIGMENTATION

Vulvar lesions that may appear pigmented are listed in Table 4.4.

NEVI

Nevi, while more common in sun-exposed areas of the body, are not rare on the vulva (Fig. 4.35). They may be asymptomatic, particularly if flat, or they may become irritated. Excision is often performed because of clinical concern, to rule out a melanoma. Vulvar nevi may either be junctional, compound, or intradermal (Fig. 4.36). Atypical nevi can also occur (21).

LENTIGO SIMPLEX

These are small, irregular, hyperpigmented areas that can occur on the vulva (Fig. 4.37). Biopsy may be performed for clinical concern of melanoma. Histologically, lentigo con-

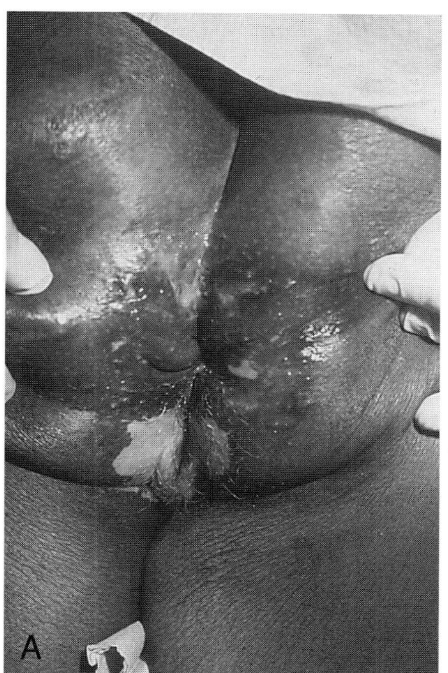

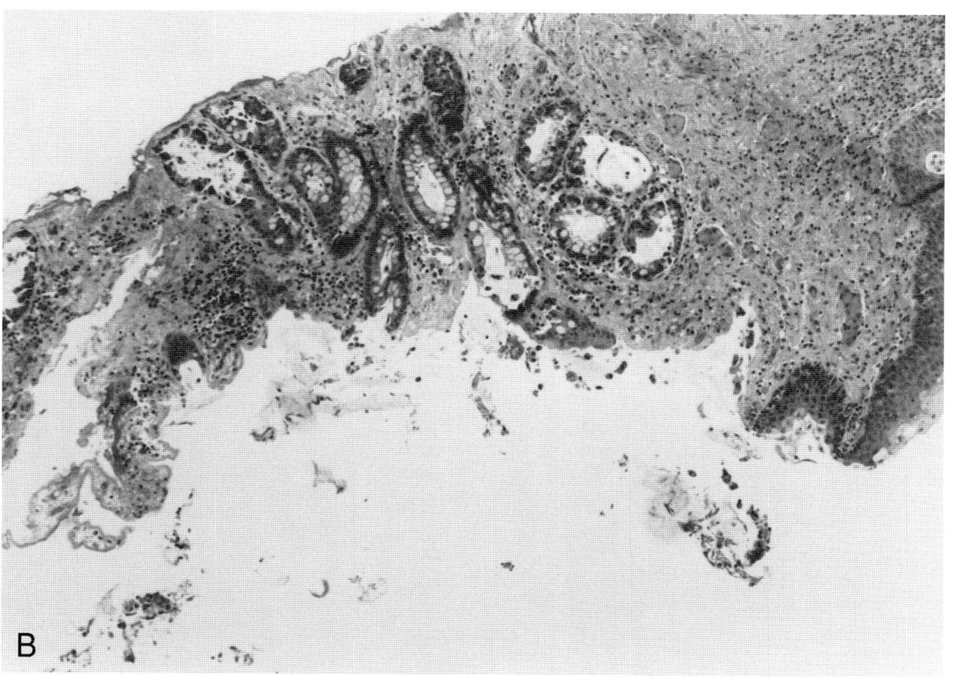

FIGURE 4.34. A. Rectoperineal and rectovaginal fistulas. These may be seen as a sequela of Crohn's disease. Reprinted with permission from Chapman & Hall, New York. **B.** Rectovaginal fistula. Rectal mucosa adjacent to vaginal mucosa.

TABLE 4.4. Lesions That May Be Pigmented (1, 2, 21)

Lentigo
Vulvar melanosis
Nevus
VIN
Postinflammatory hyperpigmentation
Seborrheic keratosis
Hemangioma
Condyloma
Verruca vulgaris
Hemosiderin deposition
Squamous cell carcinoma
Basal cell carcinoma
Melanoma
Kaposi's sarcoma

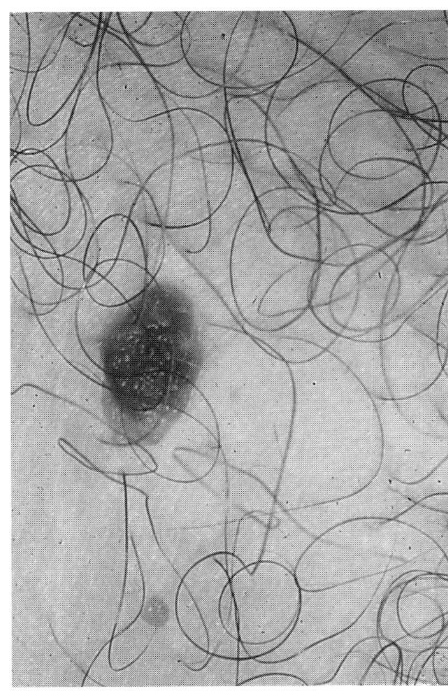

FIGURE 4.35. Vulvar nevus. Reprinted with permission from Chapman & Hall, New York.

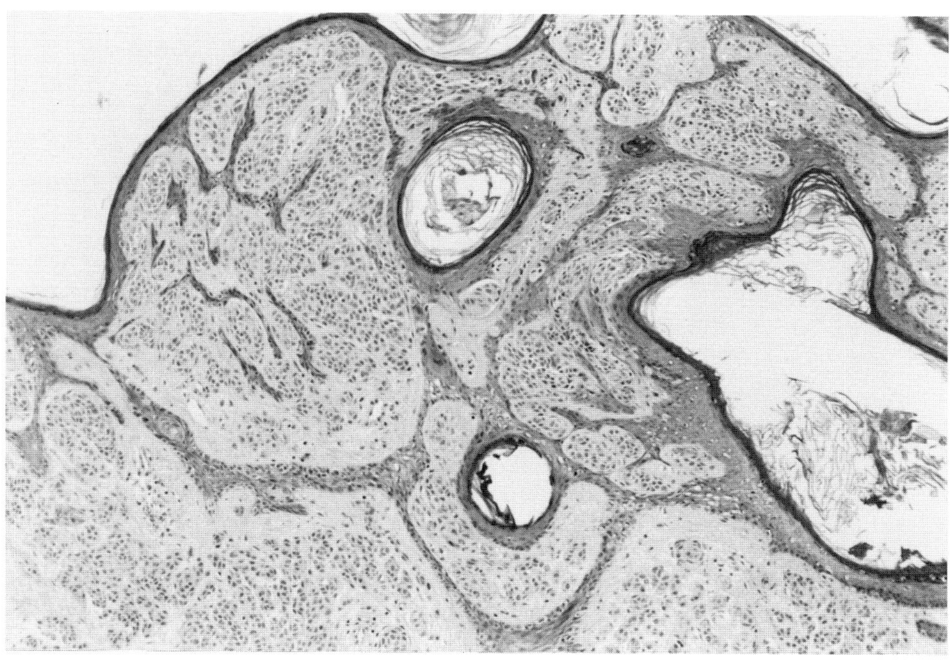

FIGURE 4.36. Nevus. Intradermal nevi such as this occur frequently on the vulva.

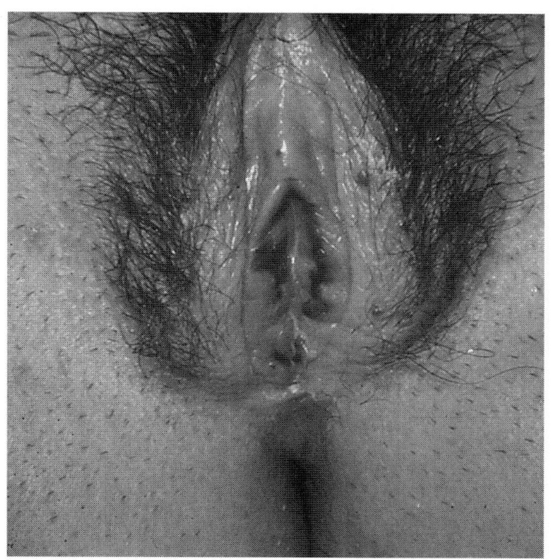

FIGURE 4.37. Lentigo. Multiple pigmented areas are seen. Reprinted with permission from Chapman & Hall, New York.

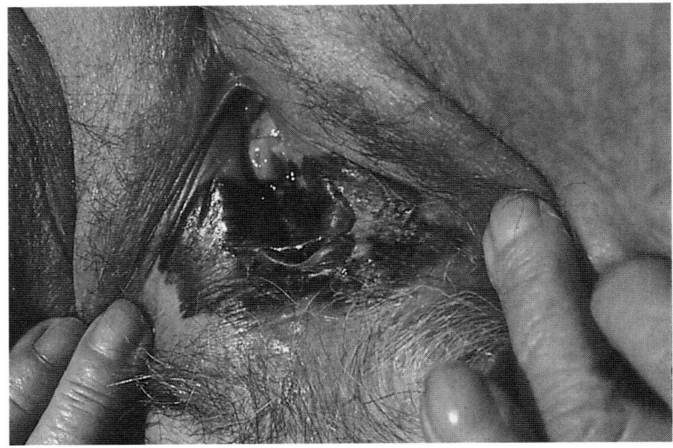

FIGURE 4.38. Melanosis of the vulva. This lesion may be biopsied out of concern to rule out melanoma. Reprinted with permission from Chapman & Hall, New York.

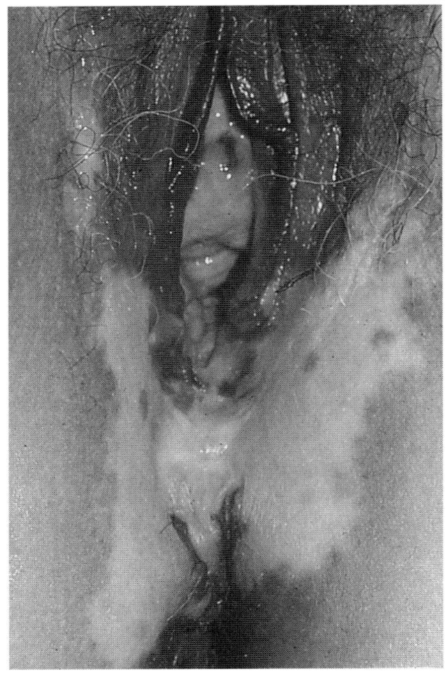

FIGURE 4.39. Vitiligo. The depigmentation of vitiligo may occur on the vulva. Reprinted with permission from Chapman & Hall, New York.

sists of increased pigmentation of the basal cell layer, sometimes with an increase in the number of melanocytes (21).

MELANOSIS

Large confluent areas of hyperpigmentation, histologically identical to lentigo simplex, are termed "melanosis" (Fig. 4.38). Biopsies may be submitted for clinical concerns (21).

VITILIGO

Vitiligo can occur on the vulva and is seen as an area of depigmentation. Histologically, decreased or absent melanocytes can be noted (Fig. 4.39)(1).

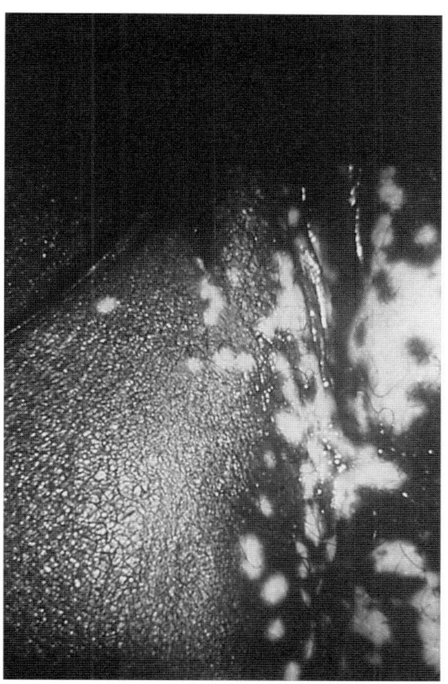

FIGURE 4.40. Postinflammatory hypopigmentation (leukoderma). The lesion is seen grossly as depigmentation. Reprinted with permission from Chapman & Hall, New York.

TABLE 4.5. Classification of Nonneoplastic Epithelial Disorders of the Vulva (22)

Lichen sclerosus
Squamous hyperplasia
Other dermatoses

POSTINFLAMMATORY CHANGES

Postinflammatory hypopigmentation (leukoderma) may appear as pale areas on the vulva after episodes of inflammatory disease (Fig. 4.40). Histologically, pigment incontinence into the dermis occurs and basal layer pigmentation decreases, but melanocytes are present. In postinflammatory hyperpigmentation, basal layer melanin increases, and melanocytes may be increased. Pigment incontinence into the dermis also exists (Fig. 4.41)(21).

NONNEOPLASTIC EPITHELIAL DISORDERS

The most recent classification of the International Society for the Study of Vulvovaginal Disease (ISSVD) eliminated the term "dystrophy" from the classification of vulvar diseases. The current classification of nonneoplastic epithelial disorders is listed in Table 4.5 (22).

LICHEN SCLEROSUS

Lichen sclerosus is most commonly seen by the gynecologist in the postmenopausal woman. It should be noted, however, that the disease can occur anywhere on the body,

FIGURE 4.41. Postinflammatory hyperpigmentation. In postinflammatory hyperpigmentation, there is an increase in basal pigmentation. There may be increased melanocytes. Pigment incontinence is seen.

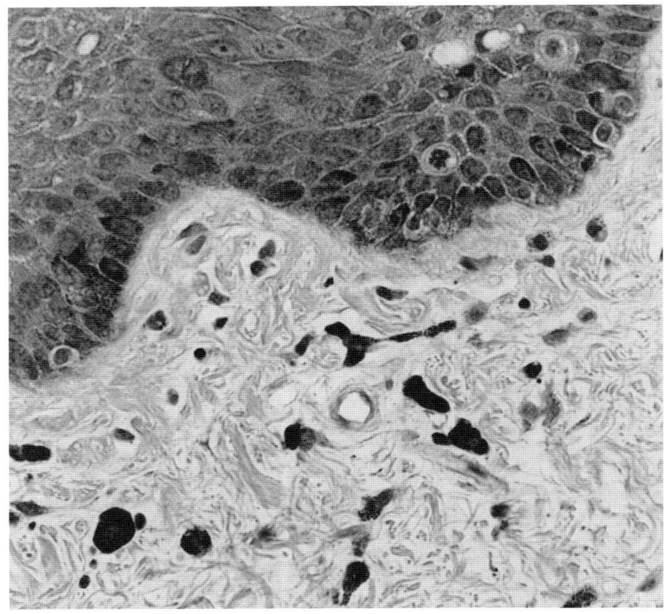

FIGURE 4.42. Lichen sclerosus. There is whitening and narrowing of the introitus. Reprinted with permission from Chapman & Hall, New York.

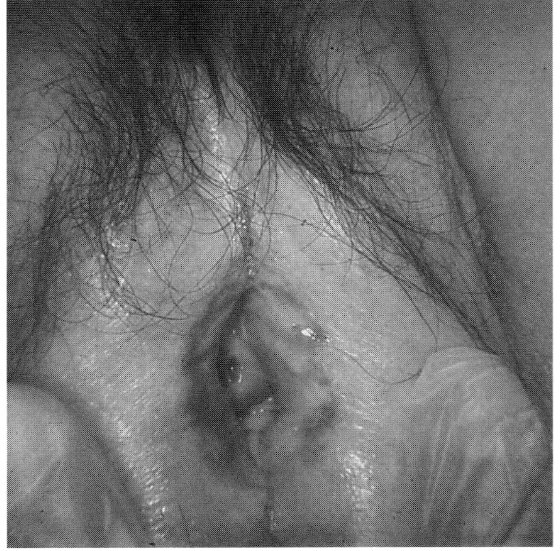

and it has also been described in the pediatric population. Some genetic predisposition to this disease exists.

Clinically, vulvar lichen sclerosus presents with severe pruritus. As the condition progresses, the labia majora and minora fuse, the introitus becomes narrowed, and the vulvar skin develops a thinned, white appearance (Fig. 4.42). Histologically, there is loss of rete pegs, dermal homogenization, and a variable chronic inflammatory infiltrate in the dermis (Fig. 4.43). Topical testosterone or topical steroids are the most common treatment modalities (22, 23).

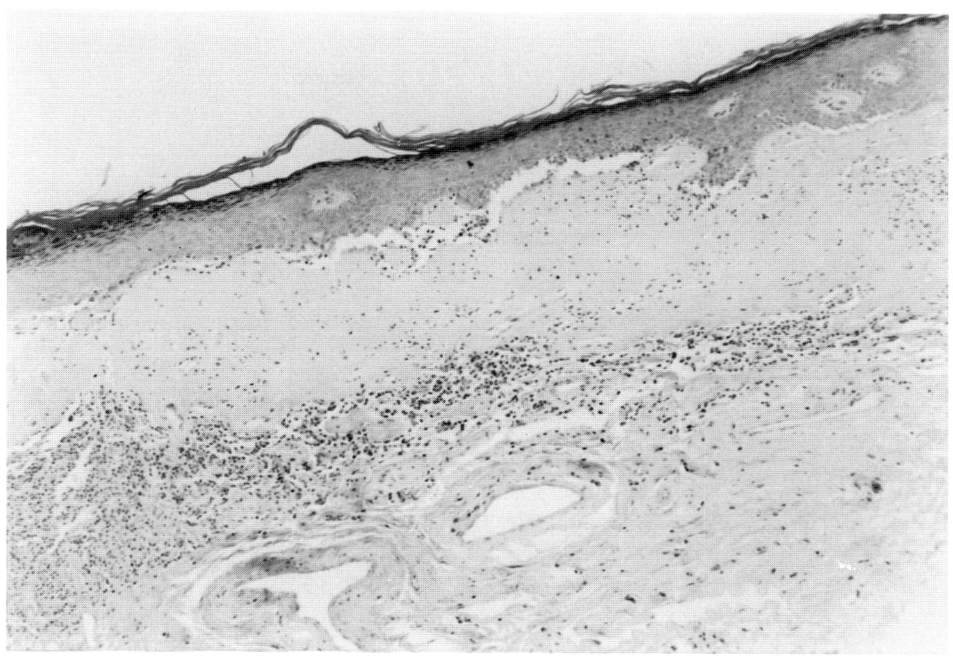

FIGURE 4.43.   Lichen sclerosus. Histologically, epithelial thinning with loss of rete pegs and dermal homogenization is seen. A variable chronic inflammatory infiltrate may be present.

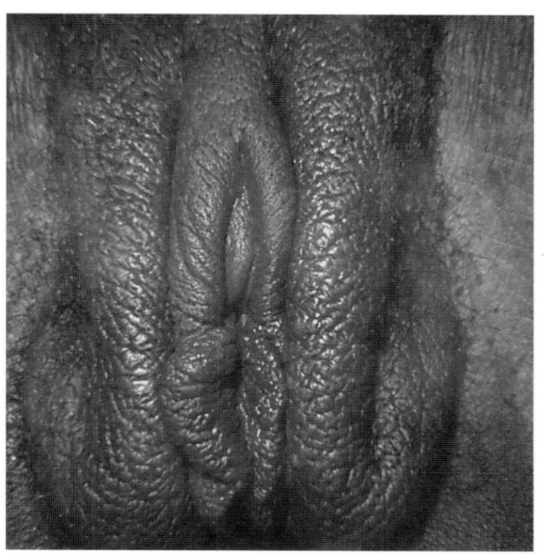

FIGURE 4.44. Squamous hyperplasia. Vulvar skin appears coarse and thickened. Reprinted with permission from Chapman & Hall, New York.

SQUAMOUS HYPERPLASIA

Squamous hyperplasia is a pruritic condition analogous to lichen simplex chronicus, and it is often the sequela of an uninterrupted itch-scratch cycle. The vulvar skin grossly appears coarse and thickened (Fig. 4.44). Histologically, acanthosis and hyperkeratosis

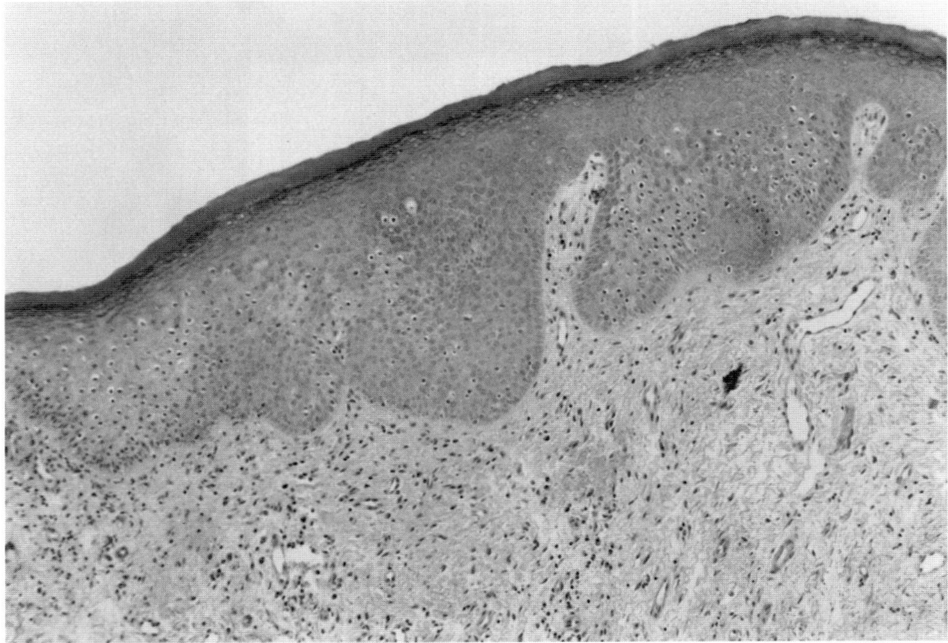

FIGURE 4.45.   Squamous hyperplasia. The condition is characterized by hyperkeratosis, acanthosis, and nonspecific chronic inflammation.

TABLE 4.6.   Cystic Lesions of the Vulva (1, 2, 24–29)

Bartholin's cyst/abscess
Epidermal inclusion cyst
Mucinous cyst
Skene's duct cyst
Ciliated cyst of the vestibule
Cyst of the Canal of Nuck
Mesonephric-like cysts
Suburethral diverticulum

exist. Mild dermal chronic inflammation may exist. The presence of epithelial atypia raises the question of VIN (Fig. 4.45). Squamous hyperplasia is generally treated with topical steroids (1, 22).

CYSTIC LESIONS OF THE VULVA

Cystic lesions of the vulva are listed in Table 4.6.

BARTHOLIN'S GLAND CYST

Obstruction of the Bartholin's duct in the absence of infection leads to a Bartholin's cyst (Figs. 4.46 and 4.47). While generally painless, these cysts can be quite large and

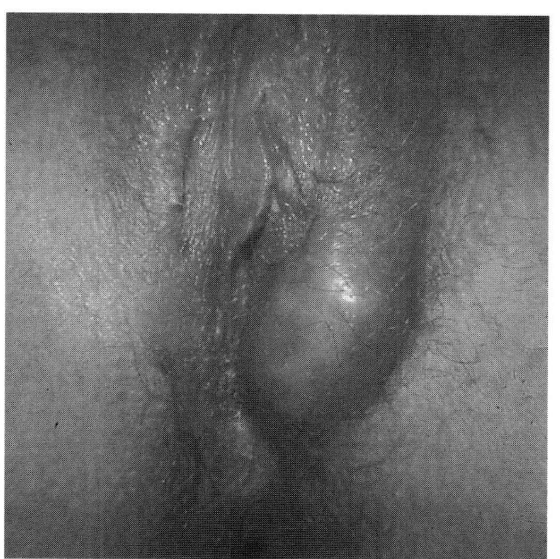

FIGURE 4.46.   Bartholin's cyst. The lesion presents as a vulvar cyst arising in the area of the Bartholin's gland. Reprinted with permission from Chapman & Hall, New York.

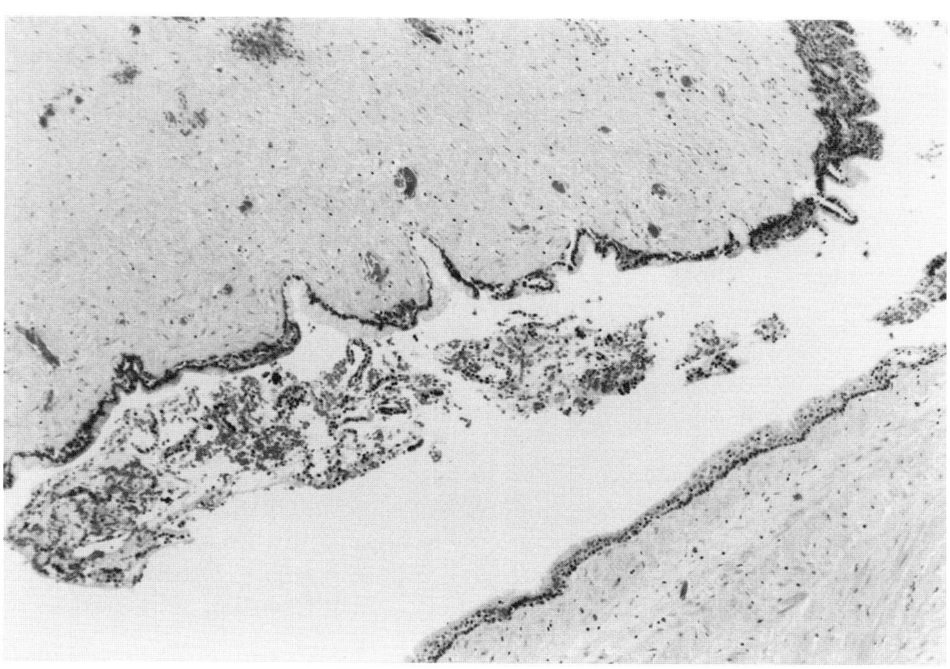

FIGURE 4.47.   Most Bartholin's cysts are duct cysts, lined by Bartholin duct epithelium. Here both transitional and mucinous epithelium are seen.

may become annoying to the patient. Bartholin's cysts usually are lined by Bartholin's duct epithelium. These are commonly treated by marsupialization, which creates a new opening that is sutured open to promote drainage. An abscess may be secondary to Neisseria gonorrheae; however, it is often due to mixed flora. Bartholin's abscesses are acutely painful, and they may be marsupialized or drained by placing a catheter to promote drainage.

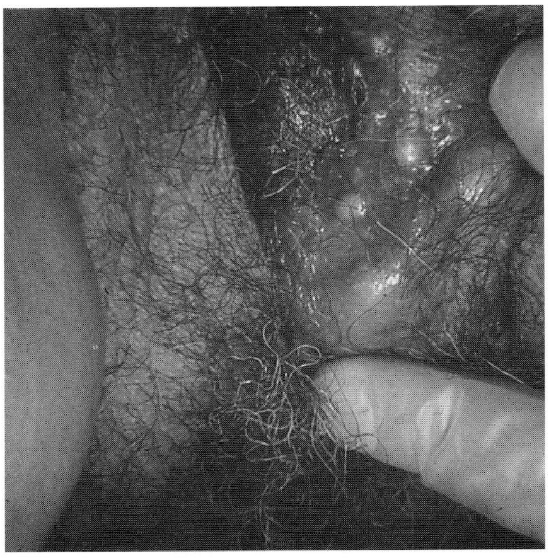

FIGURE 4.48. Epidermal inclusion cysts. These cysts may be multiple on the hair-bearing vulva. Reprinted with permission from Chapman & Hall, New York.

When women over the age of 40 present with a Bartholin's cyst or abscess, one should consider the possibility of an underlying carcinoma, and biopsies or gland excisions may be sent to the pathology laboratory to rule out this condition (24).

EPIDERMAL INCLUSION CYSTS

Usually asymptomatic unless they become infected, these lesions manifest as nodules on the vulva (Fig. 4.48). They may be excised if they become inflamed or if the patient desires it. Epidermal inclusion cysts are lined by keratinizing squamous epithelium and filled with a pale grumous material, the product of desquamation of the cyst lining (Fig. 4.49) (1).

CYSTS WITHIN THE VESTIBULE

Mucinous Cyst

These cysts arise from the minor vestibular glands and are lined by a simple mucinous epithelium (Figs. 4.50 and 4.51). If the cyst is present in the anterior vestibule, the differential includes Skene's duct cyst, which is usually lined by transitional epithelium. If the cyst arises posteriorly, a Bartholin's cyst is in the differential, but would be deeper-seated than a cyst of a minor vestibular gland (1, 25).

Periurethral (Skene's Duct) Cysts

These cysts may be lined by transitional or mucinous epithelium. Squamous metaplasia may be present in mucinous cysts. Epidermal inclusion cysts and mesonephric-like cysts also can arise in this area. Skene's duct cysts are excised if large or enlarging (Fig. 4.52) (1, 26).

Ciliated Cysts of the Vestibule

Cysts lined by tubo-endometrial epithelium have been reported secondary to Stevens-Johnson Syndrome, 5-fluorouracil therapy, or laser treatment (1).

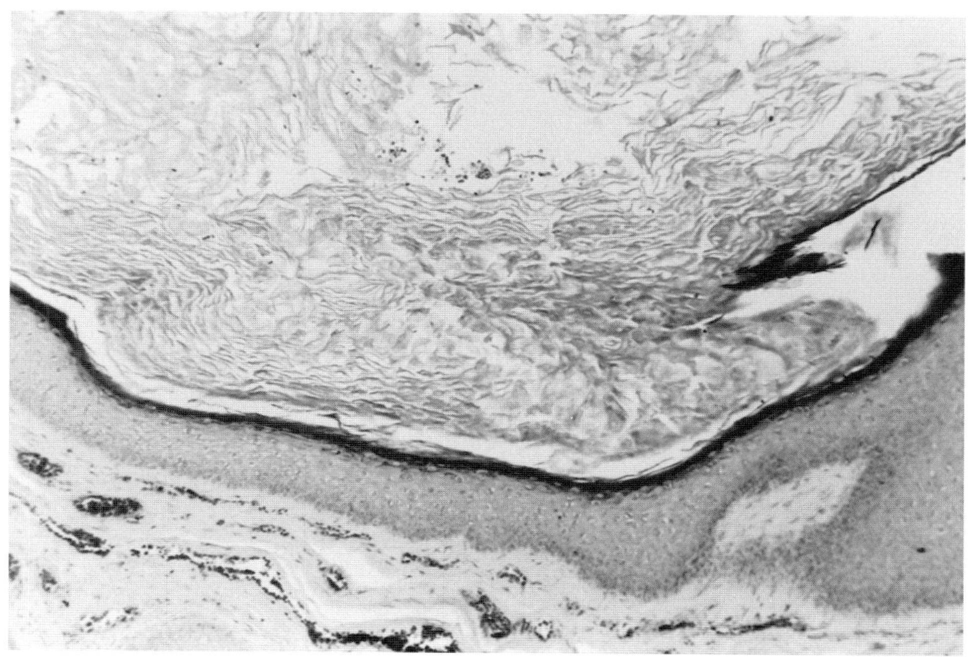

FIGURE 4.49.   Epidermal inclusion cyst. Histologically, they are lined by keratinized squamous epithelium.

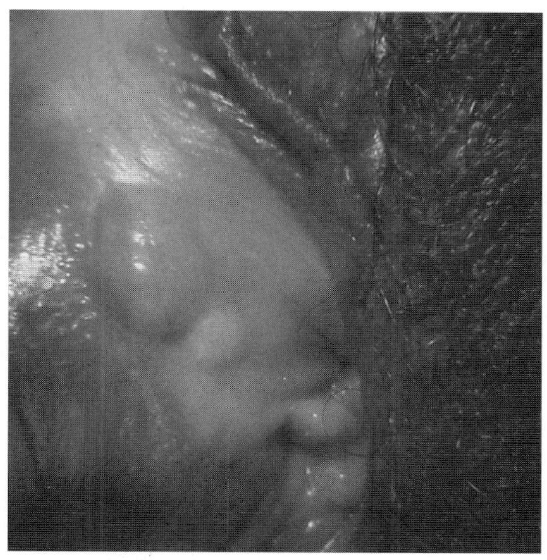

FIGURE 4.50. Vestibular mucinous cyst. Reprinted with permission from Chapman & Hall, New York.

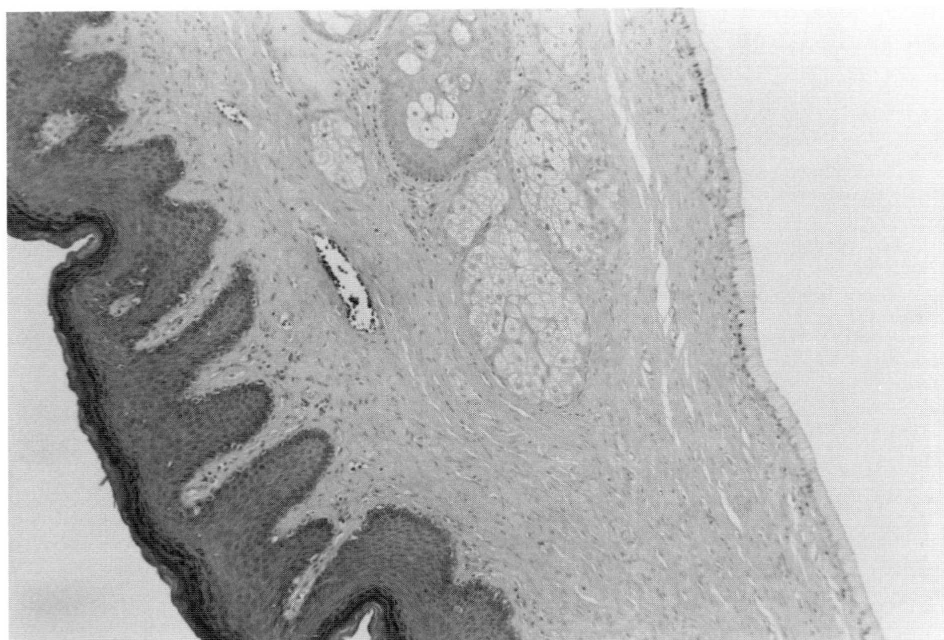

FIGURE 4.51. Mucinous cyst. Mucinous cysts arise from minor vestibular glands and are lined by a single layer of mucinous epithelium.

FIGURE 4.52. Skene's duct cyst. Reprinted with permission from Chapman & Hall, New York.

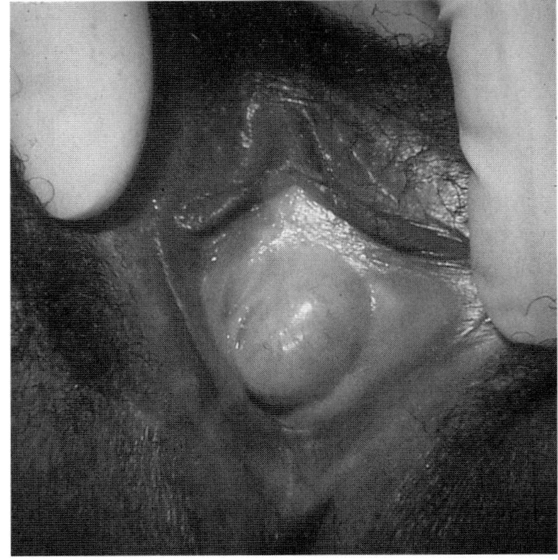

Mesonephric-like Cysts

These cysts are lined by a cuboidal or nonciliated columnar epithelium surrounded by a thin rim of smooth muscle. They are termed "mesonephric-like" rather than "mesonephric" by some, as the mesonephric ducts do not descend into the vestibule (1, 2, 27).

Suburethral Diverticulum

A lesion most often seen in postmenopausal women, suburethral diverticulum may arise from infection of paraurethral glands. Suburethral diverticula may become infected, resulting in chronic cystitis. Compression of an infected diverticulum will express purulent material per urethra. Grossly, these lesions may resemble cysts in the vestibular region (Fig. 4.53) and care must be taken by the clinician in order to avoid urethral injury during an attempted so-called cyst excision. The treatment for suburethral diverticulum is surgical repair (1, 28).

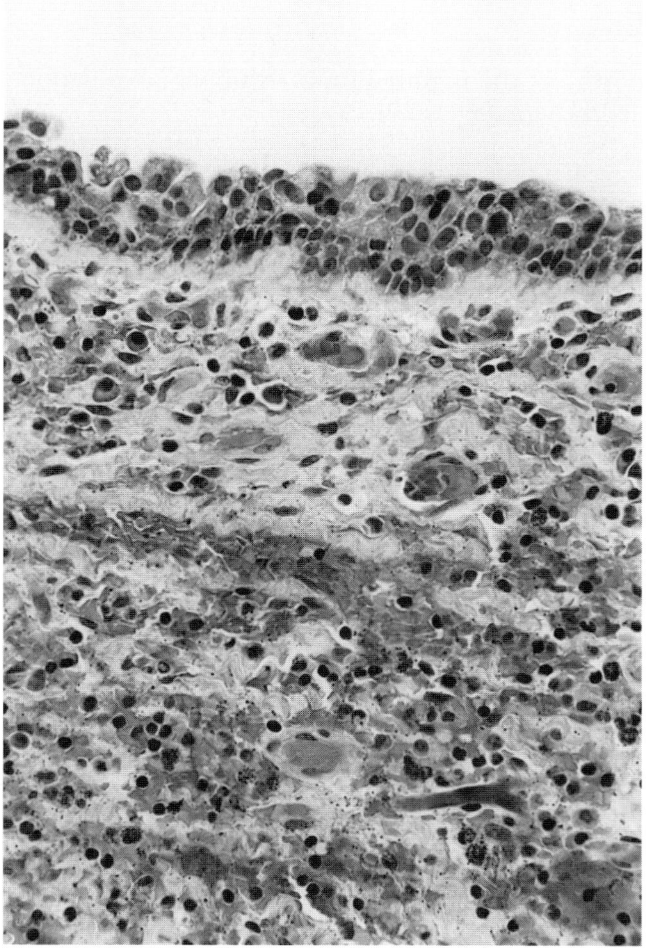

FIGURE 4.53. Suburethral diverticulum. The diverticulum is severely inflamed and is lined by transitional epithelium.

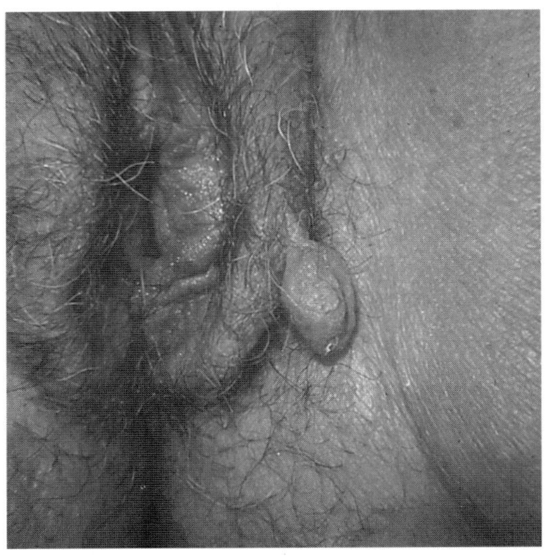

FIGURE 4.54. Fibroepithelial papilloma. The lesions may appear papillary or as skin tags. Reprinted with permission from Chapman & Hall, New York.

CYSTS OF THE CANAL OF NUCK

These mesothelial-lined cysts are located in the inguinal canal or upper labia majora, and they are analogous to hydrocele in the male (1, 29).

PAPILLARY LESIONS OF THE VULVA

Vulvar lesions with a grossly papillary appearance include condylomata (see Sexually Transmitted Diseases in this chapter), verrucous carcinoma (see Chapter 5), micropapillomatosis labialis, and fibroepithelial papillomas.

FIBROEPITHELIAL PAPILLOMAS

Fibroepithelial papillomas (acrochordons, skin tags) are commonly located on the hair-bearing vulva (Fig. 4.54). They are comprised of a fibrovascular stroma lined by keratinizing, stratified squamous epithelium (Fig. 4.55). They may be predominantly epithelial or predominantly stromal. They have not been shown to be caused by human *Papillomavirus*. They are often excised as a method of treatment (1, 2).

MICROPAPILLOMATOSIS LABIALIS (MPL)

Micropapillomatosis labialis appears as multiple delicate papillary projections, located in the vestibule, and can extend up the medial labia minora (Fig. 4.56). MPL may present with burning or pruritus, or it may be asymptomatic. Histologically, the lesion contains fibrovascular cores lined by thinly keratinized squamous epithelium (Fig. 4.57). No relationship to human *Papillomavirus* has been established (30). No therapy is generally required.

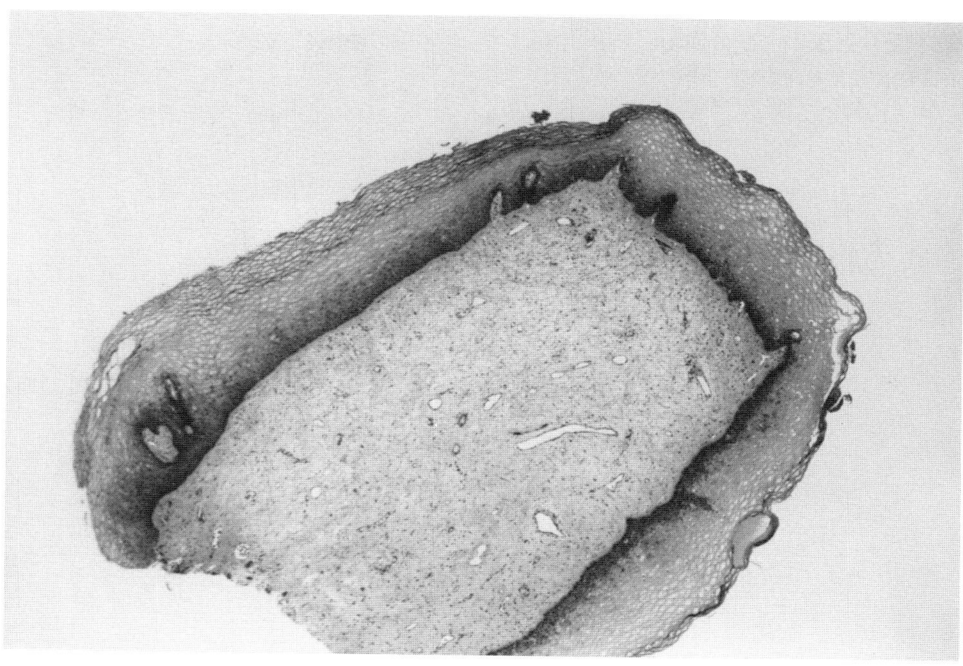

FIGURE 4.55.   Fibroepithelial papilloma. Histologically, they show no koilocytosis; they should not be mistaken for condylomas.

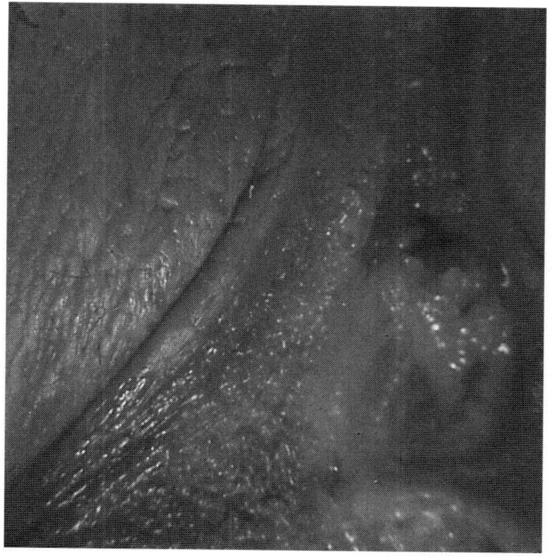

FIGURE 4.56. Micropapillomatosis labialis. The condition appears as delicate papillary "fingers" in the vestibule and sometimes extending up the inner labia minora. Courtesy of Dr. Alex Young.

FIGURE 4.57. Histologically, micropapillomatosis labialis shows no evidence of HPV infection.

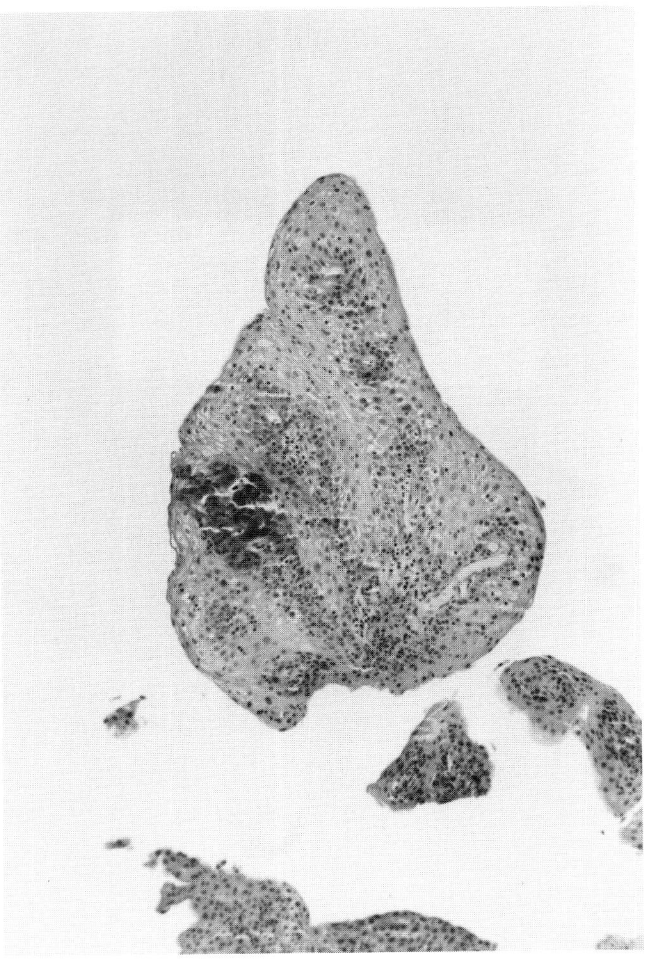

FIGURE 4.58. Endometriosis. Endometriosis in an episiotomy scar. Reprinted with permission from Chapman & Hall, New York.

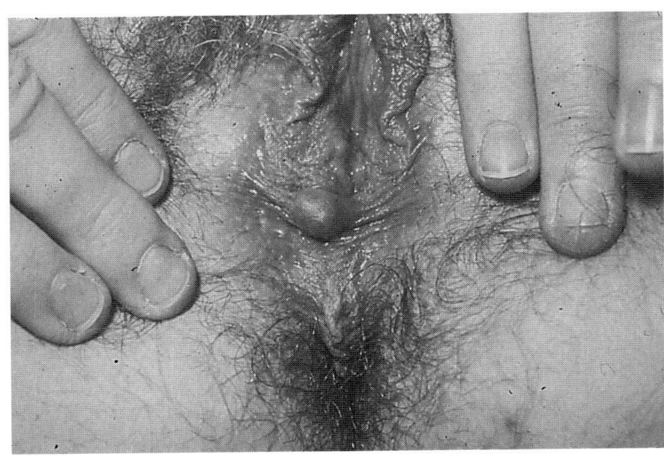

OTHER TUMOR-LIKE LESIONS OF THE VULVA
ENDOMETRIOSIS

Endometriosis, consisting of ectopic endometrial glands and stroma, may be seen on the vulva, usually secondary to implantation in an episiotomy scar (Figs. 4.58 and 4.59) (31).

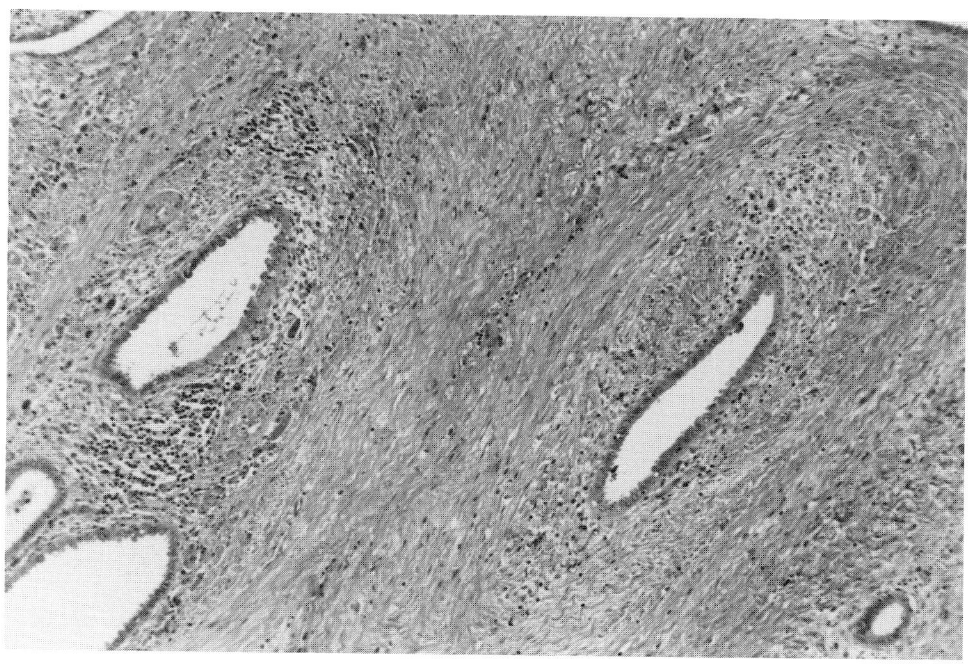

FIGURE 4.59.   Endometriosis. Endometrial glands and stroma are present, as is a dense fibrotic reaction.

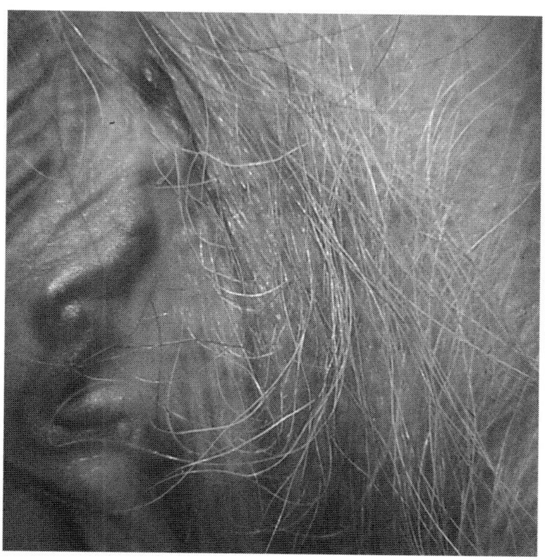

FIGURE 4.60.   Vulvar varicosities. Reprinted with permission from Chapman & Hall, New York.

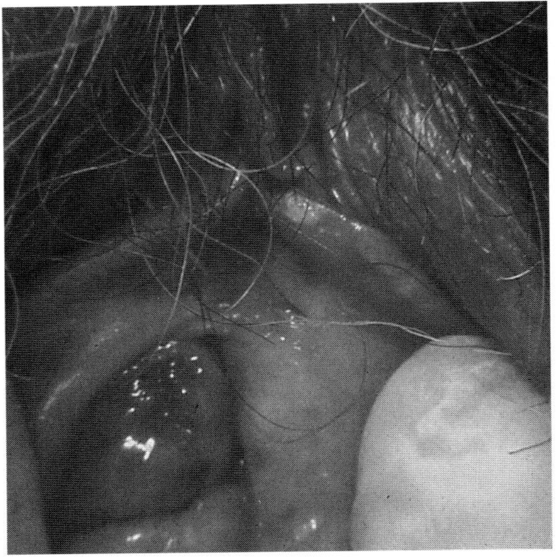

FIGURE 4.61. Urethral caruncle. The red granular tissue is probably due to urethral prolapse. Reprinted with permission from Chapman & Hall, New York.

VARICES

Vulvar varicosities become more common with increasing parity and are more prominent in the pregnant state (Fig. 4.60). Care must be taken not to traumatize them during a vaginal delivery. These are not generally excised unless thrombosed.

URETHRAL CARUNCLE

Most often seen in postmenopausal women, these lesions are probably due to partial prolapse of the urethral mucosa. Grossly, they appear as red, raised, granulation-like tissue (Fig. 4.61). Estrogen is the first line of therapy, although excision is occasionally warranted (1).

BENIGN NEOPLASMS

Tumors and tumor-like lesions of the vulva are listed in Table 4.7.

HIDRADENOMA PAPILLIFERUM

This benign neoplasm occurs almost exclusively in the genital region. It has been described as a tumor of sweat gland origin; however, it has recently been suggested that these tumors arise from mammary-like glands of the vulva (32). Hidradenomas may penetrate the epithelial surface, and the protruding erythematous papillary tissue may cause clinical concern regarding malignancy (Fig. 4.62). Histologically, these are well-circumscribed neoplasms. The low-power view of crowded glands and papillae should not be mistaken for an adenocarcinoma. Characteristically, a two-cell layer is present

TABLE 4.7.   Benign Tumors and Tumor-like
Lesions of the Vulva (1, 2, 33)

Fibroepithelial papilloma
Micropapillomatosis labialis
Seborrheic keratosis
Angiokeratoma
Keratoacanthoma
Leiomyoma
Fibroma
Lipoma
Neurofibroma
Desmoid tumor
Lymphangioma
Schwannoma
Glomus tumor
Dermatofibroma
Rhabdomyoma
Hidradenoma papilliferum
Clear cell hidradenoma
Trichoepithelioma
Tricholemmoma
Syringoma
Pleomorphic adenoma
Adenoma of minor vestibular glands
Nodular fascitis
Ectopic breast
Hemangioma
Pyogenic granuloma
Granular cell tumor
Angiomyofibroblastoma

in the tumor. The inner layer often shows secretory "snouts" at the apex of the epithelium, and the outer layer is more attenuated (Fig. 4.63) (33).

HEMANGIOMA AND RELATED LESIONS

Capillary and cavernous hemangiomas may occur on the vulva, particularly in children, but these are rarely biopsied (Fig. 4.64). Acquired hemangiomas are not infrequent on the vulva, and they present as multiple, small, purple papules (Fig. 4.65). Histologically, multiple blood-filled capillary or cavernous channels are seen in hemangiomas (Fig. 4.66A). A variant of hemangioma, angiokeratoma shows dilated vascular spaces immediately beneath hyperplastic hyperkeratotic epithelium (Fig. 4.66B). Pyogenic granulomas may also occur on the vulva. This variant of hemangioma shows ulceration of overlying epithelium with underlying granulation tissue (1, 2, 33).

FIGURE 4.62. Hidradenoma papilliferum. The lesion grossly may cause concern regarding malignancy. Reprinted with permission from Chapman & Hall, New York.

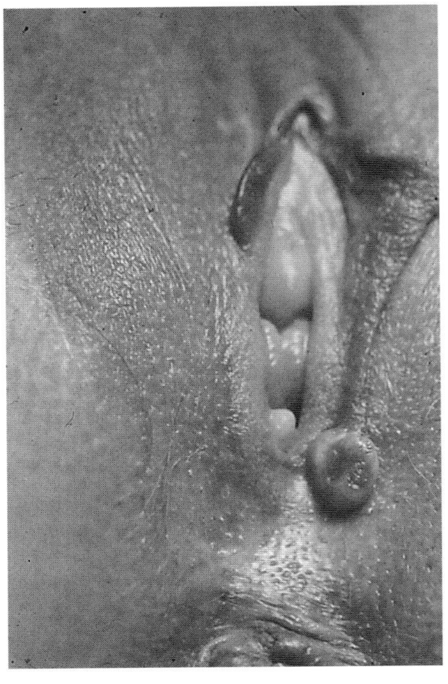

FIGURE 4.63. Hidradenoma papilliferum. Histologically, this sweat gland tumor is well-circumscribed, with papillae and glandular spaces lined by two cell layers.

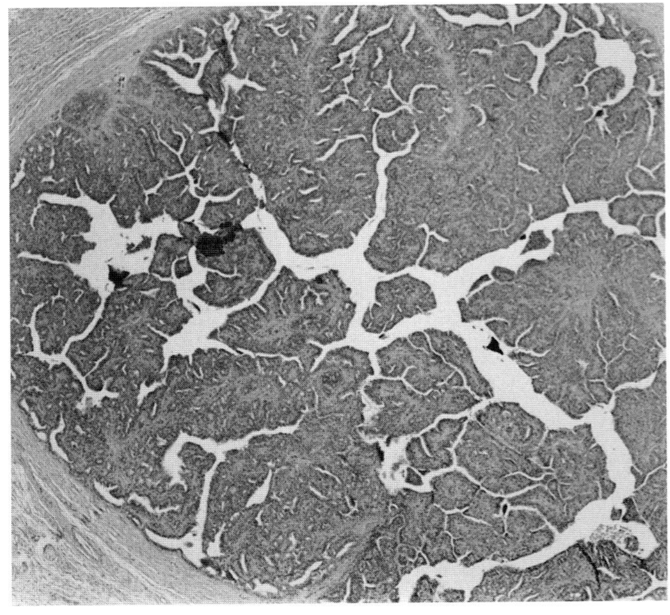

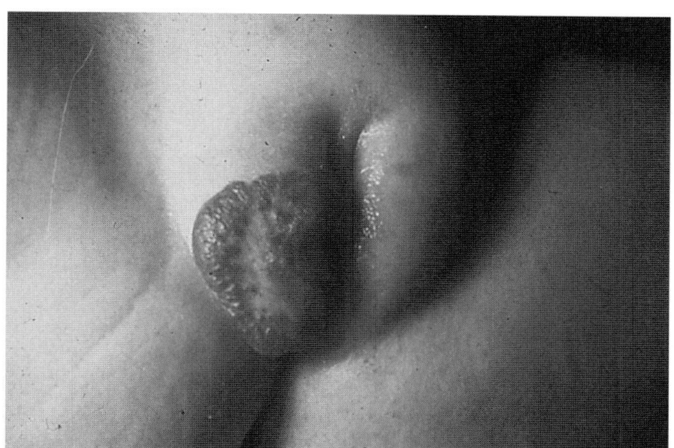

FIGURE 4.64. Hemangioma. Vulvar hemangiomas may be seen in children. Reprinted with permission from Chapman & Hall, New York.

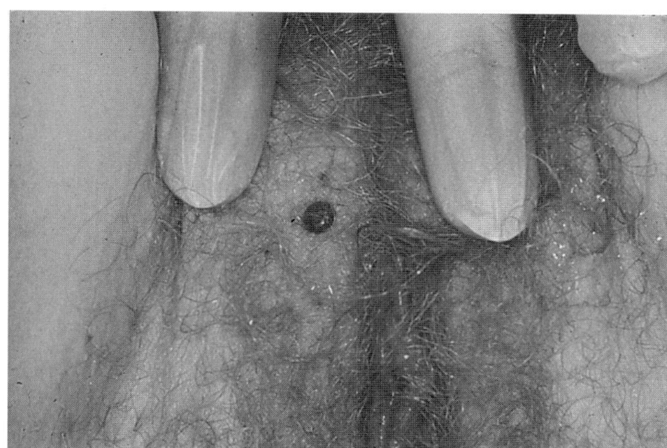

FIGURE 4.65. Hemangioma. Hemangiomas may occur as acquired lesions in older women. Reprinted with permission from Chapman & Hall, New York.

GRANULAR CELL TUMOR

Granular cell tumors are lesions of peripheral nerve sheath origin (Fig. 4.67). Although malignant behavior has been described, these tumors are usually benign. They have a nonencapsulated infiltrative margin. The cells contain small uniform nuclei and have an abundant eosinophilic granular-appearing cytoplasm, which stains for S100 protein (Fig. 4.68). Overlying epithelium often shows pseudoepitheliomatous hyperplasia. Excision is the treatment of choice (34).

SYRINGOMA

A benign tumor of eccrine sweat glands, syringomas grossly appear as papules and microscopically consist of multiple dilated tubules with comma-like tails in a fibroconnective tissue stroma. The tubules have a two-cell layer (Fig. 4.69)(35).

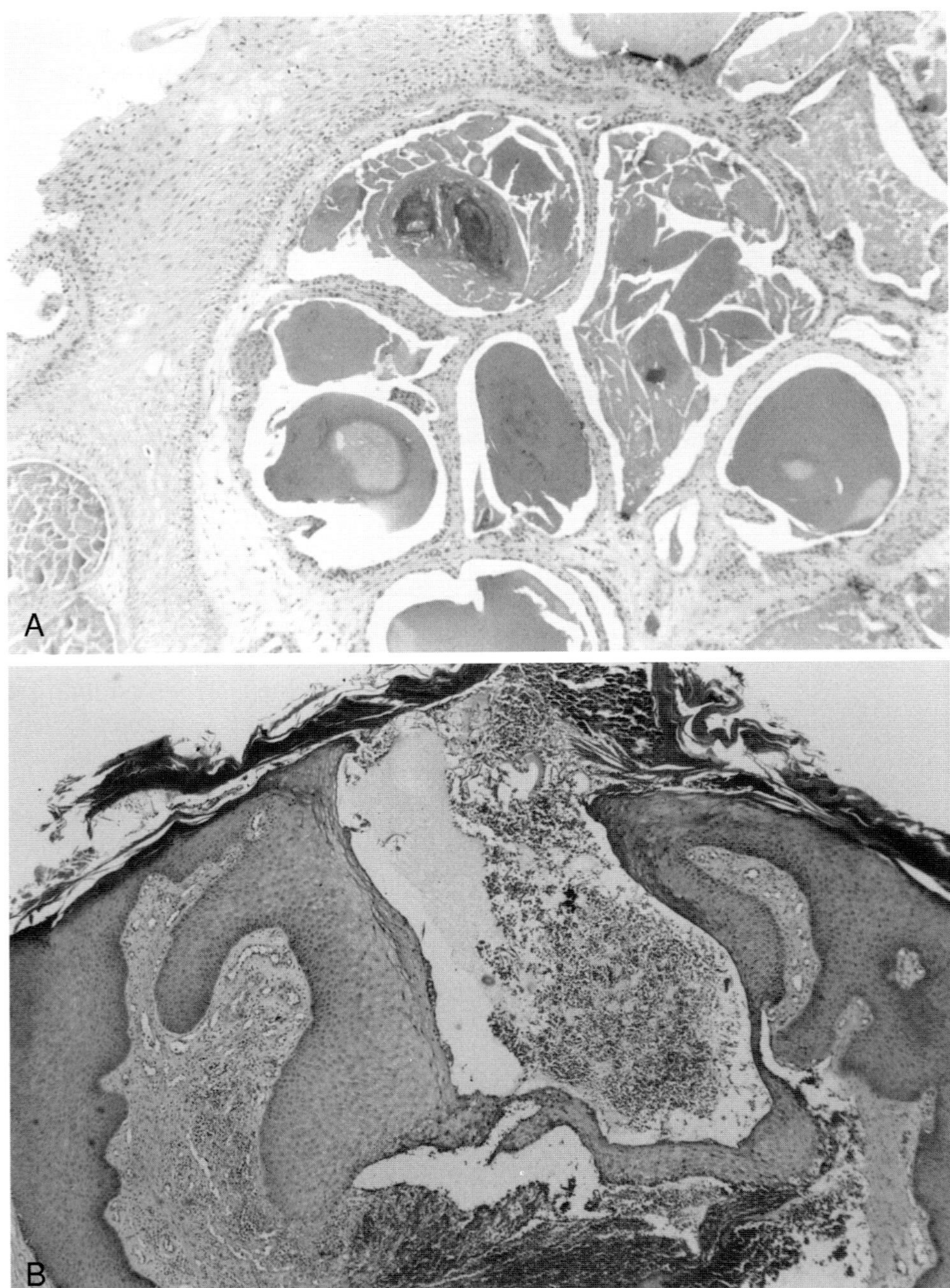

FIGURE 4.66. **A.** Hemangioma. This lesion is composed of large, dilated, blood-filled spaces. **B.** Angiokeratoma. Blood-filled spaces under a hyperkeratotic epithelium are present in this lesion.

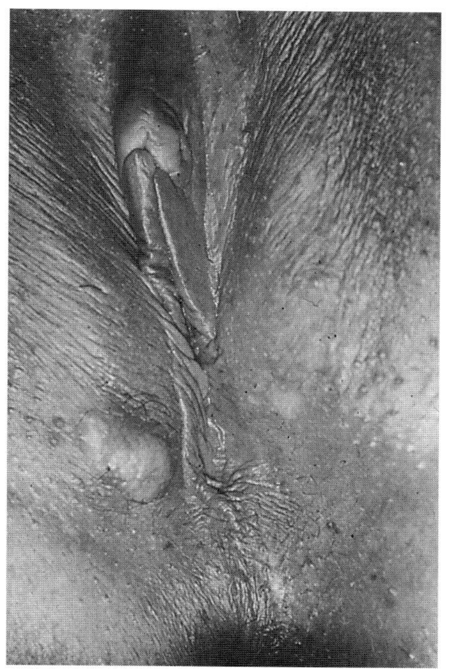

FIGURE 4.67. Granular cell tumor. Reprinted with permission from Chapman & Hall, New York.

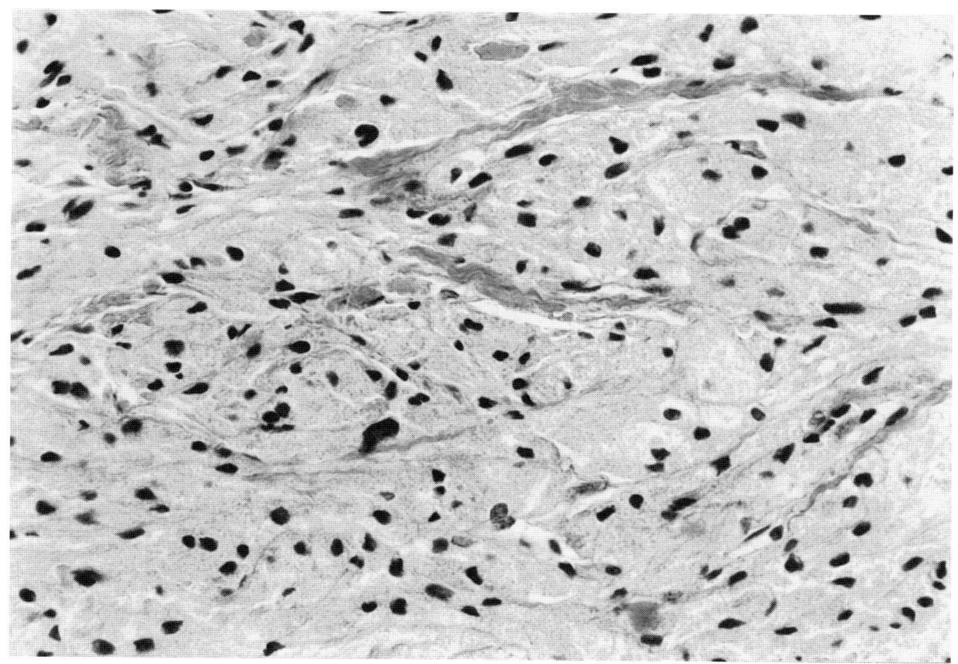

FIGURE 4.68. Granular cell tumor. The characteristic granular cytoplasm is seen.

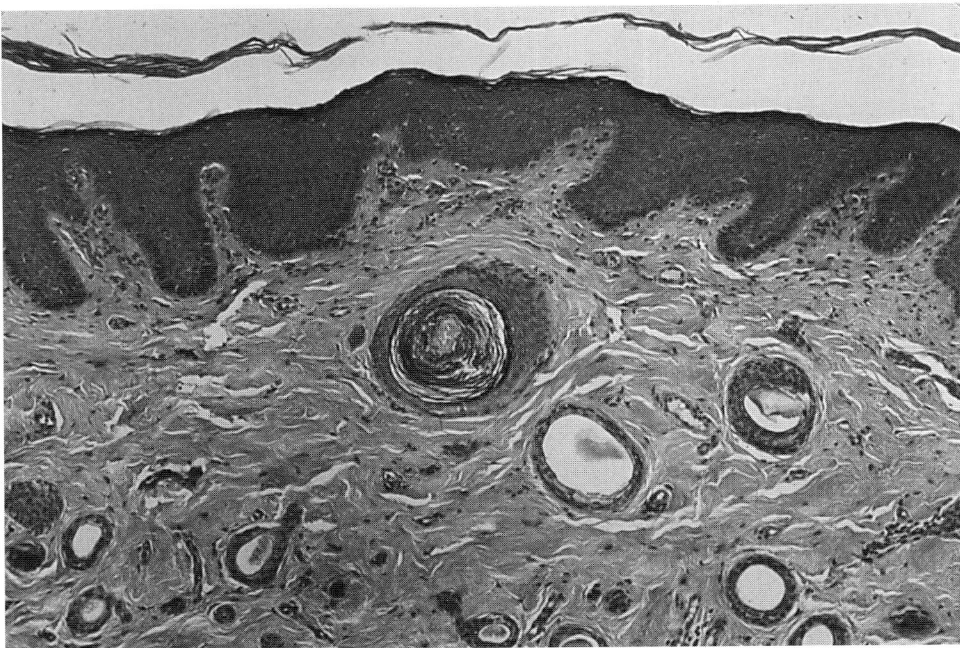

FIGURE 4.69.   Syringoma. Comma-shaped tubules are seen. Reprinted with permission from Chapman & Hall, New York.

AGGRESSIVE ANGIOMYXOMA

These lesions are discussed here to differentiate them from angiomyofibroblastomas (see next section). Aggressive angiomyxomas are locally aggressive and tend to recur after excision Grossly, the tumor is myxoid, with ill-defined margins. Histologically, the tumor is composed of fibroblasts and myofibroblasts in a myxoid mucin-containing stroma with abundant blood vessels that are often thickened or hyalinized (Fig. 4.70). Stroma is usually of low cellularity, with stellate or spindle cells, and frequent extravasation of erythrocytes . Mitoses and atypia are absent. Stromal cells stain for vimentin, but desmin reactivity varies with different reports (36–39).

ANGIOMYOFIBROBLASTOMA

This recently described lesion must be distinguished from aggressive angiomyxoma. One particular distinguishing feature is that these neoplasms are well circumscribed. In one series, the average size was 4.7 cm (38). This is in contradistinction to aggressive angiomyxomas, which are usually larger than five centimeters (39). Histologically, angiomyofibroblastomas have hypercellular and hypocellular areas. Most of the tumor cells are spindled, having some plasmacytoid and epithelioid cells. Stromal cells tend to concentrate perivascularly, and multinucleation may be present. Atypia and mitotic activity are minimal. Stromal cells stain for vimentin and desmin. Blood vessels are abundant; however, such vessels are not often hyalinized or thickened as in aggressive angiomyxoma (Fig. 4.71). Other histologic features distinguishing angiomyofibroblastoma from aggressive angiomyxoma are higher cellularity, more numerous blood ves-

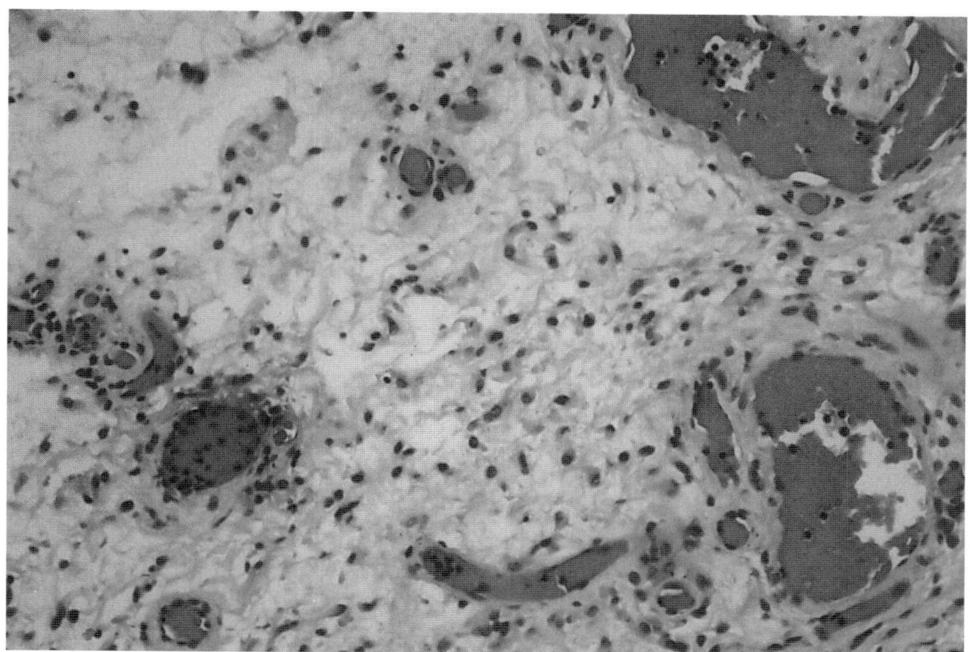

FIGURE 4.70.   Aggressive angiomyxoma. The lesion is deceptively bland histologically, with scarce spindle cells and vessels in a myxoid stroma.

sels, frequent plump stromal cells, minimal stromal mucin, and rarity of erythrocyte extravasation. Excision is usually curative for angiomyofibroblastomas (36–39).

SEBORRHEIC KERATOSIS

These lesions occur on the hairbearing vulva and are raised, brown or black, and waxy in appearance (Fig. 4.72). Microscopically, they are characterized by hyperkeratosis, acanthosis, papillomatosis, and the presence of keratin-filled horn cysts (Fig. 4.73). Excision is curative.

BENIGN LESIONS ARISING IN MAMMARY-LIKE TISSUE OF THE VULVA

In addition to the more common hidradenoma, which some feel arises from mammary-like tissue rather than sweat glands (32), lesions that histologically resemble a fibroadenoma of breast have been seen (Fig. 4.74).

LEIOMYOMA

Vulvar leiomyomas are uncommon. The distinction from leiomyosarcoma is discussed in Chapter 5.

VULVOVAGINAL SYMPTOMS IN THE PEDIATRIC AGE GROUP

Occasionally, a vulvar specimen may be received from a pediatric patient. The common symptoms and their etiologies are listed in Table 4.8.

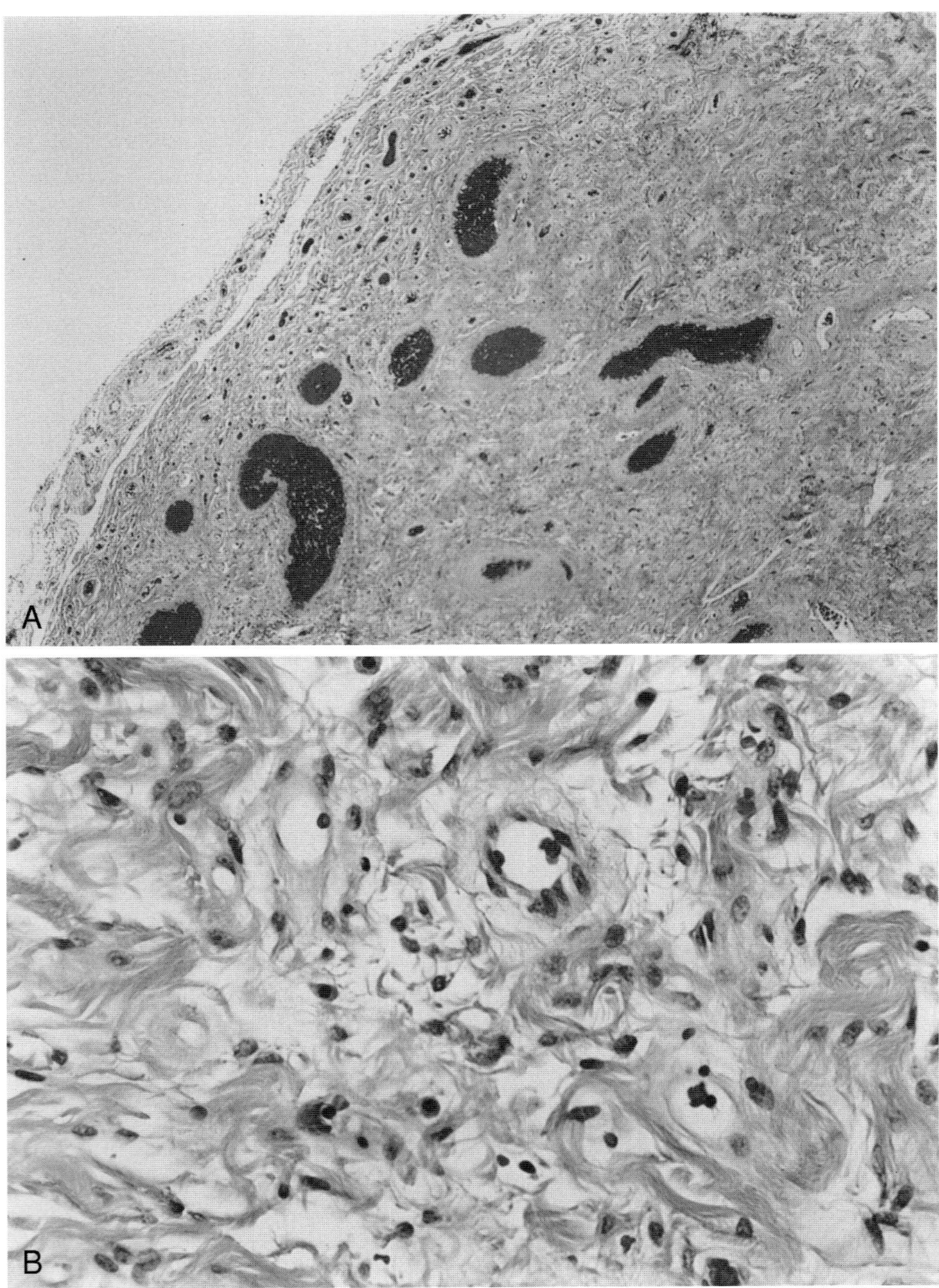

FIGURE 4.71.   Angiomyofibroblastoma. **A.** The lesion is well circumscribed. **B.** The tumor is composed of multiple thin blood vessels in a fibrous stroma containing epithelioid and plasmacytoid cells.

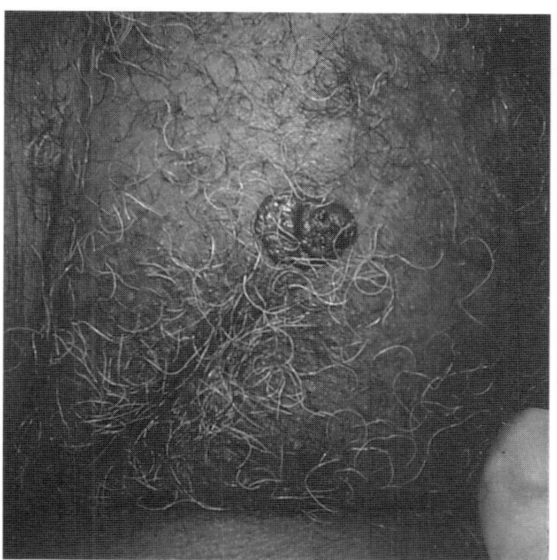

FIGURE 4.72. Seborrheic keratosis. The typical dark, "greasy" appearance of seborrheic keratosis is shown. Reprinted with permission from Chapman & Hall, New York.

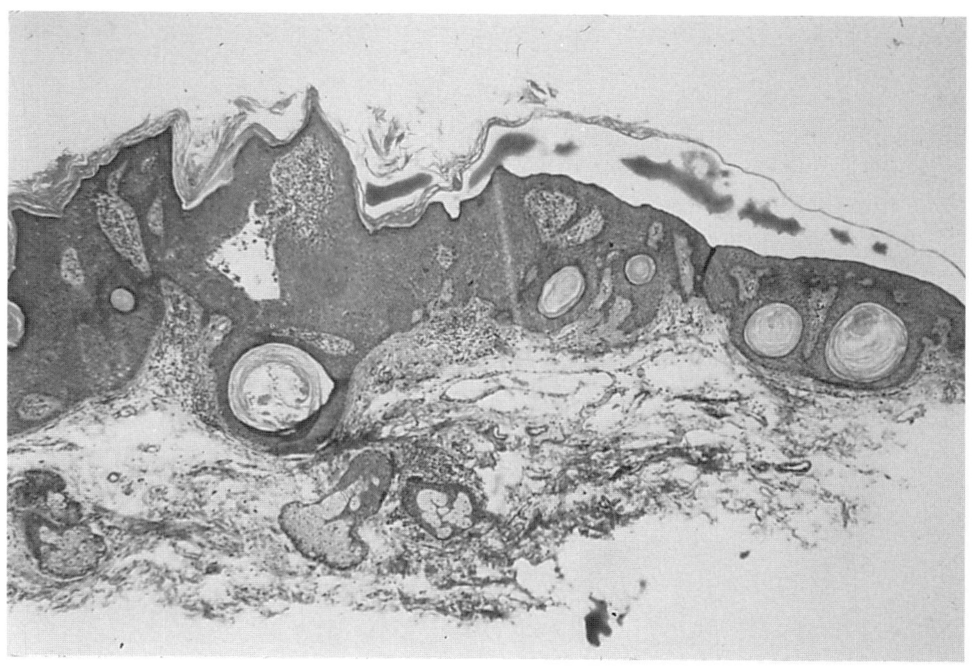

FIGURE 4.73. Seborrheic keratosis. Histologically, there is hyperkeratosis, acanthosis, papillomatosis, and keratin-filled cysts. Reprinted with permission from Chapman & Hall, New York.

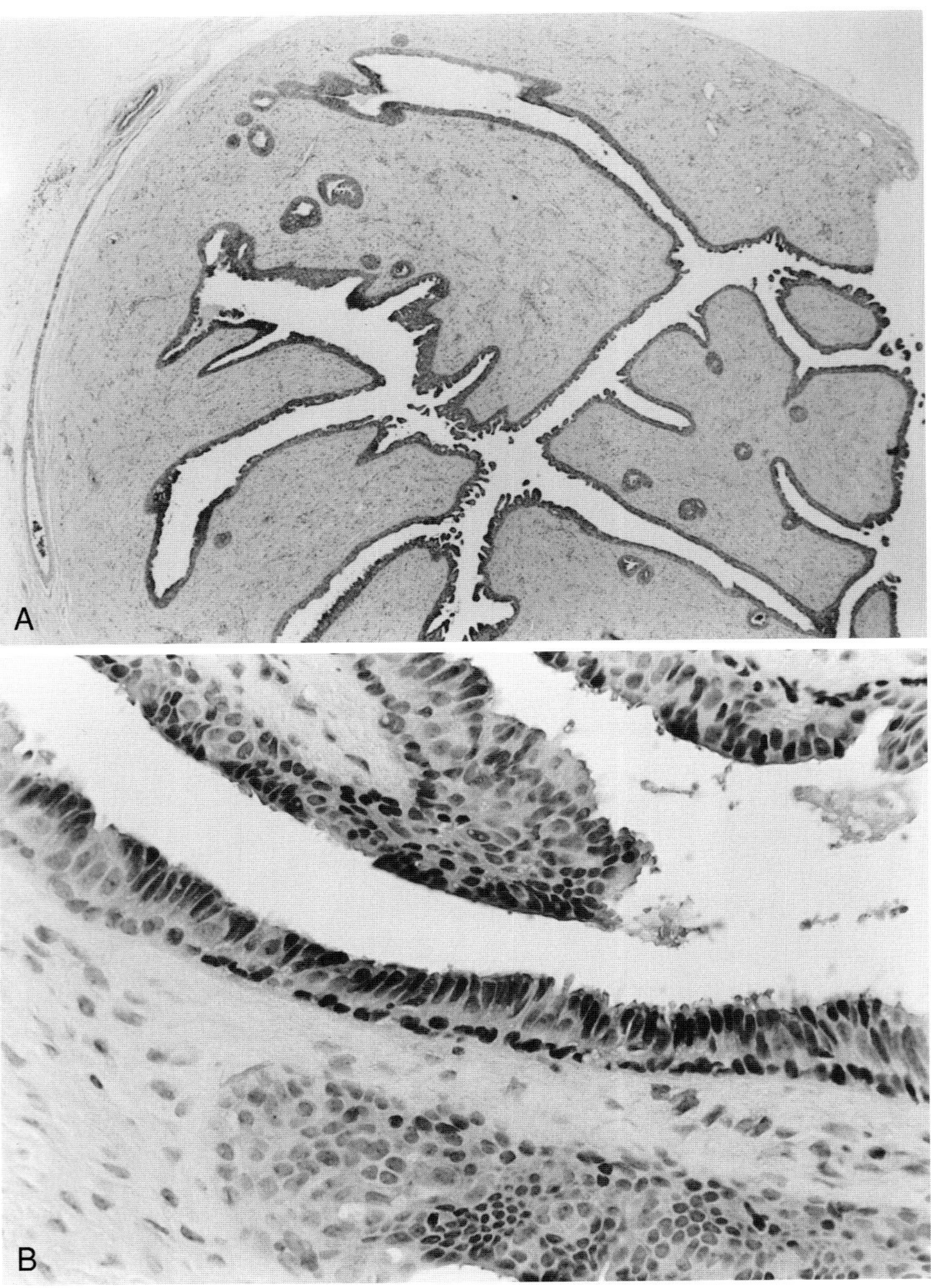

FIGURE 4.74. Fibroadenoma. Benign fibroadenoma arising in the vulva. The lesion is well-circumscribed **(A)** and contains a two-cell epithelial layer **(B)**.

TABLE 4.8.   Common Symptoms and Causes of Vulvovaginopathies (in children)

Bleeding
    Prolapsed urethra
    Infection, especially with condylomata acuminata
    Trauma, including foreign object in the vagina
    Endocrine disorders
    Benign and malignant neoplasms
    Sexual abuse
Discharge
    Infection
        Fecal flora
        Sexually transmitted diseases
        Enterobiasis
    Hygienic practices (overzealous or inadequate)
    Labial adhesions
    Foreign body
Dermatitis
    Lichen sclerosus
    Lichen planus
    Seborrheic dermatitis
    Atopic dermatitis
    Contact dermatitis
    Vulvar psoriasis

Reprinted with permission from the following: American College of Obstetricians and Gynecologists: Pediatric Gynecologic Disorders. Technical Bulletin No. 201. Washington, DC, copyright 1995.

REFERENCES

1. Wilkinson EJ, Stone IK. Atlas of Vulvar Disease. Baltimore: Williams & Wilkins, 1995.
2. Wilkinson EJ. Benign diseases of the vulva. In: Kurman RJ, ed. Blaustein's Pathology of the Female Genital Tract. 4th ed. New York: Springer-Verlag, 1994.
3. Wilkinson EJ. Normal histology and nomenclature of the vulva, and malignant neoplasms including VIN [review]. Dermatol Clin 1992;10:283–296.
4. Nuovo GJ, Friedman D, Richart RM. In situ hybridization of human *Papillomavirus* DNA segregation patterns in lesions of the female genital tract. Gynecol Oncol 1990;36: 256–262.
5. Strand A, Rylander E, Wilander E, et al. HPV infection in male partners of women with squamous intraepithelial neoplasia and/or high risk HPV. Acta Dermatol Venereol 1995; 75:312–316.
6. Hatch KD. Clinical appearance and treatment strategies for human *Papillomavirus:* a gynecologic perspective. Am J Obstet Gynecol 1995:172(4pt2):1340–1344.
7. Brock BV, Selke S, Benedetti J, et al. Frequency of asymptomatic shedding of herpes simplex virus in women with genital herpes. JAMA 1990;263:418–420.

8. Elgart ML. Sexually transmitted diseases of the vulva [review]. Dermatol Clin 1992;10: 387–403.
9. Freinkel AL. Histological aspects of sexually transmitted genital lesions. Histopathology 1987;11:819 –831.
10. Mroczkowski TF, Martin DH. Genital ulcer disease. Dermatol Clin 1994;12:753–764.
11. Joseph AK, Rosen T. Laboratory techniques used in the diagnosis of chancroid, granuloma inguinale and lymphogranuloma venereum. Dermatol Clin 1994;12:1–8.
12. McKay M. Vulvodynia: diagnostic patterns. Dermatol Clin 1992;10:423–433.
13. Prayson RA, Stoler MH, Hart W. Vulvar vestibulitis: a histopathologic study of 36 cases, including human *Papillomavirus* in situ hybridization analysis. Am J Surg Pathol 1995;19: 154–160.
14. Wilkinson EJ, Guerrero E. Daniel R, et al. Vulvar vestibulitis is rarely associated with human *Papillomavirus* types 6,11,16, or 18. Int J Gynecol Pathol 1993;12:344–349.
15. Bessim S, Heller DS, Dottino P, et al. Malakoplakia of the female genital tract causing urethral and ureteral obstruction: a case report. J Reprod Med 1991;36:691–694.
16. Morgan ED, Laszlo JD, Stumpf PG. Incomplete Behcet's syndrome in the differential diagnosis of genital ulceration and postcoital bleeding. A case report. J Reprod Med 1988; 33:844–846.
17. Stage AH, Jumeniuk JM, Easley WK. Bullous pemphigoid of the vulva: a case report. Am J Obstet Gynecol 1984:150:169–170.
18. Lim HW, Bystryn JC. Evaluation and management of diseases of the vulva: bullous disease. Clin Obstet Gynecol 1978;21:1007–1022.
19. Eisen D. The vulvovaginal-gingival syndrome of lichen planus. The clinical characteristics of 22 patients. Arch Dermatol 1994;130:1379–1382.
20. McKay M. Vulvar dermatoses: common problems in dermatological and gynaecological practice [review]. Br J Clin Prac 1990;71(Symposium Suppl):5–10.
21. Rock B. Pigmented lesions of the vulva [review]. Dermatol Clin 1992;10:361–370.
22. Wilkinson EJ. The 1989 presidential address. International Society for the Study of Vulvar Disease. J Reprod Med 1990;35:981–991.
23. Meffert JJ, Davis BM, Grimwood RE. Lichen sclerosus [review]. J Am Acad Dermatol 1995; 32:393–416.
24. Visco AG, Del Priore G. Postmenopausal Bartholin gland enlargement: a hospital-based cancer risk assessment. Obstet Gynecol 1996;87:286–290.
25. Oi RH, Munn R. Mucous cysts of the vulvar vestibule. Hum Pathol 1982;13:584–586.
26. Miller EV. Skene's duct cyst. J Urol 1984;131:966–967.
27. Junaid TA, Thomas SM. Cysts of the vulva and vagina. A comparative study. Int J Gynaecol Obstet 1981;19:239–243.
28. Ginsburg DS. Genadry R. Suburethral diverticulum in the female. Obstet Gynecol Surv 1984;39:1–7.
29. Schneider CA, Festa S, Spillet CR, et al. Hydrocele of the Canal of Nuck [review]. N J Med 1994;91:37–38.
30. Garzetti GG, Ciavattini A, Goteri G, et al. Vaginal micropapillary lesions are not related to human *Papillomavirus* infection: in situ hybridization and polymerase chain reaction detection techniques. Gyn Obstet Invest 1994;38:134–139.
31. Cheng DL, Heller DS, Oh C. Endometriosis of the perineum: report of 2 new cases and a review of the literature [review]. Eur J Obstet Gynecol Reprod Biol 1991;42:81–84.
32. van der Putte SC. Mammary-like glands of the vulva and their disorders [review]. Int J Gynecol Pathol 1994;13:150–160.
33. Hood AF, Lumadue J. Benign vulvar tumors [review]. Dermatol Clin 1992;10:371–385.
34. Guenther L, Shum D. Granular cell tumor of the vulva. Pediatr Dermatol 1993;10: 153–155.
35. Belardi MG, Maglione MA, Vighi S, et al. Syringoma of the vulva: a case report [review]. J Reprod Med 1994;39:957–959.

36. Elchalal U, Lifschitz-Mercer B, Dgani R, et al. Aggressive angiomyxoma of the vulva [review].Gynecol Oncol 1992;47:260–262.
37. Steeper TA, Rosai J. Aggressive angiomyxoma of the female pelvis and perineum: report of nine cases of a distinctive type of gynecologic soft-tissue neoplasm. Am J Surg Pathol 1983;7:463–475.
38. Neilsen G, Rosenberg A, Young R, et al. Angiomyofibroblastoma of the vulva and vagina. Mod Pathol 1996;9:284–291.
39. Fletcher CD, Tsang WY, Fisher C, et al. Angiomyofibroblastoma of the vulva: a benign neoplasm distinct from aggressive angiomyxoma. Am J Surg Pathol 1992;16:373–382.

MALIGNANT DISEASES OF THE VULVA

Debra S. Heller, MD

■

Intraepithelial Neoplasia of the Vulva
Invasive Neoplasms of the Vulva
Mesenchymal Malignancies of the Vulva
Other Malignancies of the Vulva

INTRAEPITHELIAL NEOPLASIA OF THE VULVA

VULVAR INTRAEPITHELIAL NEOPLASIA (VIN)

In 1986, the International Society for the Study of Vulvar Diseases (ISSVD) changed the terminology of intraepithelial lesions of the vulva, discarding such terms as Bowen's disease, Bowenoid papulosis, and Erythroplasia of Querat (1). Lesions are now classified as vulvar intraepithelial neoplasia I, II, or III, based on the degree of maturation abnormality; such classification is similar to the cervical intraepithelial neoplasia (CIN) terminology of the cervix. Some laboratories diagnose VIN as either low-grade VIN (VIN I) or high-grade VIN (VIN II–III), corresponding to Bethesda system diagnoses. The incidence of VIN, and notably high-grade VIN, is increasing, particularly in women under 35 years of age. The lesions present as multifocal maculopapular lesions, which may be white in appearance or pigmented (Figs. 5.1 and 5.2). The lesions may be asymptomatic, or pruritus may be a presenting complaint. Most lesions are located on the labia minora and perineum. The histologic picture is one of various degrees of abnormal epithelial maturation. Abnormalities include nuclear pleomorphism with hyperchromatic nuclei, multinucleation, increase in the nuclear/cytoplasmic ratio, mitotic activity including atypical mitotic figures, and dyskeratosis. Lesions also often show acanthosis and parakeratosis. The presence of melanophages explains the pigmentation of some of these lesions. In low-grade VIN (VIN I), the abnormal maturation is confined to the lower third of the epithelium (Fig. 5.3); in VIN II, to the lower two-thirds (Fig. 5.4), In VIN III, the abnormal epithelium extends above two-thirds of the epithelium (Fig. 5.5). High-grade VIN encompasses the latter two diagnoses. The term VIN III encompasses the older concepts of "severe dysplasia" and "carcinoma-in-situ." The distinction, if any, between flat condyloma and VIN I is unclear. HPV 16 is the most commonly identified HPV type in VIN (2). VIN commonly involves skin appendages, and this

FIGURE 5.1. High-grade VIN. Multifocal pigmented lesions are present. Reprinted with permission from Chapman & Hall, New York.

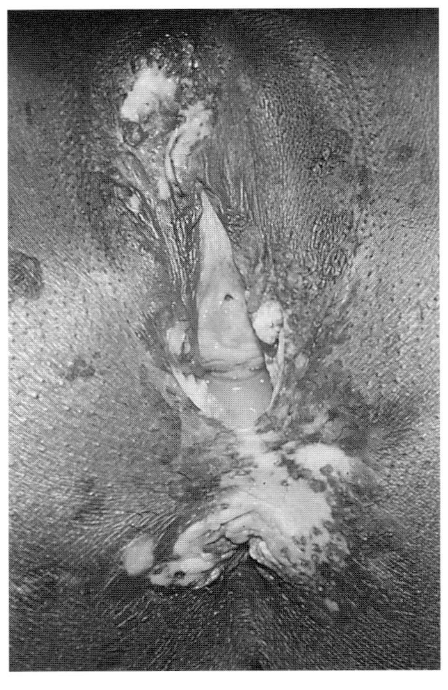

FIGURE 5.2. The lesions may appear white due to hyperkeratosis. Reprinted with permission from Chapman & Hall, New York.

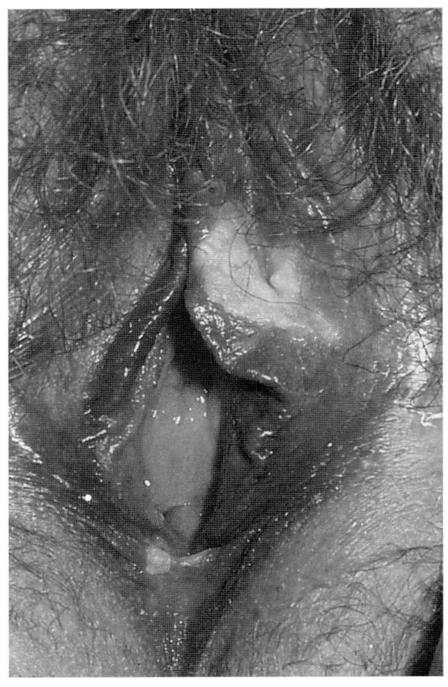

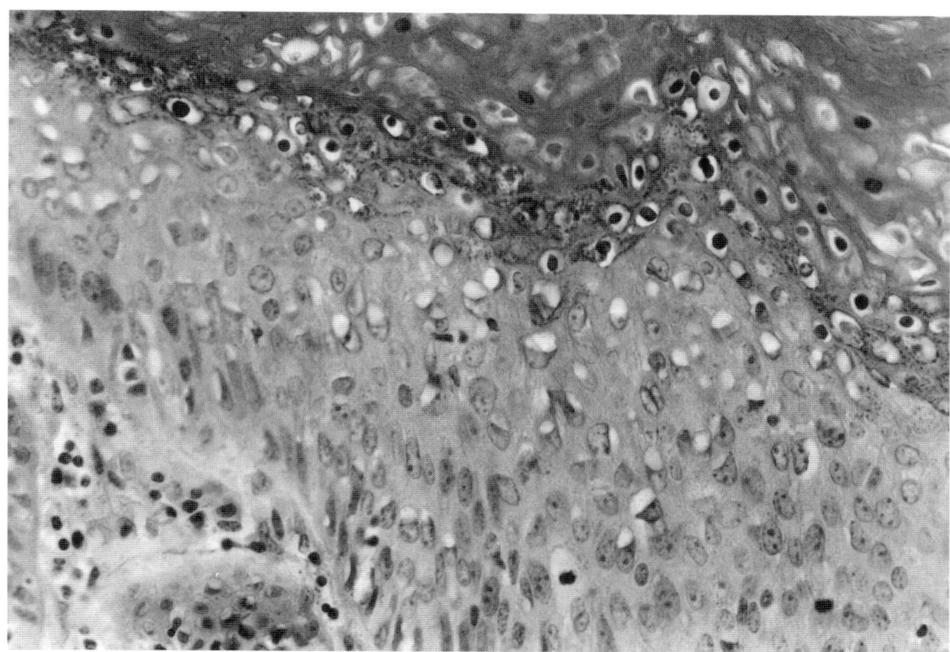

FIGURE 5.3.   VIN I (low-grade VIN). Abnormal maturation is confined to the lower third of the epithelium. Changes suggestive of HPV effect are present

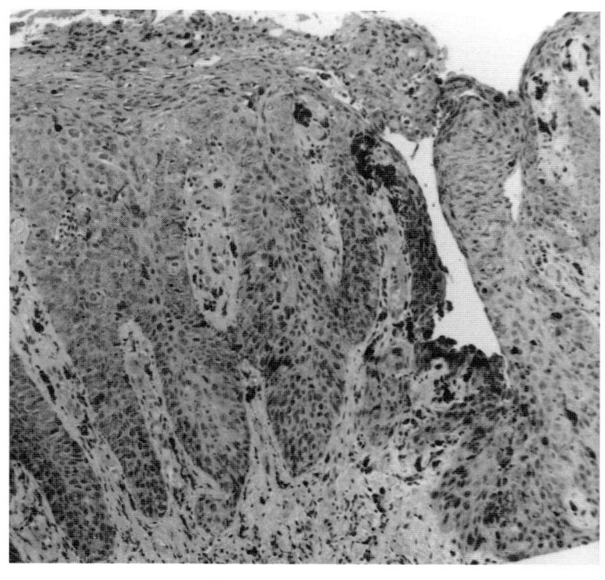

FIGURE 5.4.   Pigmented VIN II (high-grade VIN). The presence of melanophages, seen here abundantly in the dermis, explains the pigmented gross appearance of many of these lesions.

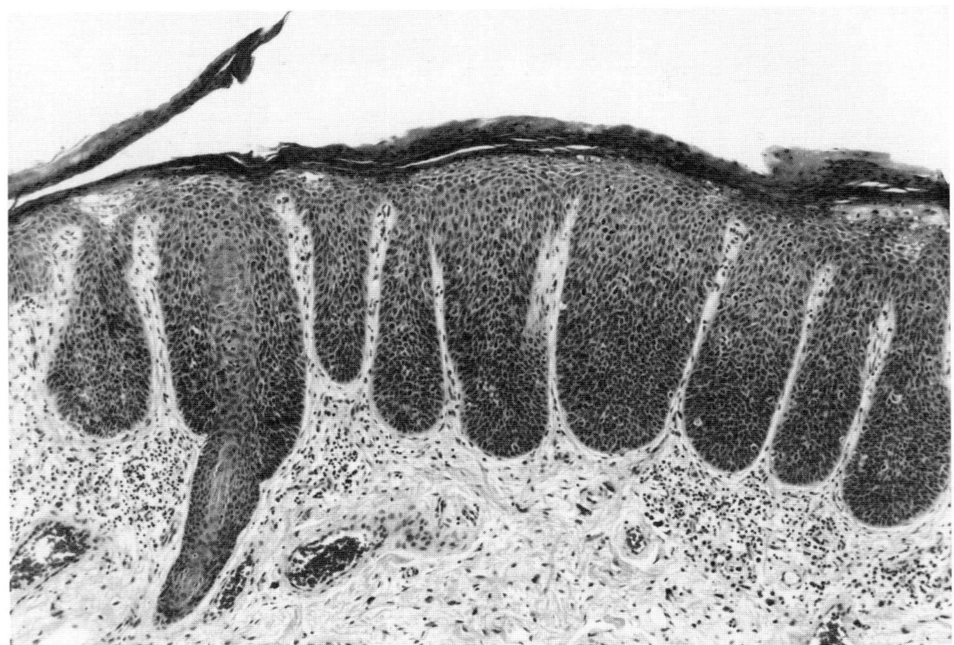

FIGURE 5.5. VIN III (basaloid VIN). There is abnormal maturation throughout the entire epithelial thickness. Cells are small and basaloid in appearance. Parakeratosis and acanthosis are seen.

should not be mistaken for invasion. Analogous to patterns recently described for invasive squamous cell carcinoma (3), high-grade VIN lesions have been described as showing basaloid and warty patterns. These patterns may coexist, and they have an increased association with HPV (4). Basaloid VIN (Fig. 5.5) is composed of small immature basal-appearing cells; warty VIN (Fig. 5.6) shows koilocytotic atypia. These distinctions were not made in the older literature. In addition, a less common pattern of VIN III, known as differentiated VIN, has been classified. In differentiated VIN, eosinophilic cells with prominent nucleoli are present in the basal and parabasal areas with variable keratinization and even occasional pearl formation (Fig. 5.7). Overlying epithelium shows enlarged nuclei with prominent nucleoli and vesicular chromatin. The apparent maturation can be misleading (5).

Therapy for VIN is usually surgical, the extent of which is individually tailored. Young women with diffuse lesions may be treated as conservatively as possible (6) with follow-up because of the low risk of associated carcinoma; however, in older women, VIN carries a much higher risk of progression (7). VIN is more likely to progress to invasive cancer in the immunosuppressed as well as the elderly (8). It is also more likely to be unifocal in the elderly, as opposed to the multifocal lesions of the reproductive aged patient. In one study, 3.8% of treated and 87.5% of untreated patients with VIN III progressed to invasive carcinoma (9).

Laser ablation is of limited use in treating high-grade or extensive VIN because it provides no specimen to rule out carcinoma. Therapy with 5-Fluorouracil has been used, but it can be extremely irritating. Excision remains the mainstay of therapy.

A finding seen on occasion in reproductive aged women that may raise the question

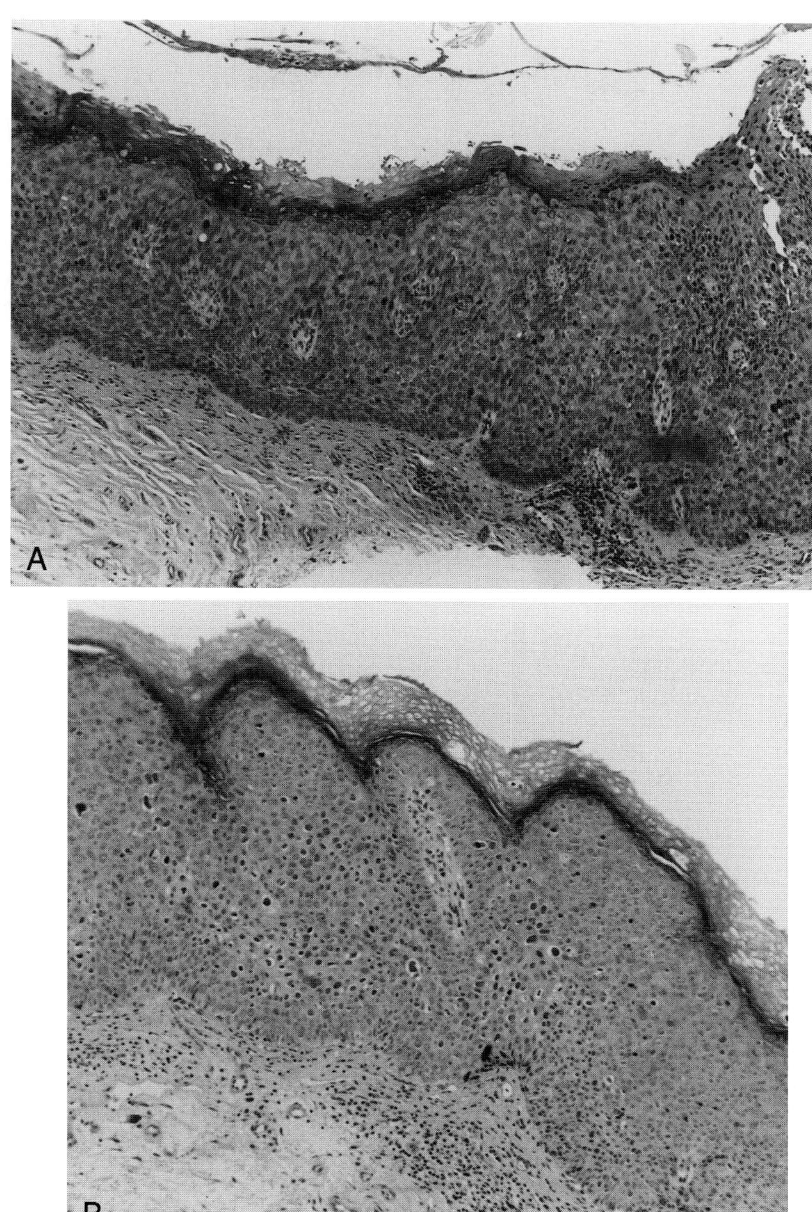

FIGURE 5.6.   Warty VIN III. **A.** The configuration of the lesion is "warty" due to papillomatosis. **B.** Koilocytotic atypia is a feature of these lesions.

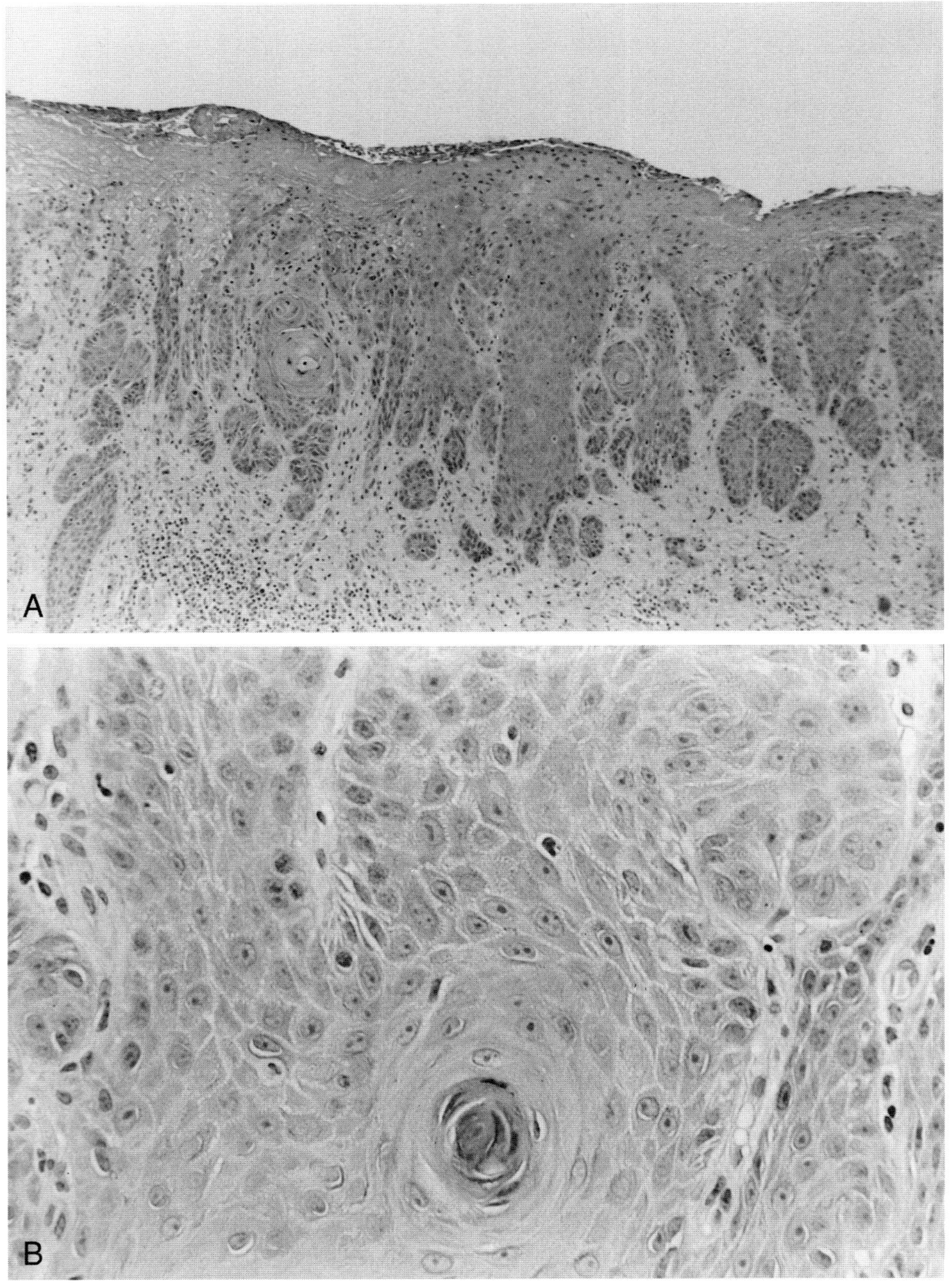

FIGURE 5.7. Differentiated VIN. **A.** There is no apparent maturation abnormality, which can be misleading. **B.** Enlarged eosinophilic cells with prominent nucleoli and keratinization are present in the parabasal and basal area. Here, a keratin pearl is seen.

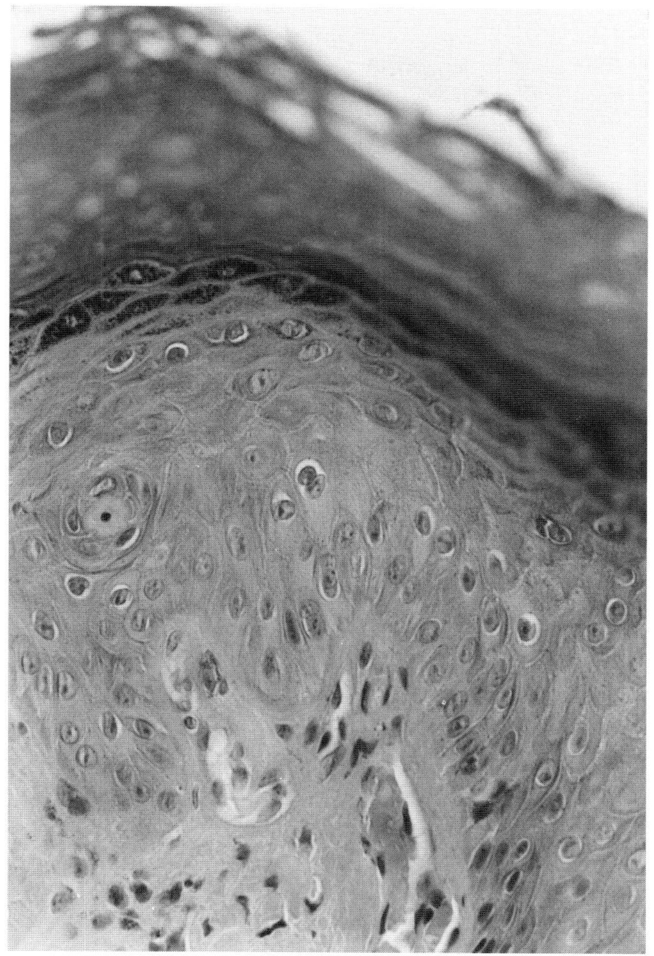

FIGURE 5.8. Multinucleated atypia. Multinucleation without atypia is seen in the lower epithelial layers.

of a VIN diagnosis is multinucleated atypia, described by McLachlin and colleagues (10). In these cases, the multinucleation is confined to the lower and middle epithelial layers. Nuclear atypia is not a feature, and nucleoli are prominent. This finding was not found to be associated with HPV (10)(Fig. 5.8).

PAGET'S DISEASE OF THE VULVA

Paget's disease is usually seen in older Caucasian women. The lesion presents with pruritus, and grossly appears red and velvety, with overlying white plaques (Fig. 5.9). Histologically, the characteristic large eosinophilic Paget cells are seen predominantly in the basal layer of the epithelium (Fig. 5.10); they also spread upward within the epidermis (Pagetoid spread) and may extend around dermal appendages. The rate of an associated underlying invasive adenocarcinoma of the vulva at the time of diagnosis varies in the literature (Fig. 5.11). In one series it was 21% (11). Extragenital malignancies may also be associated with Paget's disease of the vulva. An important distinction is between Paget's disease and a pagetoid pattern of spread of a malignant melanoma. Monoclonal antibodies have been used to distinguish the two. Bacchi et al. (12) noted

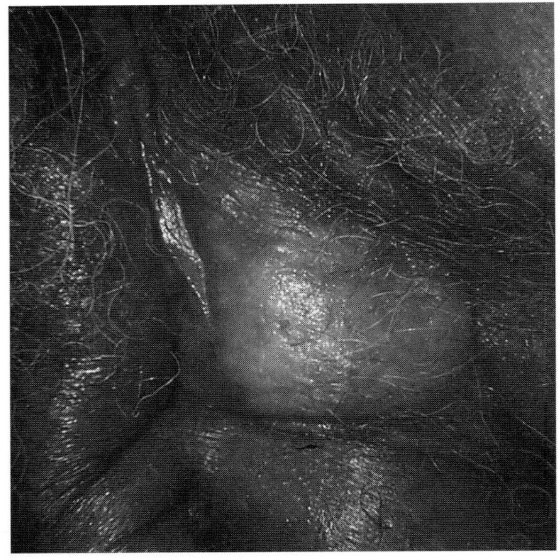

FIGURE 5.9. Paget's disease. The lesion is red and velvety with overlying white plaques. Reprinted with permission from Chapman & Hall, New York.

that HMB45 was specific for melanoma. Melanoma also stains with S100 protein. Paget's disease in Bacchi's study stained for the low molecular weight keratin 35 beta H11. Paget cells also stain for carcinoembryonic antigen, mucin, and with the Periodic Acid-Schiff reaction, and are negative for HMB45 and S100 protein. In evaluating margin involvement in Paget's disease, Bacchi's group noted that normal epithelium stained with the high molecular weight keratin 34 beta E12, as opposed to the low molecular weight keratin 35 beta H11 demonstrated in the Paget cells (12).

Therapy for noninvasive Paget's disease is local excision. Paget's disease tends to extend beyond the grossly visible margins, and frozen sections may be requested at the time of surgery. Frozen sections will not be helpful in the case of skip lesions (12).

In terms of prognosis, distinguishing noninvasive from the less common invasive Paget's disease (Fig. 5.10C,D) is important, as is searching for the presence of an underlying adenocarcinoma. In one series (13), for intraepithelial and minimally invasive Paget's disease, 4 out of 19 patients recurred locally, with a mean recurrence time of 6.3 years. These patients had all had positive margins. When there was an underlying carcinoma, prognosis was poor, with metastases frequent and early (7 out of 11 patients died from the disease) (13). Extensive lymph node metastases have occurred even with a minimally invasive occurrence of the disease (14).

Paget's disease of the vulva has also been associated with an increased risk of nonvulvar cancers, including carcinomas of breast, rectum, bladder, urethra, cervix, and basal cell carcinoma. This association has been reported as ranging from 14–54%, with 26% in Feuer's series (11). Twenty-one percent of Feuer's cases also had an invasive, underlying primary vulvar adenocarcinoma. Adenocarcinoma may arise directly from dermal appendages, from the Bartholin's glands, or from breast-like tissue in the vulva, or it may be invasive Paget's disease itself. As Paget cells often involve adnexal structures, at least a O.5cm depth of excisions is recommended (11).

The origin of Paget's disease is uncertain. Intraepithelial precursor cells have been postulated as the cells of origin, as have accessory mammary glands, or mammary-like glands of the vulva (15).

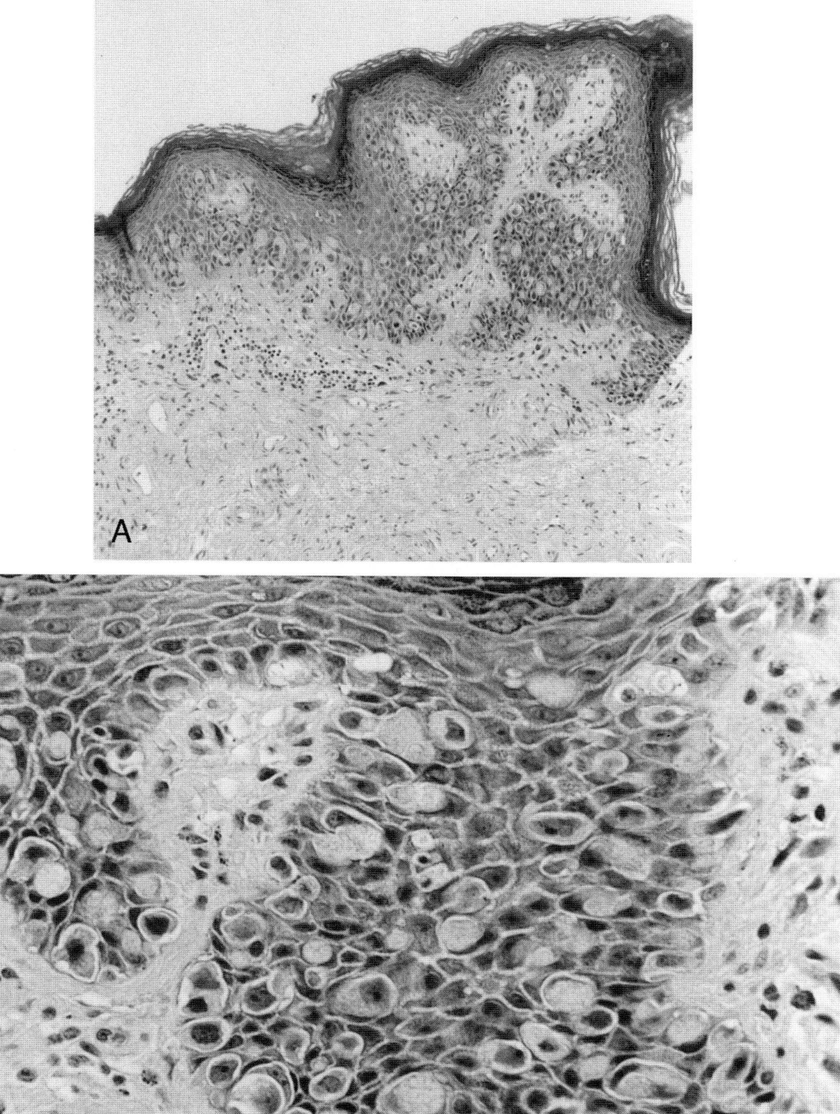

FIGURE 5.10.   Paget's disease. **A.** The neoplastic cells are seen predominantly at the dermal-epidermal junction. The cells also percolate up the epithelium ("Pagetoid spread") and sometimes surround dermal appendages. **B.** Paget cells are large with abundant eosinophilic PAS-positive cytoplasm. *(figure continues)*

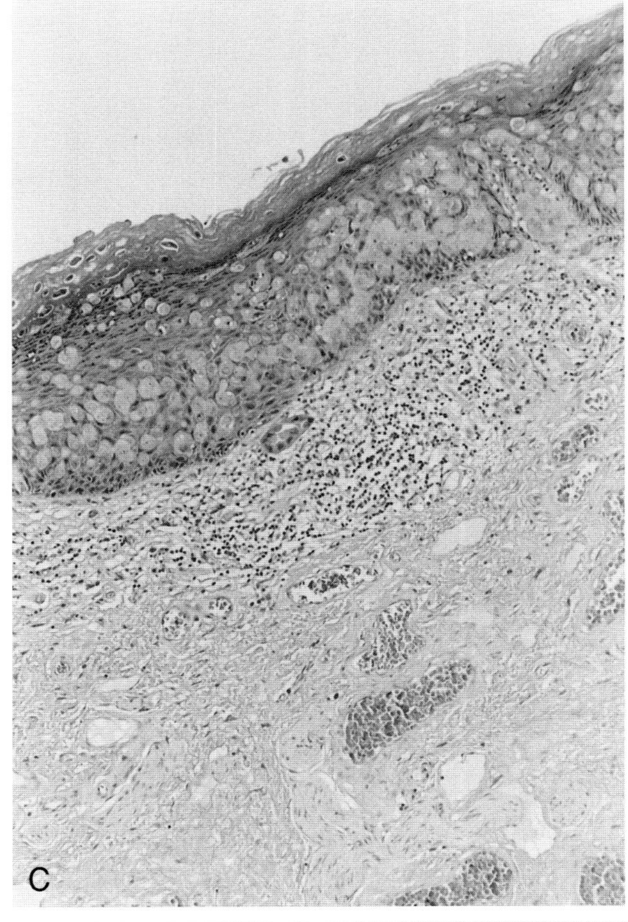

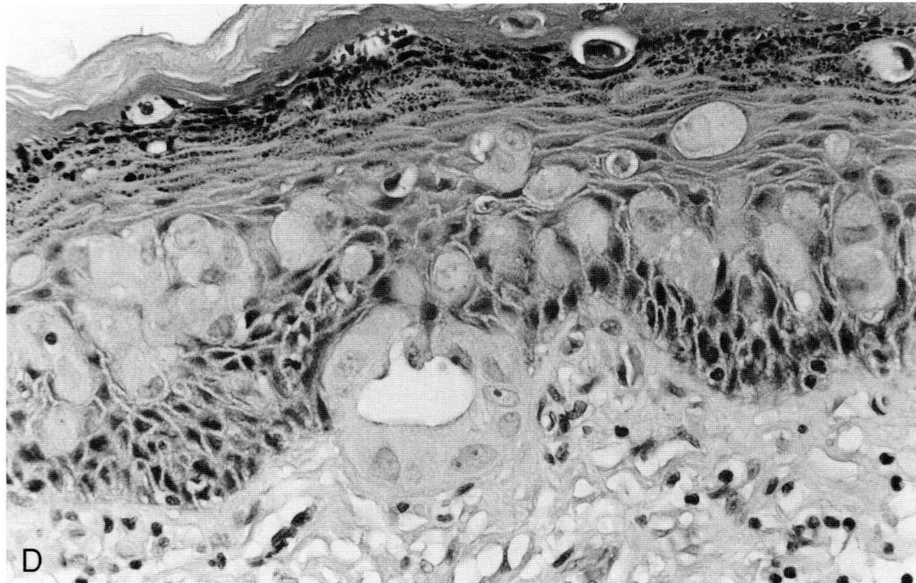

FIGURE 5.10. (*continued*) **C,D.** Paget's disease with focal invasion.

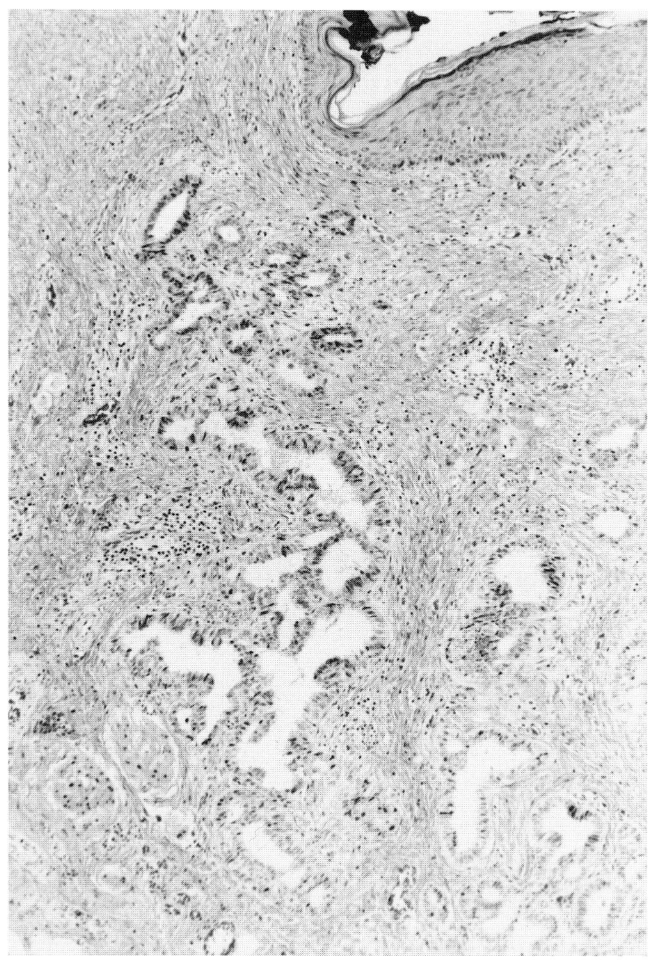

FIGURE 5.11. Invasive adenocarcinoma associated with Paget's disease (not shown). Most vulvar adenocarcinomas not associated with the Bartholin's gland are adenocarcinomas of dermal appendages arising in the presence of Paget's disease.

INVASIVE NEOPLASMS OF THE VULVA

INVASIVE EPITHELIAL NEOPLASMS OF THE VULVA

Invasive malignancies of the vulva are listed in Table 5.1. Ninety percent of invasive vulvar malignancies are squamous cell carcinomas (16). Risk factors for invasive squamous cell carcinoma of the vulva include a history of VIN, cigarette smoking, immunosuppression, and a history of granulomatous inflammation of the vulva, particularly granuloma inguinale. Some of these lesions have been associated with hypercalcemia (17).

SQUAMOUS CELL CARCINOMA

Superficially Invasive Squamous Cell Carcinoma

The concept of early invasive squamous cell carcinoma of the vulva (microinvasive, superficially invasive, stage IA) has been an evolving one, with emphasis on attempting to identify that subset of patients without risk of nodal involvement, as node involve-

TABLE 5.1. Malignant Tumors of the Vulva

Squamous cell carcinoma and variants
  Squamous cell carcinoma
  Basaloid carcinoma
  Warty carcinoma
  Verrucous carcinoma
  Lymphoepithelioma-like carcinoma
  Acantholytic (adenoid squamous) carcinoma
  Spindle cell carcinoma
  Giant cell carcinoma
Adenocarcinoma
  Paget's disease
  Adenocarcinoma of dermal appendages (sweat/sebaceous gland carcinoma)
  Adenocarcinoma of Bartholin's gland
  Adenocarcinoma in mammary-like tissue
Transitional cell carcinoma of urethra/Bartholin's gland
Small cell and other neuroendocrine carcinomas, including PNET and Merkel cell
  tumor
Malignant melanoma
Mesenchymal tumors
  Leiomyosarcoma
  Rhabdomyosarcoma
  Fibrosarcoma
  Malignant fibrous histiocytoma
  Angiosarcoma
  Epithelioid sarcoma
  Kaposi's sarcoma
  Malignant rhabdoid tumor
  Liposarcoma
  Malignant schwannoma
  Lymphangiosarcoma
  Hemangiopericytoma
Lymphoma
Endodermal sinus tumor
Histiocytosis X
Metastatic lesions

ment is the main prognosticator (18). Currently, minimally invasive squamous cell carcinomas are defined as well-differentiated lesions less than 2 cm in diameter, with less than or equal to 1-mm invasion and no nodal metastasis. Of 163 patients with superficial squamous cell carcinoma in one series (19), none had lymph node metastases. However, one patient who presented with an ipsilateral node recurrence has been described as initially having a 0.5 mm invasion treated with radical wide local excision (20).

Invasive Squamous Cell Carcinoma

Squamous cell carcinoma of the vulva had traditionally been viewed as a disease of elderly Caucasian women. It is now thought that there are two pathophysiologic mechanisms involved in the disease (3, 21). Elderly women more often get non-HPV-related well-differentiated neoplasms (Fig. 5.12). A younger group of women under 60 years of age is now presenting with HPV-related lesions that often have a basaloid or warty histology (Figs. 5.13 and 5.14) (see the following section). Therapy is currently individualized as the goal is to do the least radical surgery possible (9). There is significant

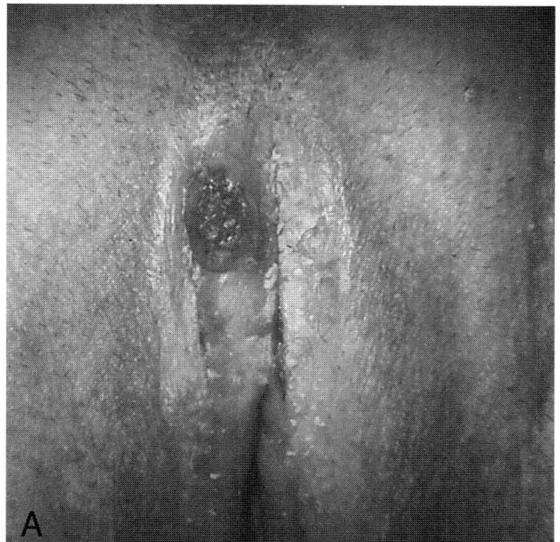

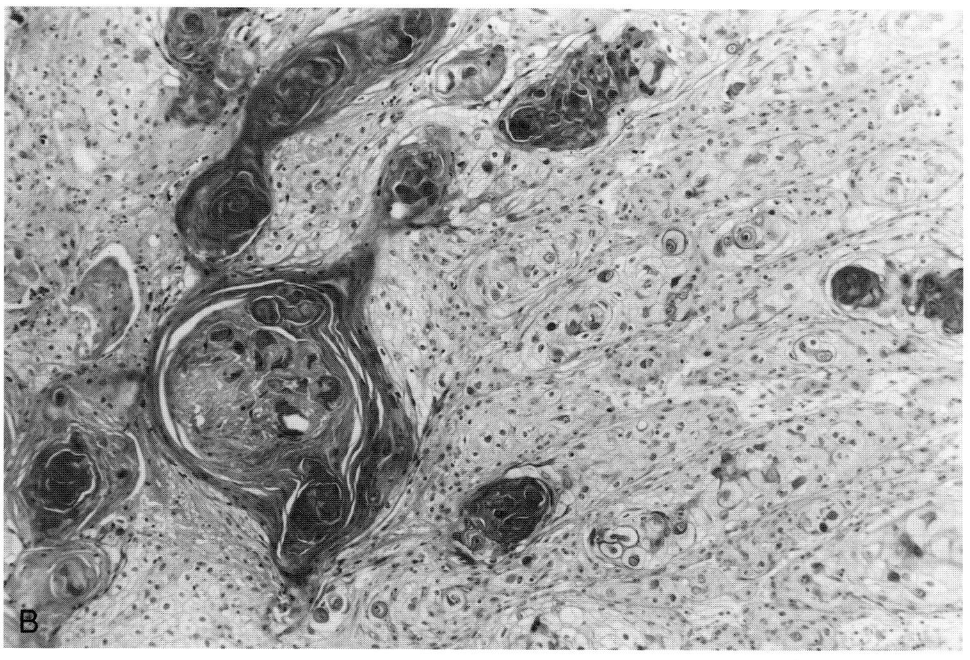

FIGURE 5.12. Well-differentiated invasive squamous cell carcinoma of the vulva. **A.** Well-differentiated squamous cell carcinoma arising in an elderly patient who also has lichen sclerosis. Reprinted with permission from Chapman & Hall, New York. **B.** Well-differentiated keratinizing squamous cell carcinoma.

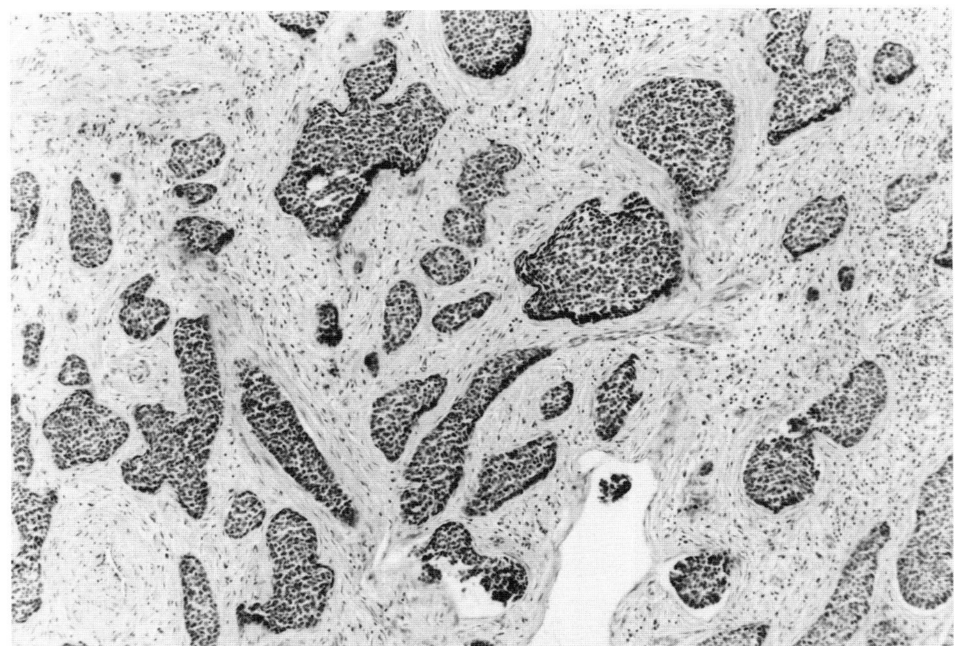

FIGURE 5.13. Basaloid carcinoma of the vulva. The cells of this invasive lesion resemble those of basaloid VIN.

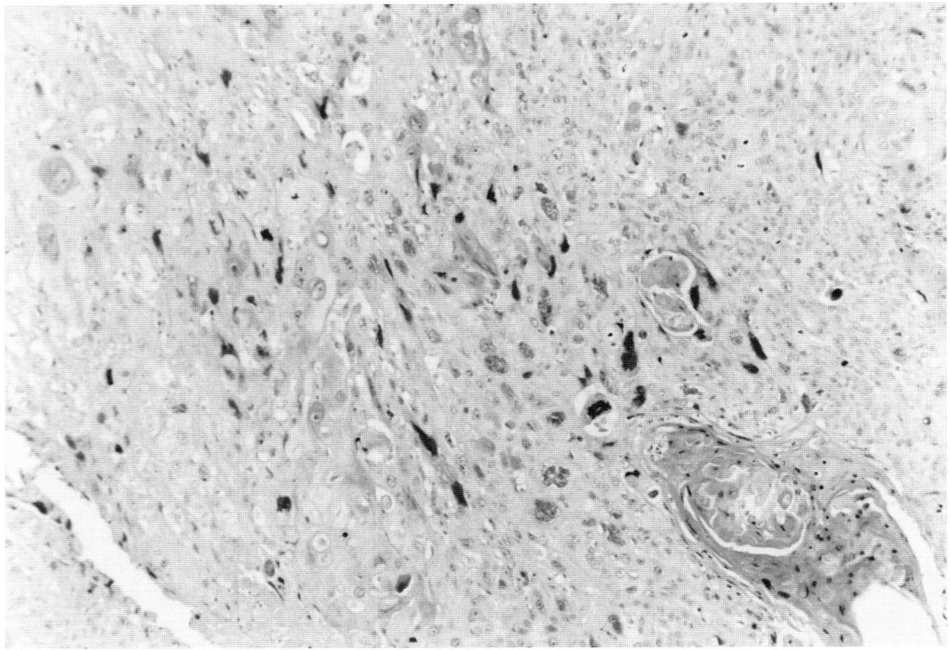

FIGURE 5.14. Warty carcinoma of the vulva. The histology is similar to well-differentiated squamous cell carcinoma, with the additional finding of koilocytotic atypia.

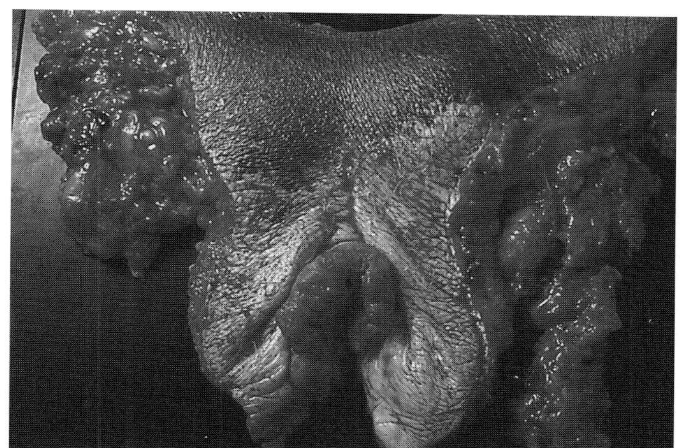

FIGURE 5.15. Resection, squamous cell carcinoma of the vulva. This "butterfly" excision, which includes inguinal lymph nodes, has been associated with significant postoperative morbidity. More recently, making separate incisions has decreased postoperative problems. Note the carcinoma arising in the clitoral region.

morbidity (wound breakdown, lymphedema) to the older "butterfly" incision that includes an en bloc radical vulvectomy and inguinal lymphadenectomy (Fig. 5.15). More recently, triple incisions with skin bridges have been performed, as have even less extensive surgical procedures in selected cases. In 1988, the International Federation of Gynecology and Obstetrics (FIGO) adopted a staging system for vulvar cancer (modified in 1995) that uses surgical rather than clinical lymph node evaluation (Table 5.2). More accurate prediction of outcome has been obtained with surgical versus clinical lymph node evaluation (22). Spread of vulvar squamous cell carcinoma is by direct extension and involvement of regional lymph nodes. Positivity of lymph nodes is related to depth of invasion, tumor grade, presence of lymphvascular space involvement, clinical node status, and patient age (23). Depth of invasion is measured from the nearest dermal papillae to the deepest point of invasion. Some authors (5) also recommend reporting tumor thickness. Thickness is measured from the bottom of the granular layer (or from the surface in nonkeratinized epithelium) to the deepest point of invasion (Fig. 5.16). Tumor grading tends to be subjective. Well-differentiated squamous cell carcinomas show keratinization and/or well-developed intercellular bridges. Poorly differentiated squamous cell carcinomas are barely recognizable as squamous lesions, and they are composed of sheets and nests of undifferentiated cells. Moderately differentiated tumors fall in the middle. The pathologist should include mention of all relevant variables in the report (Table 5.3).

Basaloid and Warty Carcinoma

Recently, Kurman and colleagues (3) have described particular histologic features seen in squamous cell carcinomas of the vulva associated with younger age, which they have termed basaloid and warty carcinomas. An increased prevalence of HPV in basaloid and warty carcinomas exists as compared with conventional keratinizing squamous cell carcinoma. Basaloid carcinoma is composed of smaller less-mature-appearing cells, resembling the cells of a VIN III lesion (Fig. 5.13). Warty carcinomas are similar to conventional squamous cell carcinomas but have changes resembling koilocytotic atypia (Fig. 5.14). Eighty-three percent of keratinizing squamous cell carcinomas had adjacent squamous hyperplasia in Kurman and colleagues' series (3), while 77% of basaloid and warty tumors had adjacent basaloid or warty VIN. A greater number of patients with the

---

TABLE 5.2. Staging of Vulvar Carcinoma (FIGO)

Stage 0
  Tis intraepithelial carcinoma
Stage I
  T1N0M0 confined to vulva/perineum, ≤2 cm in size, negative nodes
    Stage IA confined to vulva/perineum; ≤2 cm in size, negative nodes; stromal
      invasion ≤1 mm
    Stage IB confined to vulva/perineum; ≤2 cm in size, negative nodes; stromal
      invasion >1 mm
Stage II
  T2N0M0 confined to vulva/perineum; >2 cm, negative nodes
Stage III
  TNM includes the following:
    T3N0M0   Tumor of any size with adjacent spread
    T3NIM0   to lower urethra and/or vagina and/or
    T1N1M0   anus (T3), and/or unilateral regional lymph
    T2N1M0   node metastasis (N1)
Stage IVa
  TMN includes the following:
    T1N2M0   Tumor invades upper urethra and/or bladder
    T2N2M0   mucosa and/or rectal mucosa, and or pelvic
    T3N2M0   bone (T4), and/or bilateral regional lymph node
    T4anyNM0   metastases (N2)
Stage IVb
  any T distal metastases (includes pelvic nodes)
  any NM1

TNM classification:
T = Primary tumor; T1-confined to vulva/perineum, ≤2 cm; T2-confined to vulva/perineum, >2 cm; T3-
Any size, adjacent spread to lower urethra, vagina, or anus; T4-Any size, spread to upper urethra, bladder
or rectal mucosa or pelvic bone; N = regional lymph nodes; N0-no metastases (surgical); N1-unilateral
inguinal nodes; N2-bilateral inguinal nodes; M = distal metastases; M0-no metastases; M1a-pelvic lymph
node involvement; M1b-other distal metastases.
Modified from Anonymous. Modifications in the staging of Stage I vulvar and Stage I cervical cancer:
Report of the FIGO Committee on Gynecologic Oncology. Int J Gynaecol Obstet 1995;50:215–216.

TABLE 5.3. Elements to Include in the Pathology Report of a Vulvar Carcinoma

---

Diameter of tumor
Depth of invasion
Tumor thickness
Presence of any lymphvascular space involvement
Confluence
Tumor grade
Node status, including number of positive nodes (if nodes submitted)

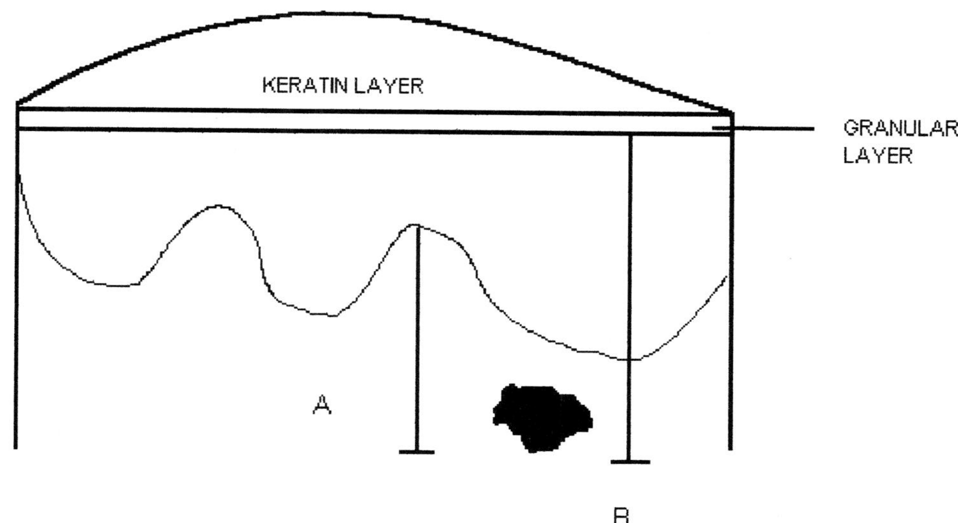

FIGURE 5.16.   Measuring depth of invasion and tumor thickness. Depth of invasion is measured from the nearest dermal papilla to the deepest point of the tumor **(A)**. Tumor thickness, used in malignant melanoma, as well as by some for squamous cell carcinoma, is measured from the bottom of the granular layer, or epithelial surface if not keratinized, to the deepest portion of the tumor **(B)**.

basaloid or warty type of carcinoma had an in-situ or invasive tumor of the cervix or vagina as well.

The differential diagnosis of a basaloid carcinoma includes basal cell carcinoma, Merkel cell tumor, or metastatic small cell carcinoma. Basal cell carcinoma can be distinguished by peripheral palisading of the cells in the tumor nests. Merkel cell tumors are rare in the vulva and are distinguished by characteristic perinuclear cytoplasmic dot-like staining with antibodies to keratin. Merkel and small cell tumors stain with neuroendocrine markers. Warty carcinoma may be confused with verrucous carcinoma; however, well-developed fibrovascular cores are seen in warty carcinoma, as opposed to verrucous carcinoma. In addition, warty carcinomas infiltrate in nests, but verrucous carcinomas have "pushing" margins (5).

Recurrence rates for squamous cell carcinoma of the vulva vary, and these have been reported to be as high as 20–30% (24). Long-term follow-up is required. While most recurrences appear within two years, a significant number occur later (25). There does not appear to be a difference in prognosis as assessed by recurrence after primary therapy between HPV-related and HPV-unrelated neoplasms (25).

Verrucous Carcinoma

Verrucous carcinoma of the vulva is a rare variant of invasive squamous cell carcinoma. Grossly, the lesion is warty and fungating in most cases (Fig. 5.17) although occasionally it is ulcerative. It presents with pruritus and/or a mass. Infection with its accompanying induration and reactive lymph nodes may clinically mimic more advanced disease (26). Histologically, verrucous carcinoma resembles a large condyloma, with minimal atypia and scant mitotic activity (Fig. 5.18); however, fibrovascular cores are not a prominent feature of verrucous carcinoma.

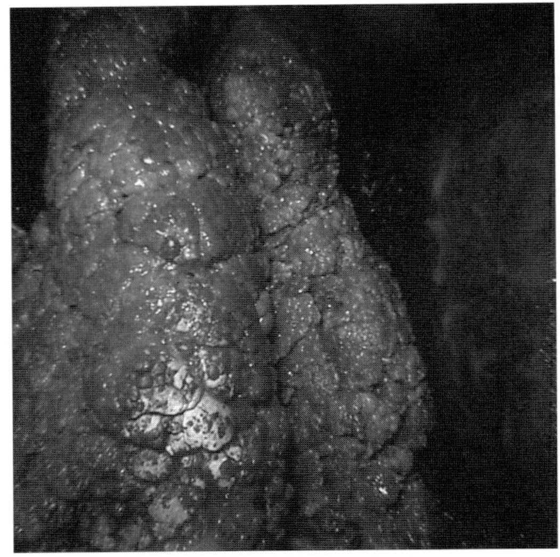

FIGURE 5.17. Verrucous carcinoma of the vulva. Verrucous carcinoma usually grows in an exophytic warty pattern. Reprinted with permission from Chapman & Hall, New York.

The lesion is characterized by a "pushing" deep border rather than by invasive nests of tumor. Brisigotti and colleagues (27) studied verrucous and squamous cell carcinomas with immunohistochemical stains. They found that AE1 and AE3 stained both types of tumors, but that the staining of the verrucous tumors was uniform whereas in the squamous cell carcinomas, staining was patchy and disorganized. They interpreted this finding as supporting the fact that verrucous carcinomas are well differentiated while squamous cell carcinomas are heterogeneous in terms of differentiation. Therapy for verrucous carcinoma is wide local excision. Verrucous carcinomas tend to recur locally, and they have been associated with HPV 6 (5).

Spindle Cell Carcinoma

Poorly differentiated squamous cell carcinomas may have a spindle cell appearance, mimicking a sarcoma (Fig. 5.19). Immunohistochemistry is helpful in the distinction since these tumors stain for keratin (28).

Acantholytic (Adenoid Squamous) Carcinoma

Pseudoglandular spaces may be seen due to acantholysis in some squamous cell carcinomas. This may be a focal change and is of no prognostic significance (17).

Lymphoepithelioma-like Carcinoma

Similar to the uncommon cervical lesion, a lymphoepithelioma-like pattern, with a dense lymphoid infiltrate between epithelial nests of tumor, may rarely occur.

Giant Cell Carcinoma

An aggressive variant of squamous cell carcinoma, this pattern contains bizarre eosinophilic giant cells, which may be multinucleated. The large nuclei may contain prominent nucleoli (17)(Fig. 5.20).

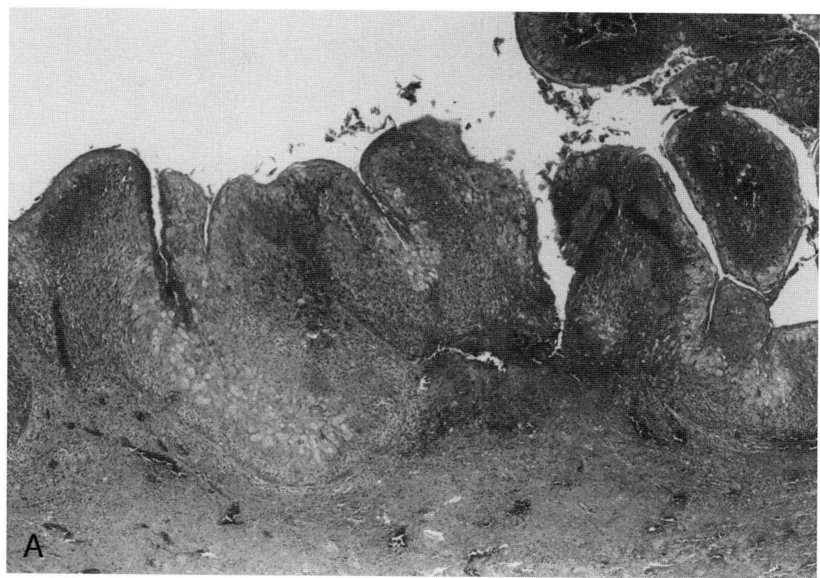

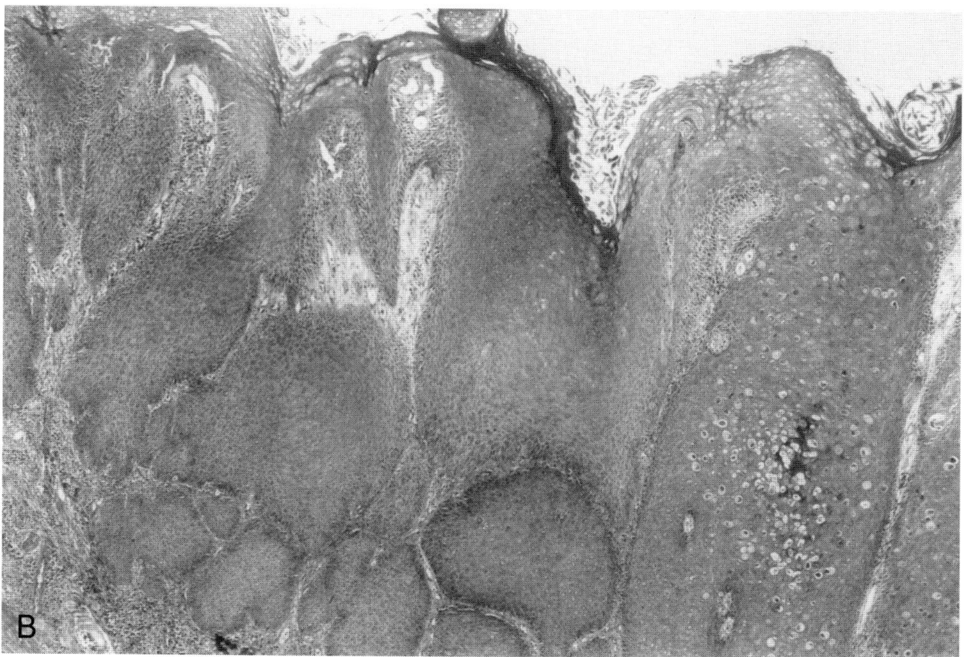

FIGURE 5.18. Verrucous carcinoma of the vulva. **A.** Verrucous carcinoma invades with a "pushing" rather than infiltrating front. **B.** Lesions are well differentiated and histologically resemble giant condylomata.

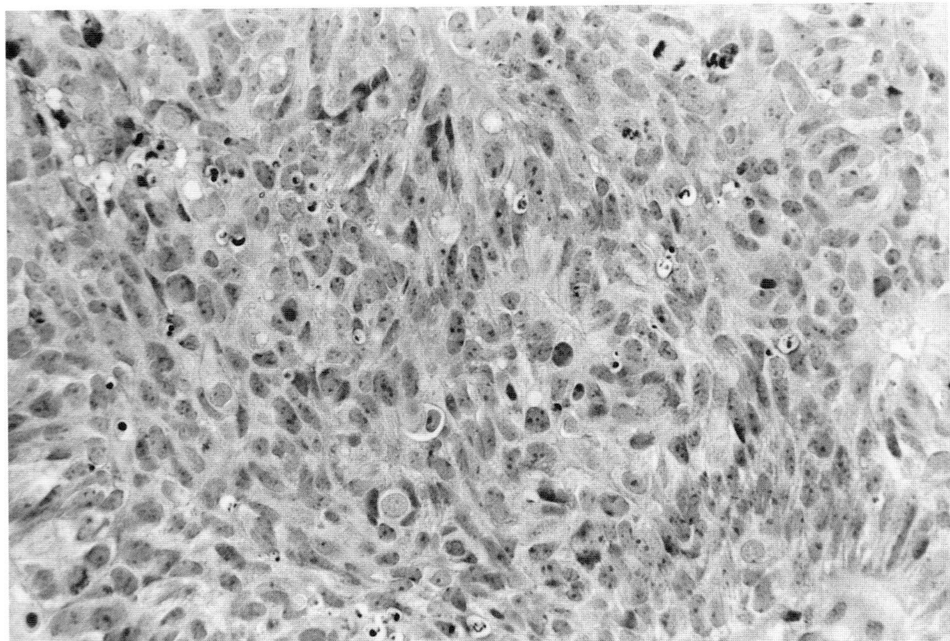

FIGURE 5.19. Spindle cell variant of squamous cell carcinoma of the vulva. Squamous cell carcinoma may have a spindle cell pattern and be confused with a sarcoma. Immunohistochemical stain for keratin can help make the distinction.

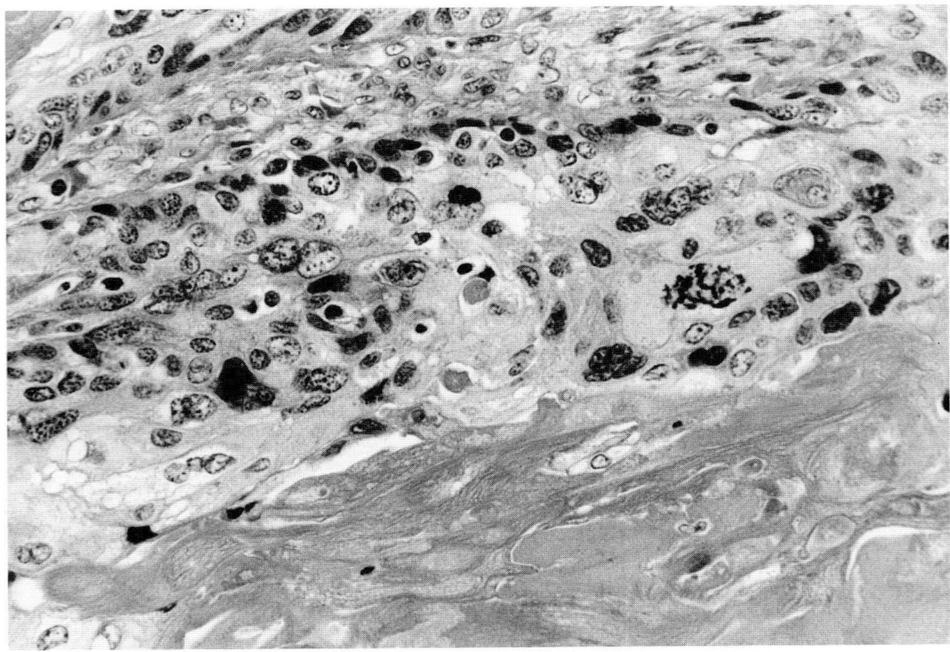

FIGURE 5.20. Giant cell variant of squamous cell carcinoma of the vulva. An aggressive variant characterized by bizarre giant cells, multinucleation, marked atypia, and atypical mitoses.

ADENOCARCINOMA OF THE VULVA

There are four types of invasive adenocarcinoma of the vulva: Bartholin's adenocarcinomas, invasive Paget's disease, sweat gland adenocarcinomas, and adenocarcinomas arising in accessory breast tissue.

Invasive Paget's Disease

Intraepithelial Paget's disease itself may progress to invasion (Fig. 5.10C,D) without an underlying apocrine carcinoma. Prognosis is poor in these cases (14).

Bartholin's Gland Carcinoma

These tumors are uncommon. They present as a persistent mass in the area of the Bartholin's gland, and this finding, particularly in women over 40 years old, requires investigation. Criteria for making the diagnosis of a Bartholin's carcinoma (29) include the following: a transition from normal to neoplastic areas histologically, a tumor in the area of the Bartholin's gland, a tumor with a compatible histology, and no evidence of a primary tumor elsewhere. Felix and colleagues (30) include in their criteria that the tumor arises deep to vulvar skin, with overlying normal vulvar skin, and that the tumor is a distinct nodule. Histologic patterns include squamous cell carcinoma, adenocarcinoma (Fig. 5.21), adenosquamous carcinoma, adenoid cystic carcinoma, transitional cell carcinoma, and undifferentiated carcinoma. In the series of cases evaluated by Felix and colleagues, HPV 16 was detected in 6 out of 7 squamous cell carcinomas, but 0/2 adenoid cystic and 0/1 adenocarcinoma. Therapy for carcinoma of the Barthol-

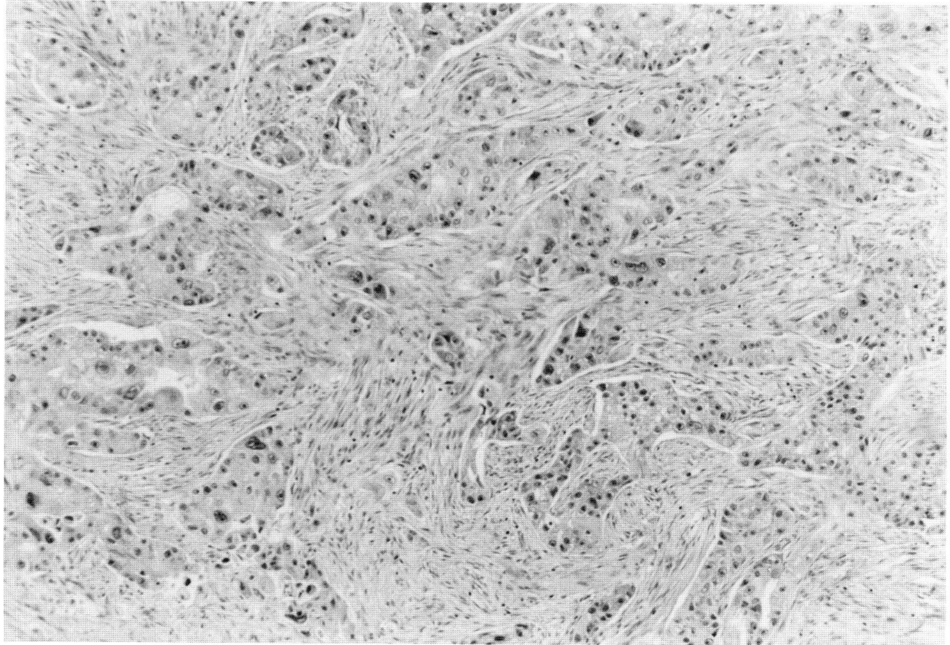

FIGURE 5.21.   Adenocarcinoma of Bartholin's gland. This tumor arose in the area of the Bartholin's gland, and no other primary neoplasm was identified.

in's gland is surgical, with radiation therapy used as adjunctive treatment at times. These tumors tend to behave aggressively.

Sweat Gland Carcinoma

Most adenocarcinomas of dermal appendages arise in association with Paget's disease (Fig. 5.11). Sweat gland carcinomas not associated with Paget's disease are rare (6). A variety of apocrine and eccrine adenocarcinomas have been described (31).

Adenocarcinoma Arising in Breast-like Tissue

Adenocarcinomas histologically similar to breast carcinomas have occurred in the vulva, and have been attributed to the presence of ectopic breast tissue or breast-like tissue in the vulva (15).

BASAL CELL CARCINOMA

Basal cell carcinomas represent 2–3% of vulvar malignancies. Lesions may be single (Fig. 5.22) or multifocal. Most occur on the inner labia in Caucasian women over 50 years of age. Histologically, the tumor is composed of basaloid cells with characteristic peripheral palisading of the cells (Fig. 5.23). Therapy is by wide local excision (32). Although generally regarded as locally aggressive tumors at worst, basal cell carcinomas of the vulva occasionally metastasize (33).

MALIGNANT MELANOMA

Malignant melanomas represent 5–10% of vulvar malignancies and usually occur in elderly Caucasian women. Unlike cutaneous melanomas, sun exposure is not a factor, and the etiology is unknown (34). Lesions present with pruritus, bleeding, and/or a mass. Histologic features are identical to cutaneous melanomas (Fig. 5.24). Lesions may

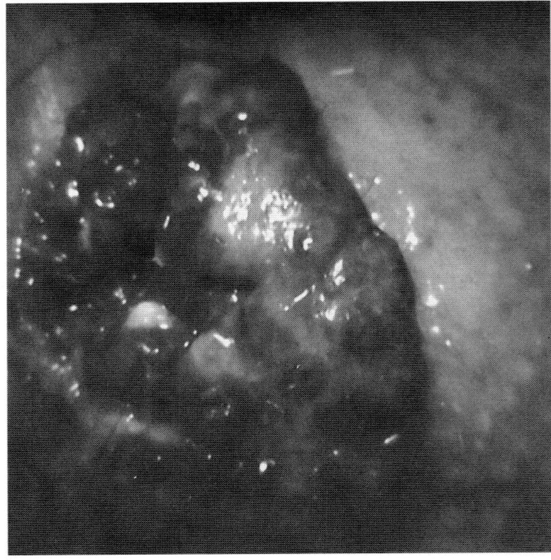

FIGURE 5.22. Basal cell carcinoma of the vulva. Reprinted with permission from Chapman & Hall, New York.

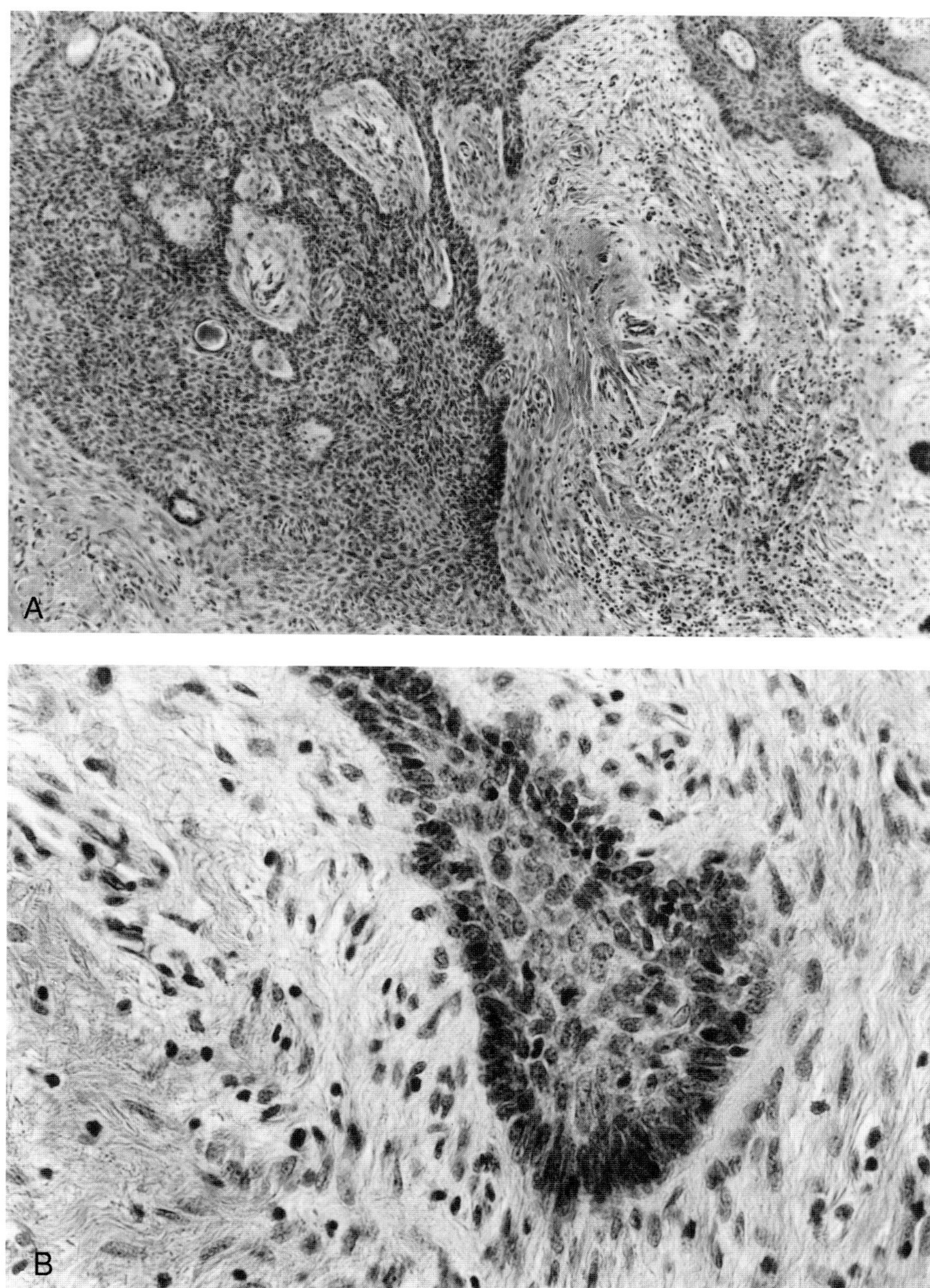

FIGURE 5.23. **A,B.** Basal cell carcinoma. Cells resembling the basal cells of the epithelium comprise this tumor. The lesion is characterized by palisading of the peripheral cells in tumor nests.

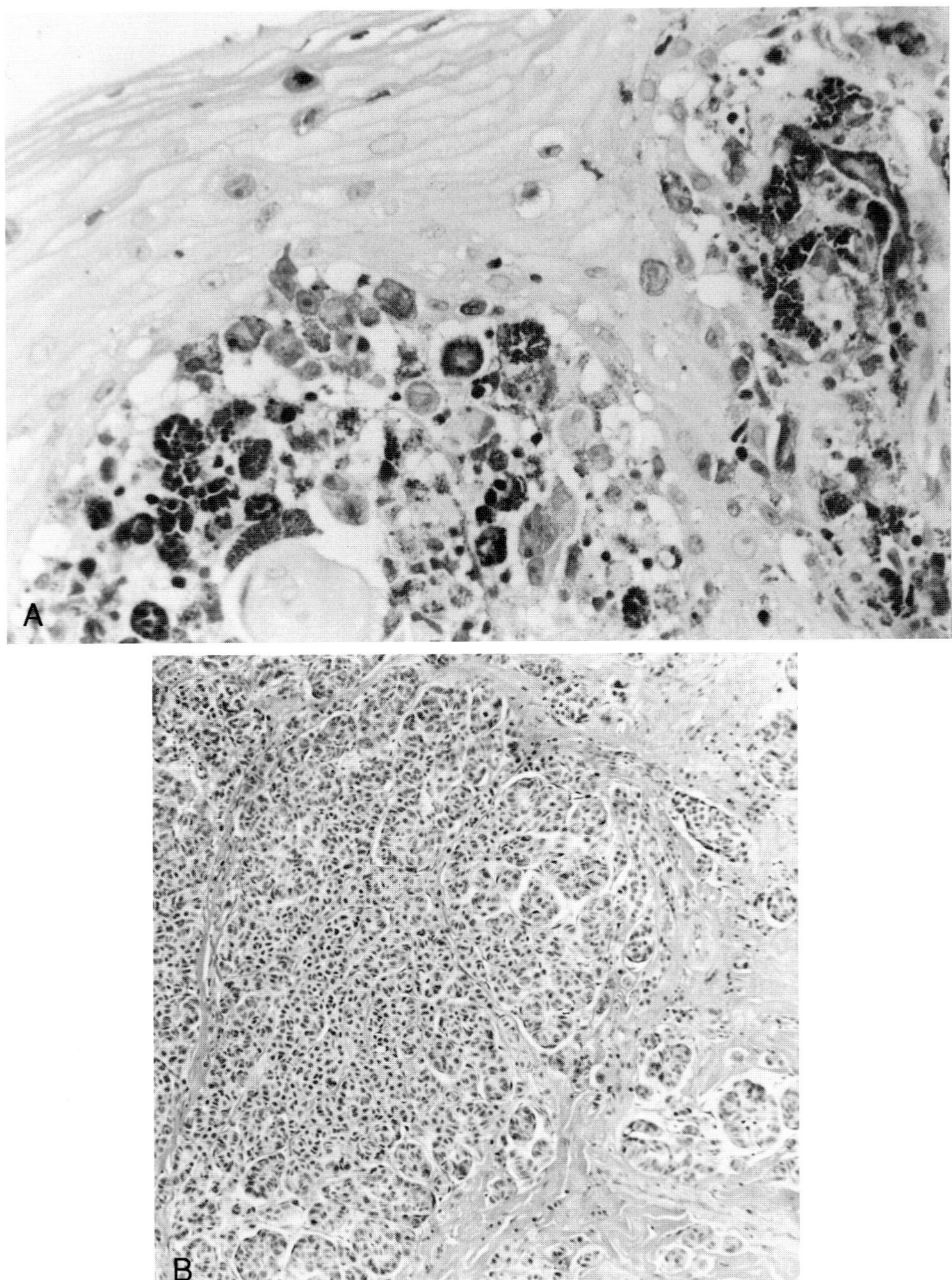

FIGURE 5.24. Malignant melanoma of the vulva. **A.** Lesions may be markedly pigmented. **B.** Malignant melanoma infiltrating in nests. The tumor was positive for HMB45 and S100 protein.

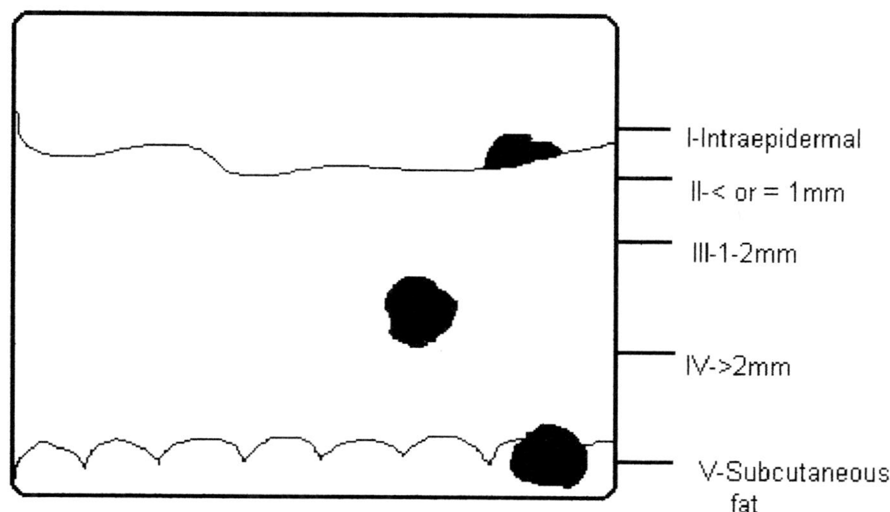

FIGURE 5.25.   Chung level measurements for melanoma of the vulva and vagina (35).

be amelanotic. Vulvar melanomas usually are diagnosed in an advanced stage, which accounts for their poor prognosis. The FIGO staging for vulvar carcinoma is not applicable to melanoma. Currently, two measurements are used in evaluating vulvar and vaginal melanoma. Chung levels (35) are a modification of the Clark level system, taking into account the difficulties in identifying a papillary and reticular dermis in the vulvovaginal area. The Chung classification is shown in Figure 5.25. The other significant information that should be reported is the thickness, as suggested by Breslow (36) (Fig. 5.16), which is measured from the bottom of the granular cell layer (or surface in nonkeratizing epithelium) to the deepest point of invasion of the tumor. For melanomas less than 0.75 mm in thickness, there is an essentially 100% 5-year survival although this drops to 48% at 10 years (37). With deeper lesions, the survival rate plummets. Initially, melanomas of the vulva were treated with radical surgery, but in view of the poor prognosis, which is not significantly improved by this type of surgery, less aggressive approaches have been used more recently.

MESENCHYMAL MALIGNANCIES OF THE VULVA
LEIOMYOSARCOMA

Sarcomas of the vulva represent about 2% of vulvar malignancies (38). The vast majority are leiomyosarcomas (39) (Fig. 5.26), with most other sarcomas appearing in the literature as case reports. Leiomyosarcomas of the vulva are rapidly growing tumors. Histologically, they are similar to leiomyosarcomas of the uterus, with mitotic activity, variable atypia, and infiltrating borders. Epithelioid patterns have also occurred. The distinction between leiomyoma and leiomyosarcoma is difficult to determine in the vulva. Lesions larger than 5 cm, with over 10 mitoses per 10 high-power fields, nuclear abnormalities,

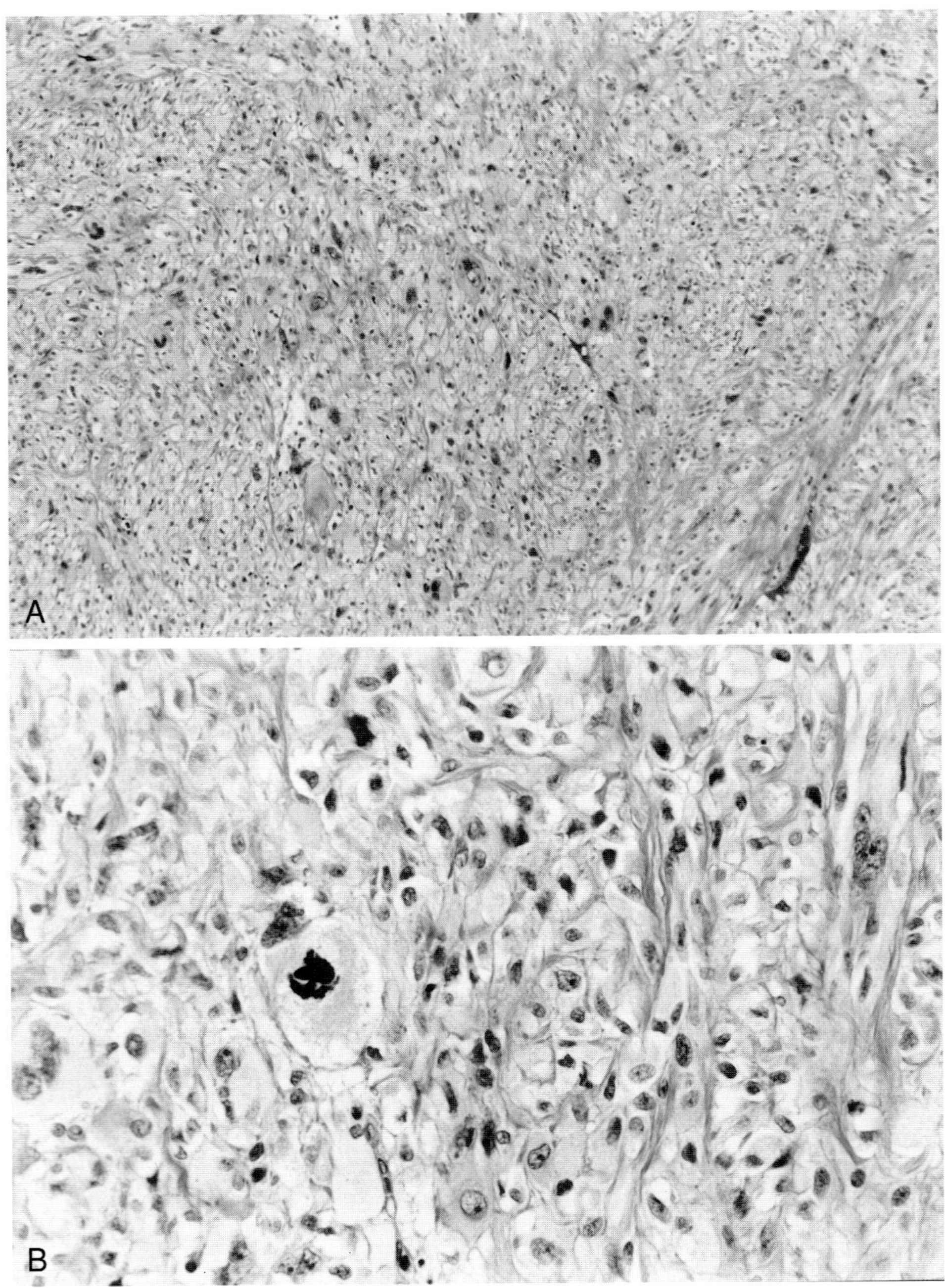

FIGURE 5.26. Leiomyosarcoma of the vulva. **A.** The lesion shows marked atypia. **B.** Areas of the tumor are epithelioid. An atypical mitosis is seen.

and infiltrative borders behave aggressively. However, lesions with between 6–10 mitoses per 10 high-power fields but with other histologically negative prognostic features have also metastasized (5). In a recent study, Nielsen and colleagues (40) proposed that the following prognostic criteria be used in evaluating vulvar smooth muscle neoplasms: size greater than 5 cm, infiltrating margins, 5 or more mitoses per 10 high-power fields, and moderate to severe cytologic atypia. If three or more of the criteria were present, they diagnosed the tumors as leiomyosarcomas. If two criteria were present, they diagnosed atypical leiomyoma, and if one risk factor was present, leiomyoma. Resection with wide margins has been used as primary therapy (40). Vulvar leiomyosarcoma is characterized by a protracted course of local recurrences terminating in fatal distal metastases.

RHABDOMYOSARCOMA

Rhabdomyosarcomas occur rarely on the vulva. Histologically, embryonal rhabdomyosarcoma is characterized by a poorly differentiated spindle cell neoplasm with interspersed primitive rhabdomyoblasts (Fig. 5.27). The polypoid variant, sarcoma botryoides, occurs rarely on the vulva in infants, and it is most often seen arising from the vagina (see Chapter 7).

AGGRESSIVE ANGIOMYXOMA

Aggressive angiomyxoma has been discussed in the previous Chapter 4.

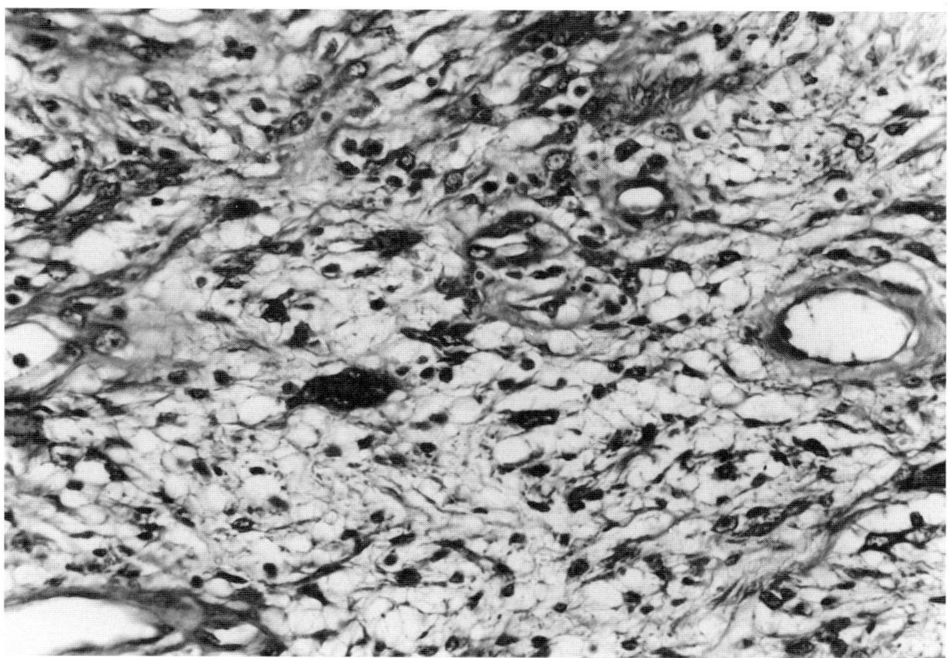

FIGURE 5.27.   Rhabdomyosarcoma of the vulva. A primitive rhabdomyoblast is present. Tumors will often stain for skeletal muscle markers.

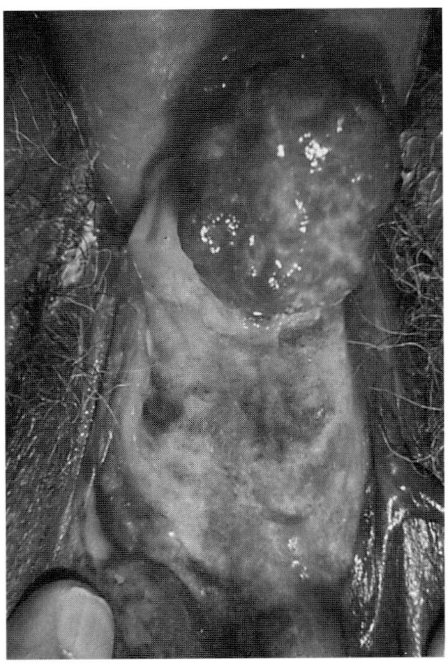

FIGURE 5.28. Urethral carcinoma. Reprinted with permission from Chapman & Hall, New York.

OTHER MALIGNANCIES OF THE VULVA
ENDODERMAL SINUS TUMOR

Endodermal sinus tumor occurs rarely on the vulva. Like the ovarian lesion, the tumor is recognizable by the Schiller-Duval bodies present and may contain PAS-positive alpha-fetoprotein-containing globules (41). Prognosis for vulvar endodermal sinus tumor is poor.

METASTATIC LESIONS

Most commonly, metastatic lesions to the vulva arise from the genital tract and spread from cervical, endometrial, and ovarian primaries. In addition, metastases from a number of remote primary sites have also occurred. A good clinical history and review of any available previous pathology slides are helpful in these cases.

URETHRAL CARCINOMA

Carcinomas arising from the urethra (Fig. 5.28) may be squamous, transitional, adenocarcinoma, or undifferentiated (42).

REFERENCES

1. Wilkinson EJ, Kneale B, Lynch PJ. Report of the ISSVD terminology committee. J Reprod Med 1986;31:973–977.
2. Buscema J, Naghashfar Z, Sawada E, et al. The predominance of human *Papillomavirus* type 16 in vulvar neoplasia. Obstet Gynecol 1988;71:601–606.

3. Kurman RJ, Toki T, Schiffman MH. Basaloid and warty carcinomas of the vulva. Distinctive types of squamous cell carcinoma frequently associated with human *Papillomaviruses.* Am J Surg Pathol 1993;17:133–134.

4. Prat J. Pathology of vulvar intraepithelial lesions and invasive carcinoma [review]. Hum Pathol 1991;22:877–883.

5. Kurman RJ, Norris HJ, Wilkinson E. Tumors of the cervix, vagina and vulva. AFIP atlas of tumor pathology, third series, fascicle 4. AFIP Washington, DC, 1992, pg 189.

6. Mulling DL, Wilkinson EJ. Pathology of the vulva and vagina [review]. Curr Opin Obstet Gynecol 1994;6:351–358.

7. Barbero M, Michelletti L, Preti M, et al. Biologic behavior of vulvar intraepithelial neoplasia. Histologic and clinical parameters. J Reprod Med 1993;38:108–112.

8. Homesley MD. Management of vulvar cancer. Cancer 1995;76:2159–2170.

9. Jones RW, Rowan DM. Vulvar intraepithelial neoplasia III: a clinical study of the outcome in 113 cases with relation to the later development of invasive vulvar carcinoma. Obstet Gynecol 1994;84:741– 745.

10. McLachlin CM, Mutter GL, Crum CP. Multinucleated atypia of the vulva-report of a distinct entity not associated with human *Papillomavirus.* Am J Surg Pathol 1994;18: 1233–1239.

11. Feuer GA, Shevchuk M, Calanog A. Vulvar Paget disease: the need to exclude an invasive lesion. Gynecol Oncol 1990;38:81–89.

12. Bacchi CE, Goldfogel GA, Greer BE, et al. Paget's disease and melanoma of the vulva. Use of a panel of monoclonal antibodies to identify cell type and to microscopically define adequacy of surgical margins. Gynecol Oncol 1992;46:216–221.

13. Kodama S, Kaneko T, Saito M, et al. A clinicopathologic study of 30 patients with Paget disease of the vulva. Gynecol Oncol 1995;56:63–70.

14. Fine BA, Fowler LJ, Valente PT. Minimally invasive Paget disease of the vulva with extensive lymph node metastases. Gynecol Oncol 1995;57:262– 265.

15. Van der Putte SC, Van Gorp LH. Adenocarcinoma of mammary-like glands of the vulva: a concept unifying sweat gland carcinoma of the vulva, carcinoma of supernumerary mammary glands, and extramammary Paget's disease. J Cutan Pathol 1994;21:157– 163.

16. Ansink AC, Kagie MJ. Benign and malignant pathology of the vulva [review]. Curr Opin Obstet Gynecol 1993;5:474–479.

17. Wilkinson EJ. Premalignant and malignant tumors of the vulva. In: Kurman R, ed. Blaustein's Pathology of the Female Genital Tract. 4th ed. New York: Springer-Verlag, 1994.

18. Garcia Inglesias A, Tejerizo Lopez LC, Garcia Sanchez MH, et al. Prognosis factors in carcinoma of the vulva. Eur J Gynaecol Oncol 1993;14:38–91.

19. Hacker NF, Van der Velden J. Conservative management of early vulvar cancer. Cancer 1993;71(Suppl):1673–1677.

20. Hicks ML, Hempling RE, Piver MS. Vulvar carcinoma with 0.5 mm of invasion and associated inguinal node metastasis. J Surg Oncol 1993;54:271–273.

21. Hording U, Junge J, Daugaard S. Vulvar squamous cell carcinoma and *Papillomaviruses:* indications for two different etiologies. Gyncol Oncol 1994;52:241– 246.

22. Hopkins MP, Reid GC, Johnston CM, et al. A comparison of staging systems for squamous cell carcinoma of the vulva. Gynecol Oncol 1992;47:34–37.

23. Homesley HD, Bundy BN, Sedlis A, et al. Prognostic factors for groin node metastases in squamous cell carcinoma of the vulva (a GOG study). Gynecol Oncol 1993;49:279–283.

24. Podratz KC, Symmonds RE, Taylor WF. Carcinoma of the vulva: analysis of treatment failures. Am J Obstet Gynecol 1982;143:34–51.

25. Tilmans AS, Sutton GP, Look KY, et al. Recurrent squamous cell carcinoma of the vulva. Am J Obstet Gynecol 1992;167:1383–1389.

26. Dvoretsky PM, Bonfiglio TA. The pathology of vulvar squamous cell carcinoma and verrucous carcinoma. Path Annual 1986;21(pt2):23–45.

27. Brisigotti M, Moreno A, Murcia C, et al. Verrucous carcinoma of the vulva. A clinicopathologic and immunohistochemical study of 5 cases. Int J Gynecol Pathol 1989; 8:1–7.

28. Santeusanio G, Schiaroli S, Aneomona L, et al. Carcinoma of the vulva with sarcomatoid features: a case report with immunohistochemical study [review]. Gynecol Oncol 1991;40: 160–163.

29. Chamlian DL, Taylor HG. Primary carcinoma of the Bartholin's gland: a report of 24 patients. Obstet Gynecol 1972;39:489– 494.

30. Felix JC, Cote RJ, Kramer EE, et al. Carcinomas of the Bartholin's gland. Histogenesis and the etiological role of human *Papillomavirus.* Am J Pathol 1993;142:925– 933.

31. Rich PM, Okagaki T, Clark B, et al. Adenocarcinoma of the sweat gland of the vulva: light and electron microscopic study. Cancer 1981;47:1352–1357.

32. Basal cell carcinoma of the vulva-a report of 4 cases. J Reprod Med 1996;41:283– 285.

33. Mizushima J, Ohara K. Basal cell carcinoma of the vulva with lymph node and skin metastasis. Report of a case and review of 20 Japanese cases [review]. J Derm 1995;22: 36–42.

34. Heller DS, Moomjy M, Koulos J et al. Vulvar and vaginal melanoma. A clinicopathologic study. J Reprod Med 1994;39:945–948.

35. Chung AF, Woodruff JM, Lewis JL Jr. Malignant melanoma of the vulva: a report of 44 cases. Obstet Gynecol 1975;45:638–646.

36. Breslow A. Tumor thickness, level of invasion and node dissection in stage I cutaneous melanoma Ann Surg 1975;182:572–575.

37. Trimble EL, Lewis JL, Jr., Williams LL, et al. Management of vulvar melanoma. Gynecol Oncol 1992;45:25–28.

38. Nirenberg A, Ostor AG, Slavin J, et al. Primary vulvar sarcomas. Int J Gynecol Pathol 1995; 14:55–62.

39. Aartsen EJ, Albus-Lutter CE. Vulvar sarcoma: clinical implications [review]. Eur J Obstet Gynecol Reprod Biol 1994;56:181–189.

40. Nielsen G, Rosenberg A, Koerner F, et al. Smooth muscle tumors of the vulva: a clinicopathological study of 25 cases and review of the literature. Am J Surg Pathol 1996; 20:779–793.

41. Penkar SJ, Irani S, Prabhu VL, et al. Endodermal sinus tumor of the vulva [case report]. J Postgrad Med 1992;38:44–45.

42. Mostofi FK, Davis CJ, Jr., Sesterhenn IA. Carcinoma of the male and female urethra [review]. Urol Clin North Am 1992;19:347–358.

6

BENIGN DISEASES OF THE VAGINA

Debra S. Heller, MD

■

Normal Histology
Congenital Anomalies
Infections and Inflammations
Benign Tumors and Tumor-like Conditions
Benign Neoplasms

NORMAL HISTOLOGY

The vagina is lined by nonkeratinizing squamous epithelium. The underlying lamina propria is composed of loose fibroconnective tissue containing abundant nerve and elastic fibers (Fig. 6.1). Some women have a discernible subepithelial zone of loose fibroconnective tissue containing stellate or spindle cells, many multinucleated. It is from this region that fibroepithelial polyps of the vagina may arise (1). The vaginal tube is bounded by a muscularis propria composed of an inner circular and outer longitudinal layer, and a thin fibroconnective tissue adventitia. The vagina normally does not contain glands. Occasionally, women have melanocytes in the basal layer of the epithelium, which explains the rare occurrence of melanocytic lesions in this area (Fig. 6.2).

CONGENITAL ANOMALIES

Congenital anomalies of the vagina are uncommon. Many arise due to abnormalities in the fusion of the paired mullerian ducts, or failure of resorption of the septum after fusion of the mullerian ducts, or failure of the fused paired mullerian ducts to meet the urogenital sinus.

ADENOSIS

In addition to structural changes of the uterus, cervix, and vagina, intrauterine exposure to diethystilbestrol (DES) is associated with adenosis, the presence of glandular epithelium in the vagina (Fig. 6.3). While usually mucinous, vaginal adenosis may also be

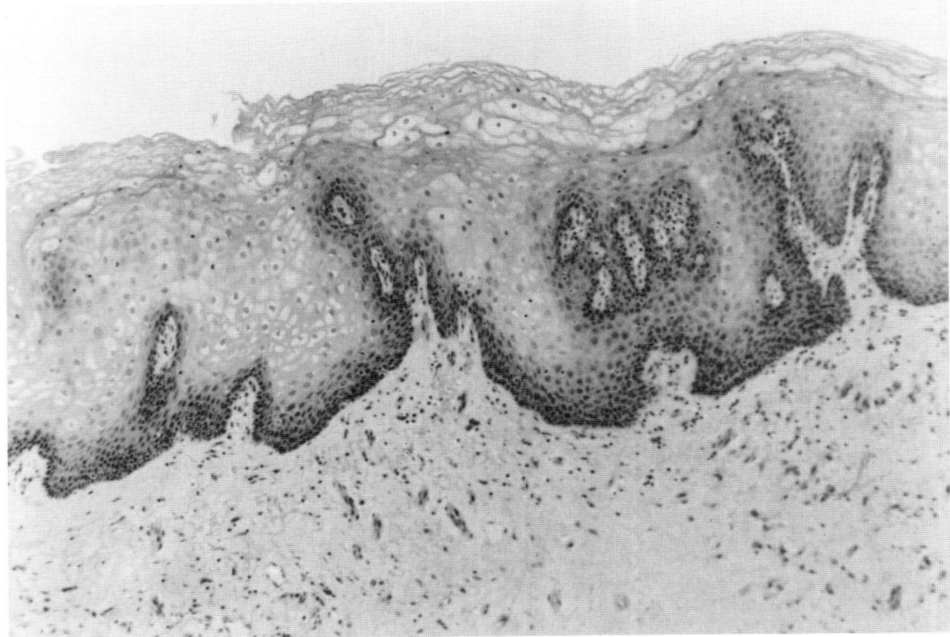

FIGURE 6.1. Normal vaginal mucosa. The vagina is lined by stratified nonkeratinizing squamous epithelium, which overlies a fibroconnective tissue lamina propria rich in elastic fibers. Vaginal epithelium is very responsive to reproductive hormones and is well glycogenated in the presence of estrogen.

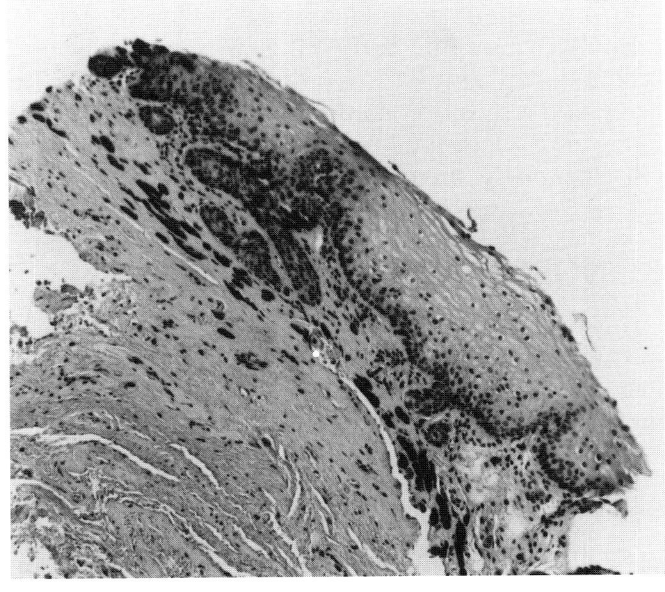

FIGURE 6.2. Blue nevus of the vagina. Spindled melanocytes containing abundant melanin are present in the lamina propria.

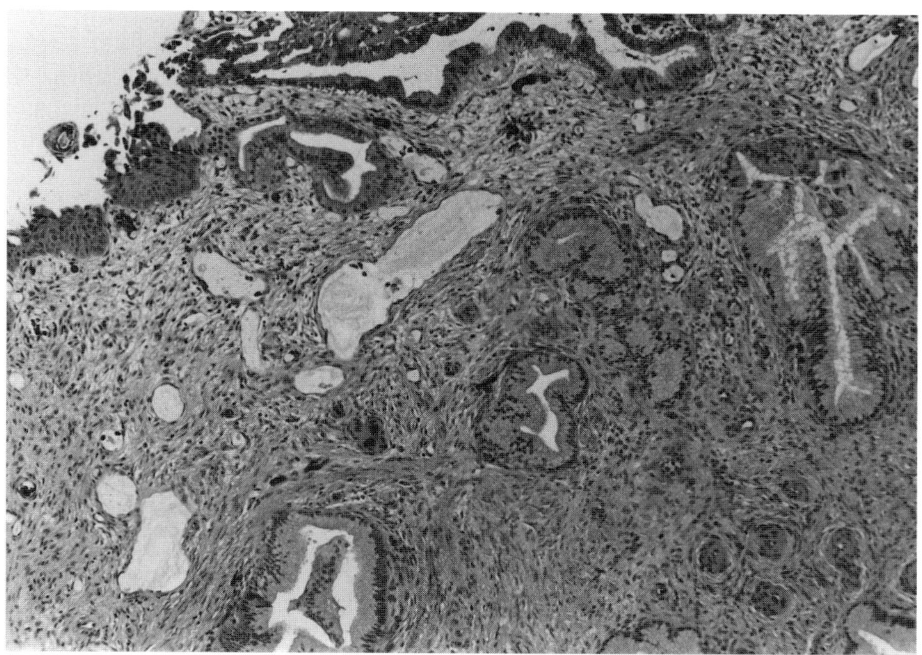

FIGURE 6.3.   Vaginal adenosis. Mucinous glands are present in the lamina propria of the vagina. There is adjacent squamous metaplasia.

tuboendometrial. Usually, squamous metaplasia is present. See chapter 10 for a detailed discussion of the effects of DES on the lower female genital tract.

VAGINAL AGENESIS

Vaginal agenesis may be an isolated finding, or it may occur in association with the absence of the uterus and fallopian tubes (Mayer-Rokitansky-Kuster-Hauser syndrome), which is often associated with urologic anomalies. Surgical creation of a neovagina can be performed, and occasional neoplasms have been reported in neovaginas (2).

VAGINAL DUPLICATION AND LONGITUDINAL SEPTUM

Vaginal duplication usually occurs in association with duplication of the cervix and uterus, as a result of a defect in mullerian duct fusion. Each vagina has a muscular layer. This is in distinction to the more common longitudinal septum, which lacks muscle, on account of the lack of resorption of the intervening septum after mullerian fusion (3).

TRANSVERSE SEPTUM

Transverse vaginal septums are one of the most common anomalies of the female genital tract. They are often lined on the upper surface with mucinous columnar epithelium, sometimes with squamous metaplasia, and lined on the lower surface with nonkeratinized squamous epithelium (3).

IMPERFORATE HYMEN

Although occasionally presenting in early childhood, this condition often presents in puberty with hematocolpos and is easily corrected surgically.

INFECTIONS AND INFLAMMATIONS
VAGINITIS

The common causes of vaginitis are discussed in Chapter 1. Aside from patient morbidity, some forms of vaginitis can have serious sequelae. For example, an association between bacterial vaginosis and premature rupture of placental membranes has been suggested. Causes of vaginal inflammatory disease are listed in Table 6.1.

TABLE 6.1. Common and Uncommon Vaginal Infections and Inflammations

Candida/Torulopsis
Bacterial vaginosis
Trichomonas
Atrophic vaginitis
Shigella sp.
Group B streptococcus
Staphlococcus aureus
Ureaplasma urealyticum
Mycoplasma hominis
Escherichia coli
Haemophilus influenzae
Corynebacterium diphtheria
Neisseria meningitidis
Neisseria gonorrhoeae
Herpes simplex
Treponema pallidum
Saccharomyces cerevisiae
Entamoeba histolytica
Enterobius vermicularis
Trichiuris trichiuria
Schistosoma mansoni
Desquamative inflammatory vaginitis
Ligneous vaginitis
Crohn's disease
Erythema multiforme
Giant cell arteritis
Thrombotic thrombocytopenic purpura
Lichen Planus
Cytomegalovirus
Tuberculous vaginitis
Malakoplakia
Actinomyces

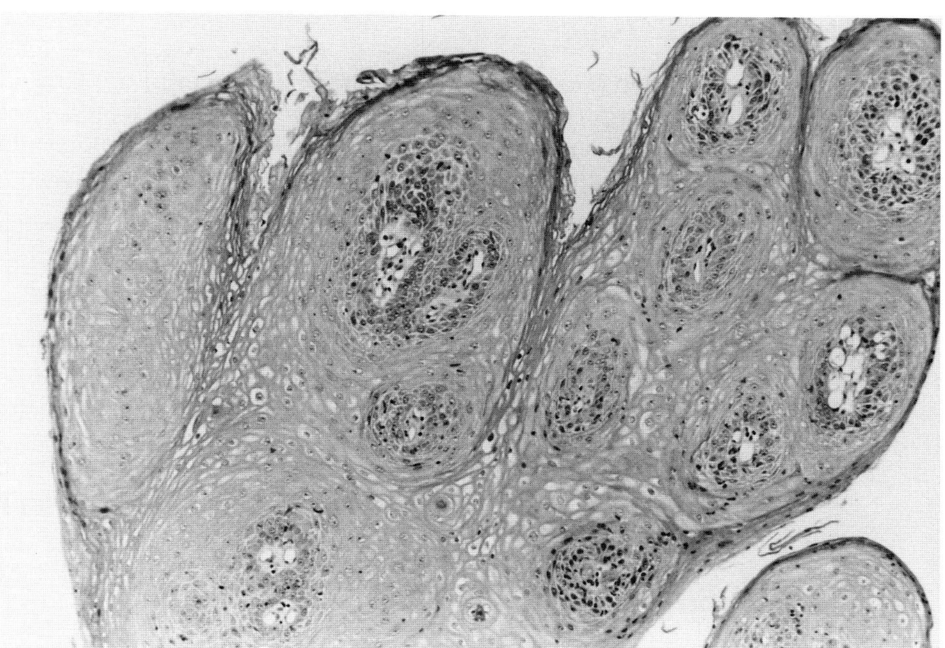

FIGURE 6.4.   Vaginal condyloma. The lesion shows papillomatosis. Koilocytosis may be subtle in vaginal and vulvar condylomata.

ULCERS

Vaginal ulcers may be seen secondary to mechanical abrasion from pessaries or tampons, and in cases of uterine prolapse. The mucosal ulceration associated with tampon usage may facilitate the development of toxic shock syndrome (see the following section).

TOXIC SHOCK SYNDROME

Toxic shock syndrome is a systemic illness usually secondary to a toxin produced by some strains of *Staphlococcus aureus;* however, other bacteria and their toxins have also been implicated. *Staphlococcus aureus* has been shown to be associated with tampon use, particularly with superabsorbant types. The myriad symptoms include fever, erythematous skin rash with desquamation, vomiting, diarrhea, hypotension, and oliguria. Treatment consists of antibiotics and hemodynamic support (4, 5).

CONDYLOMA

Vaginal condylomas may be so small as to only be visible colposcopically. The histologic hallmark of HPV infection, koilocytosis, can be seen. Lesions may be flat, or papillomatosis may be present (Fig. 6.4). HPV 6 and 11 have been identified in many of these lesions (6).

VAGINITIS EMPHYSEMATOSA

This rare condition of unknown etiology consists of air-filled spaces in the lamina propria of the vagina. Vaginitis emphysematosa may be asymptomatic or produce a discharge. The patient may notice a popping sound during intercourse. Histologically, the cystic spaces may contain hyaline material and foreign body giant cells. Lymphocytes and histiocytes are seen in the wall (7).

FISTULAS

Tracts from fistulas such as rectovaginal or vesicovaginal fistulas may be received by the pathology laboratory. These fistulas are often secondary to previous surgery, malignancy, or radiation. In cases of malignancy, ruling out neoplasia in the specimen is important. In benign cases, although a fistula tract and/or the two tissue types of the communicating areas may be identifiable, often only inflamed fibroconnective tissue is seen.

BENIGN TUMORS AND TUMOR-LIKE CONDITIONS
CYSTS

Vaginal cysts are uncommon. If large enough, they may present as a symptomatic mass. In a study of 41 cases (8) Pradhan and colleagues found that 44% were mucin-secreting cysts of mullerian origin, 23% were epidermal inclusion cysts, 11% were Gartner's duct cysts, 7% were Bartholin's duct cysts, 7% were endometriotic in origin, and 3 patients could not be classified.

Squamous Inclusion Cysts

Epidermal inclusion cysts identical to those seen on the vulva can occur in the vagina as sequelae of operations such as episiotomy (Fig.6.5).

Mullerian (Mucinous) Cysts

Mullerian-derived cysts can arise in adenosis, and these are lined by tuboendometrial or mucinous epithelium (9).

Gartner's Duct (Mesonephric) Cysts

Cysts arising in mesonephric remnants are fairly common. They are usually small and found incidentally; however, they may be large enough to produce a symptomatic mass. Gartner's duct cysts usually occur laterally. These cysts are lined by cuboidal to columnar nonciliated epithelium (Fig. 6.6). The cells contain pale nuclei with bland chromatin. The cytoplasm is mucicarmine-negative. Eosinophilic material may be seen within the cyst (9).

PROLAPSED FALLOPIAN TUBE

Occasionally after hysterectomy, particularly vaginal hysterectomy, a residual fallopian tube prolapses into the vaginal apex. It may present with postcoital bleeding, or it may

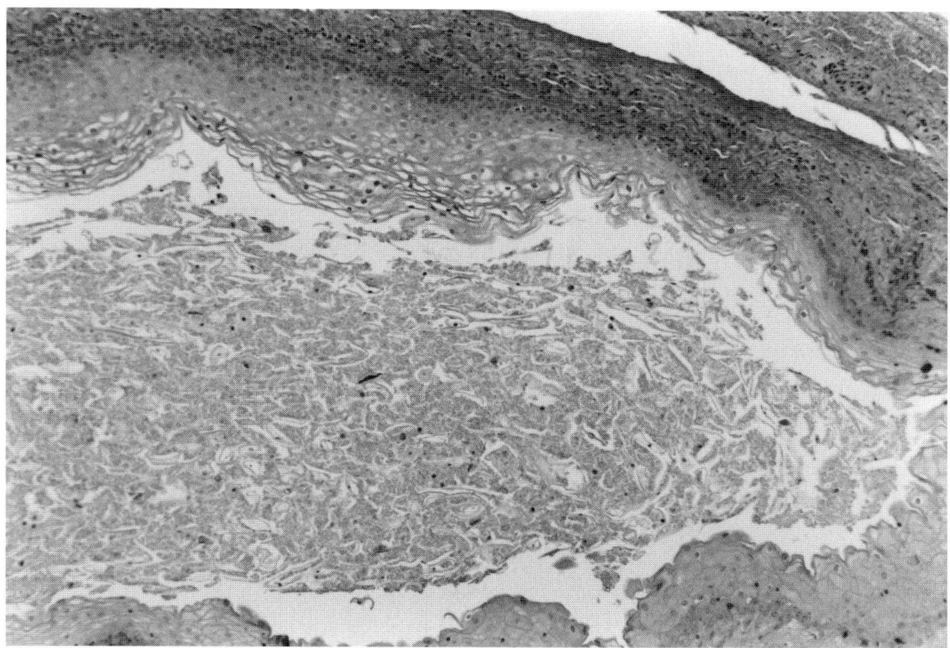

FIGURE 6.5. Epidermal inclusion cyst. The cyst is lined by squamous epithelium. These cysts can occur after a surgical procedure such as episiotomy.

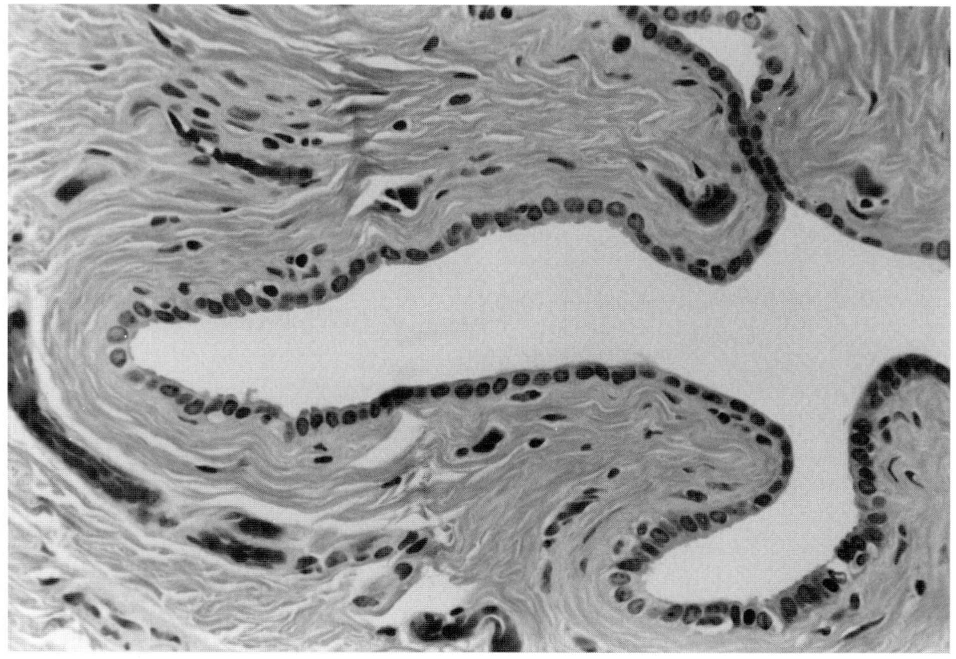

FIGURE 6.6. Gartner's duct cyst. The cyst is lined by a single layer of cuboidal nonciliated epithelium.

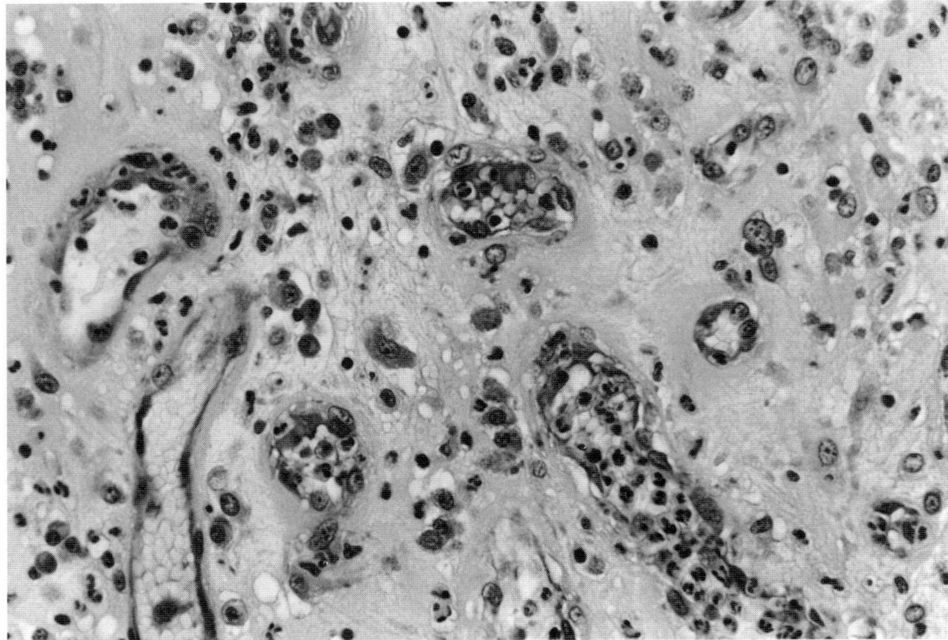

FIGURE 6.7. Granulation tissue. The lesion is composed of new capillaries, fibrovascular tissue, and a mixed acute and chronic inflammatory infiltrate.

be detected incidentally by the clinician on examination. Grossly, the prolapsed tissue at the vaginal vault is red and friable, resembling granulation tissue. In distinction to granulation tissue, tenderness in the area may be experienced. Histologically, inflamed fallopian tube mucosa may be identified and should not be mistaken for adenocarcinoma. Lack of atypia and mitoses and the presence of ciliated cells should help correctly identify a prolapsed fallopian tube.

GRANULATION TISSUE

Granulation tissue often is seen at the vaginal vault after hysterectomy. It may present with vaginal bleeding. Because of concern regarding recurrent malignancy, such tissue may be examined by biopsy. Histologically, the lesion is composed of fibroblasts and new capillary formation in a background of acute and chronic inflammation (Fig. 6.7).

POSTOPERATIVE SPINDLE CELL NODULE

Spindle cell nodules may occur in surgical sites in the female genital tract. A vaginal postoperative spindle cell nodule may present with bleeding. Histologically, the lesion is composed of spindle cells (myofibroblasts). The postoperative spindle cell nodule is mitotically active and may be very vascular. Features distinguishing the benign postoperative spindle cell nodule from a malignant spindle cell lesion include the lack of nuclear atypia and absence of atypical mitoses in the former (10). A recent history of regional surgery is also helpful.

VAGINAL POLYPS

Benign fibroepithelial polyps of the vagina often arise in a clinical background of pregnancy or hormonal therapy (8), suggesting stimulation of hormonally receptive stroma. These polyps may arise from reactive hyperplasia of the loose subepithelial zone of the vaginal wall (1). Fibroepithelial polyps may bleed or may be found incidentally. The lower vagina is the most common site of occurrence (3). Histologically, the polyps are lined by normal squamous epithelium. The stroma is composed of loose fibroconnective tissue containing scattered plump spindle cells. Large atypical stellate cells, sometimes multinucleated, may also be seen (Fig. 6.8), leading to concern of malignancy. Because of the atypical cells, these polyps have also been termed pseudosarcoma botryoides. Distinction can be made from a true sarcoma botryoides by the lack of mitotic activity, strap cells, or a cambium layer in fibroepithelial polyps. In Halvorsen's study (11), the spindle cells of the polyp stained for desmin. Ostor and colleagues evaluated vulvar and vaginal fibroepithelial polyps with atypical cells, detected staining with alpha-1 antitrypsin and alpha-1 antichymotrypsin, but did not find myoglobin positivity in stained cases (12). Two incompletely excised cases in this series recurred locally. Robboy and colleagues report vimentin, desmin, and estrogen and progesterone receptor positivity in these lesions (9). Electron microscopy of the stromal cells reveals features of both fibroblasts and myofibroblasts (9).

SQUAMOUS PAPILLOMA

Papillomas similar histologically to vestibular micropapillomatosis labialis may be seen in the vagina.

ENDOMETRIOSIS

Endometriosis may occur on the vaginal surface, or deep to the surface, particularly in the rectovaginal septum (Fig. 6.9). Endometrioid carcinomas have arisen from these lesions (13).

BENIGN NEOPLASMS

Benign neoplasms of the vagina are occasionally encountered. Benign neoplasms are listed in Table 6.2.

MULLERIAN PAPILLOMA

This uncommon lesion usually occurs in children. Immunohistochemistry supports a mullerian origin. Grossly, the lesions are polypoid and may be papillary. Histologically, the tumor is composed of fibrovascular cores covered by benign-appearing mucin-secreting hobnail cells or cells containing eosinophilic cytoplasm (Fig. 6.10) (3, 14).

LEIOMYOMA

Leiomyomas are the most common mesenchymal neoplasm of the vagina . Histologically, they resemble their uterine counterpart. Most vaginal smooth muscle neoplasms

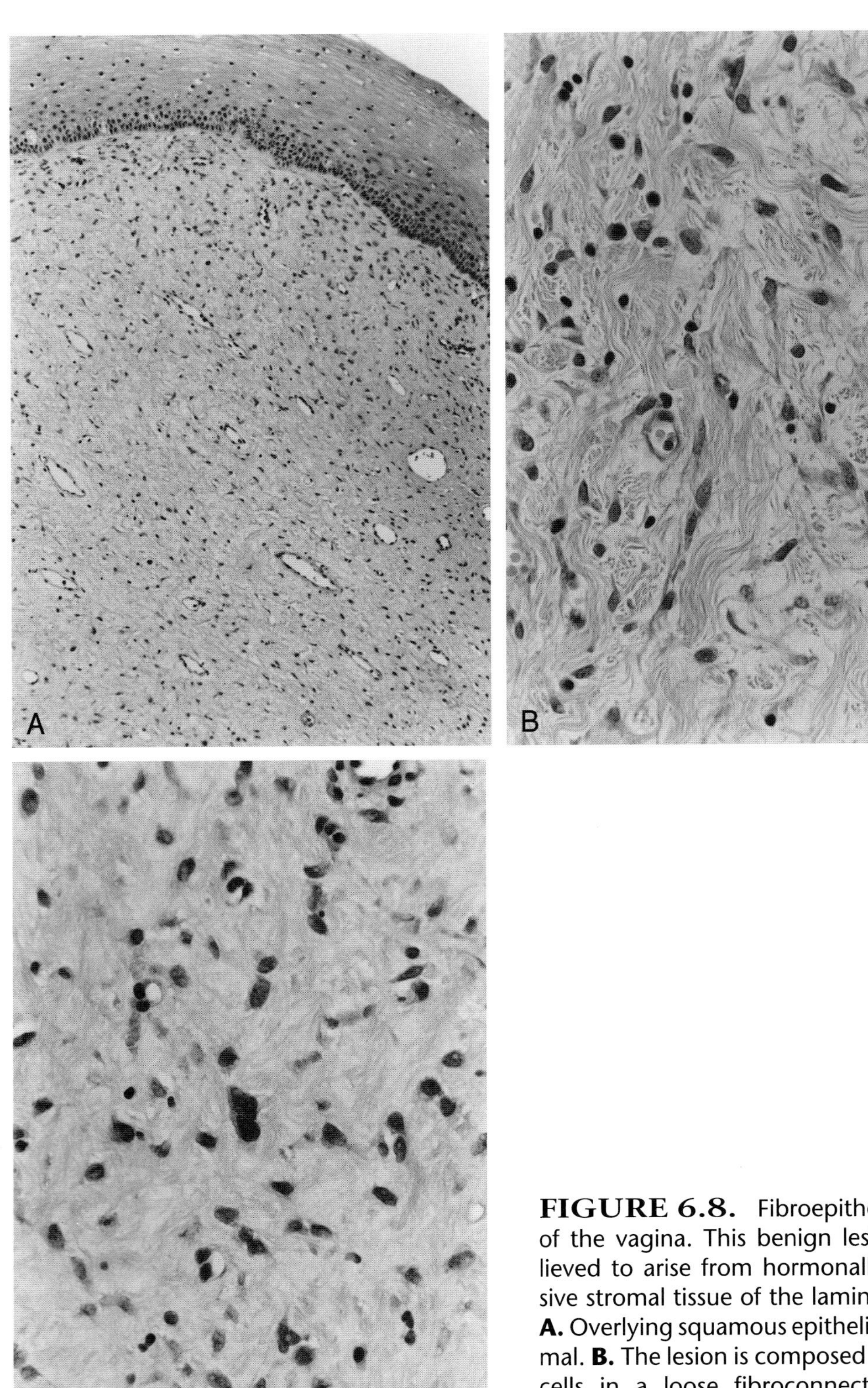

FIGURE 6.8. Fibroepithelial polyp of the vagina. This benign lesion is believed to arise from hormonally responsive stromal tissue of the lamina propria. **A.** Overlying squamous epithelium is normal. **B.** The lesion is composed of spindle cells in a loose fibroconnective tissue stroma. **C.** Atypical cells, some multinucleated, may be present and should not be interpreted as a sign of malignancy.

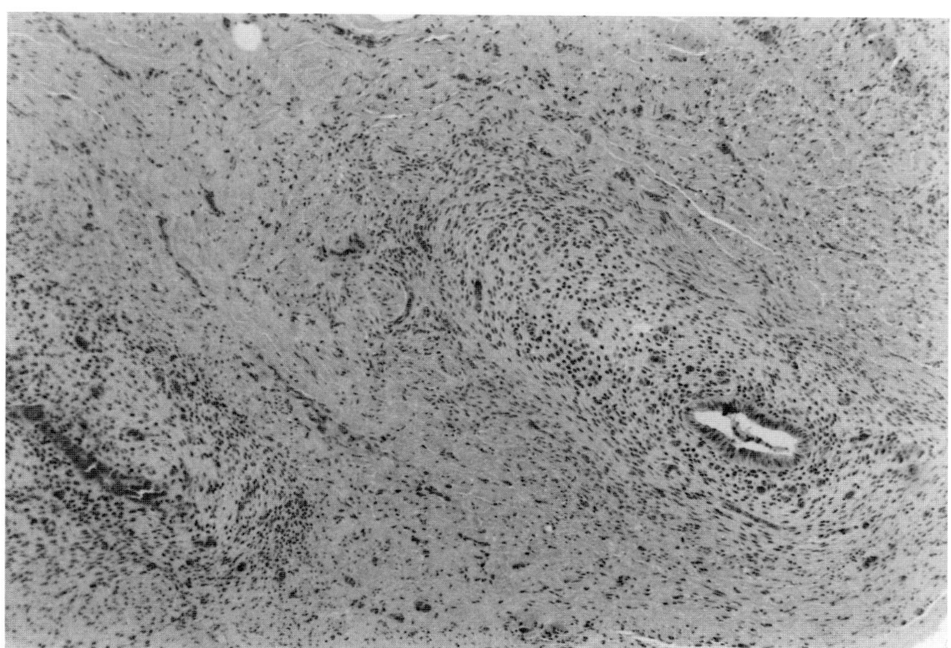

FIGURE 6.9.   Endometriosis of the rectovaginal septum. Endometrial glands and stroma are present in a background of dense fibrous tissue.

TABLE 6.2.   Benign Vaginal Neoplasms
Leiomyoma
Mullerian papilloma
Mixed tumor
Rhabdomyoma
Adenomatoid tumor
Villous adenoma
Benign cystic teratoma
Brenner tumor
Angiomyolipoma
Granular cell tumor
Hemangioma
Neurofibroma
Paraganglioma
Blue nevus
Glomas tumor
Schwannoma
Myxoma

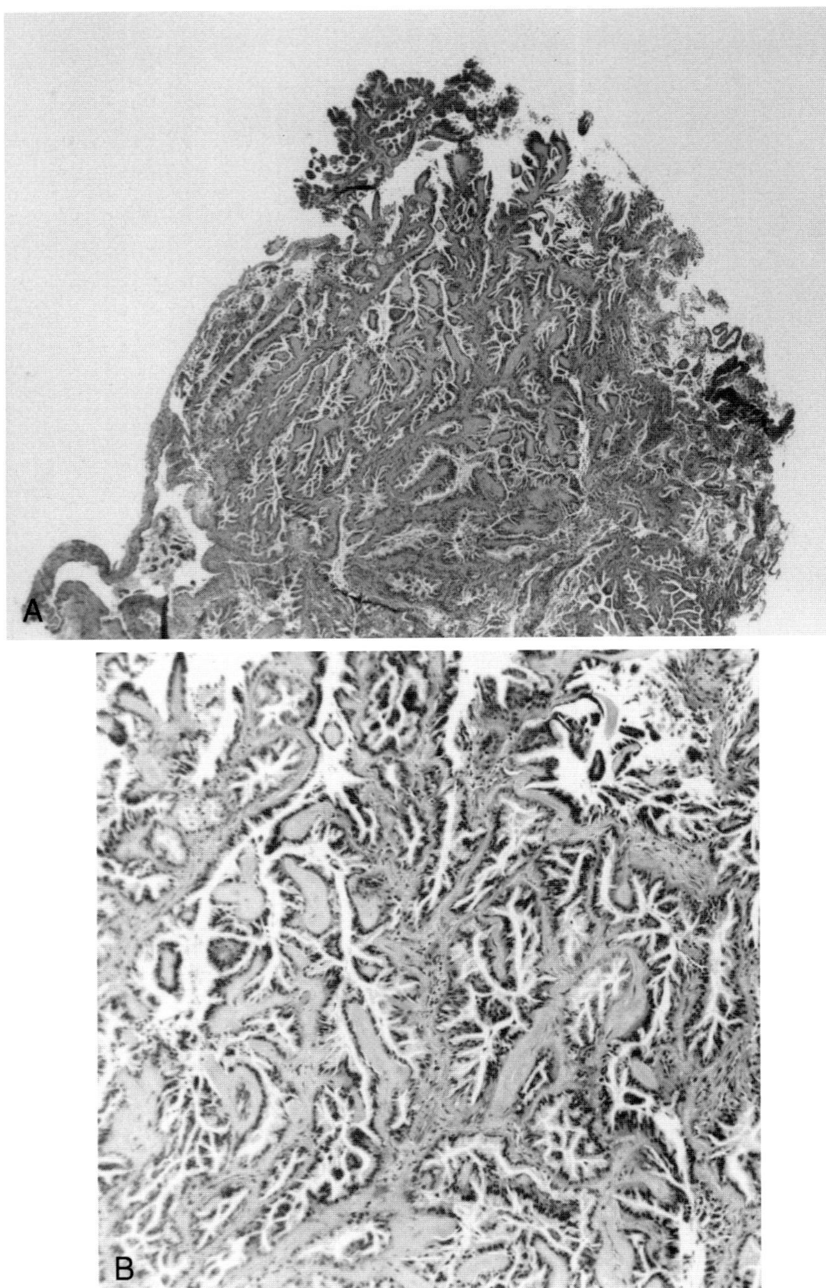

FIGURE 6.10. Mullerian papilloma. The lesion is composed of a complex structure of arborizing fibrovascular cores **(A)** lined by a single layer of epithelium **(B)**, which may be mucinous, hobnail, or eosinophilic.

are benign. Tumors with 5 or more mitoses per 10 high-power fields and significant nuclear atypia are classified as leiomyosarcomas (15).

MIXED TUMOR

This tumor occurs most often in women of reproductive age and is often located just above the hymen. The tumor is well circumscribed, nonencapsulated, and composed of bland oval-to-spindle stromal cells with focal islands of squamous or glandular epithelium. Hyaline globules are also present. Immunohistochemistry and electron microscopy support an epithelial derivation of the spindle cells, which has led Branton and Tavassoli to propose the name "vaginal spindle cell epithelioma" for these lesions (16).

REFERENCES

1. al-Nafussi AI, Rebello G, Hughes D, et al. Benign vaginal polyp: a histological, histochemical, and immunohistochemical study of 20 polyps with comparison to normal vaginal subepithelial layer. Histopathol 1992;20:145–150.
2. Wheelock JB, Schneider V, Goplerud DR. Malignancy arising in the transplanted vagina. South Med J 1986;79:1585–1587.
3. Zaino RJ, Robboy SJ, Bentley R, et al. Diseases of the vagina. In: Blaustein's Pathology of the Female Genital Tract. 4th edition. New York: Springer-Verlag, 1994:131–183.
4. Schlievert PM. Role of superantigens in human disease [review]. J Infect D 1993;167: 997–1002.
5. Wright SW, Trott AT. Toxic shock syndrome: a review [review]. Ann Emerg Med 1988;17: 268–273.
6. DiBonito L, Falconieri G, Bonifacio-Gori D. Multicentric *Papillomavirus* infection of the female genital tract: a study of morphologic pattern, possible risk factors and viral prevalence. Pathol Res Pract 1993;189:1023–1029.
7. Kramer K, Tobon H. Vaginitis emphysematosa. Arch Pathol Lab Med 1987;111:746–749.
8. Pradhan S, Tobon H. Vaginal cysts: a clinicopathological study of 41 cases. Int J Gynecol Pathol 1986;5:35–46.
9. Robboy SJ, Welch WR. Selected topics in the pathology of the vagina. Hum Pathol 1991; 22:868–876.
10. Guillou L, Gloor E, De Grandi P, et al. Postoperative pseudosarcoma of the vagina. A case report. Pathol Res Prac 1989;185:245–248.
11. Halvorsen TB, Johannesen E. Fibroepithelial polyps of the vagina: are they old granulation tissue polyps? J Clin Pathol 1992;45:235–240.
12. Ostor AG, Fortune DW, Riley CB. Fibroepithelial polyps with atypical stromal cells (pseudosarcoma botryoides) of the vulva and vagina. A report of 13 cases. Int J Gynecol Pathol 1988;7:351–360.
13. Haskel S, Shen SS, Spiegel G. Vaginal endometrioid adenocarcinoma arising in vaginal endometriosis: a case report and literature review [review].Gyncol Oncol 1989;34: 232–236.
14. Luttges JE, Lubke M. Recurrent benign Mullerian papilloma of the vagina. Immunohistochemical findings and histogenesis. Arch Gynecol Obstet 1994;255:157–160.
15. Tavassoli FA, Norris HJ. Smooth muscle tumors of the vagina Obstet Gynecol 1979;53: 689–693.
16. Branton PA, Tavassoli FA. Spindle cell epithelioma, the so-called mixed tumor of the vagina. A clinicopathologic, immunohistochemical, and ultrastructural analysis of 28 cases. Am J Surg Pathol 1993;17:509–515.

MALIGNANT DISEASES OF THE VAGINA

Debra S. Heller, MD

■

Vaginal Intraepithelial Neoplasia (VAIN)
Invasive Neoplasms of the Vagina

VAGINAL INTRAEPITHELIAL NEOPLASIA (VAIN)

VAIN is uncommon. It is estimated that there is 1 case of VAIN for every 100 cases of cervical intraepithelial neoplasia (1). Many women with VAIN have previous history of preinvasive or invasive squamous neoplasia of other genital organs, particularly the cervix (2).

As with squamous intraepithelial neoplasia in other genital sites, human *Papillomavirus* is an important etiologic factor in the development of VAIN. Risk factors include immunosuppression, previous radiation to the area, low socioeconomic status, and a history of genital warts or other HPV-related genital neoplasia. Controversy exists as to whether women with in-utero diethylstilbestrol exposure have a greater risk of developing VAIN. Whether the metaplastic squamous epithelium present in these women is more easily infected is unclear; however, exposure to the virus must occur. Most VAIN lesions arise in the upper vagina, and the condition is frequently multifocal (2). Patients present with VAIN at an older age than patients with cervical intraepithelial neoplasia. In one study, the mean age of patients with VAIN was 50.2 years (3). Most lesions in this series were in the upper vagina, and most were detected by cytology. A small but real risk of progression to invasive carcinoma exists. Twenty-three patients with VAIN were studied for at least 3 years, during which they did not undergo therapy (4). The mean age of the patients was 41 years. Lesions were often multifocal and frequently associated with VIN or CIN. Two cases (9%) progressed to invasive carcinoma, three cases (13%) persisted, and 18 cases (78%) regressed. The authors stressed the importance of vaginal colposcopy with biopsy of all lesions.

Laser ablation, excision, and 5-fluorouracil are the most often used treatment modalities. Because 5-fluorouracil can be extremely irritating to the vulva, precautions to protect the area must be undertaken with therapy.

Grossly, VAIN usually is not visible, and most lesions are detected colposcopically. Microscopically, the criteria are the same as intraepithelial neoplasia of the cervix and vulva. Some pathologists classify the lesions as VAIN I, II, or III, depending on the degree of maturation abnormality, and some divide the lesions into low-grade and high-grade squamous intraepithelial lesions corresponding to Bethesda system diagnoses (Figs. 7.1 and 7.2).

The differential diagnosis of VAIN includes atrophy, radiation effect, squamous metaplasia in adenosis, and inflammatory/reparative changes (Figs. 7.3–7.5). VAIN shows varying degrees of abnormality of maturation, with irregularities of nuclear outline, hyperchromatic nuclei, and clumping of chromatin. Mitotic activity is usually present, and atypical mitoses may be seen. In contrast, metaplastic and atrophic epithelium do not show disorderly maturation or nuclear atypia. Radiation effect does not include mitotic activity. In radiated epithelium, enlarged nuclei with smudgy chromatin, multinucleation, and cytoplasmic vacuolization may be seen. Inflammatory atypia is composed of regularly enlarged nuclei, vesicular chromatin, and often prominent nucleoli (5).

Rare references to in-situ glandular lesions of the vagina in association with previous cervical adenocarcinoma-in-situ exist (6, 7). However, since glands are usually not present in the vagina except in DES daughters, in-situ glandular neoplasia in this region is a rarity.

INVASIVE NEOPLASMS OF THE VAGINA

Invasive primary malignancies of the vagina are uncommon. Those entities that are more likely to be encountered are discussed in the following, and rare tumors are listed in Table 7.1.

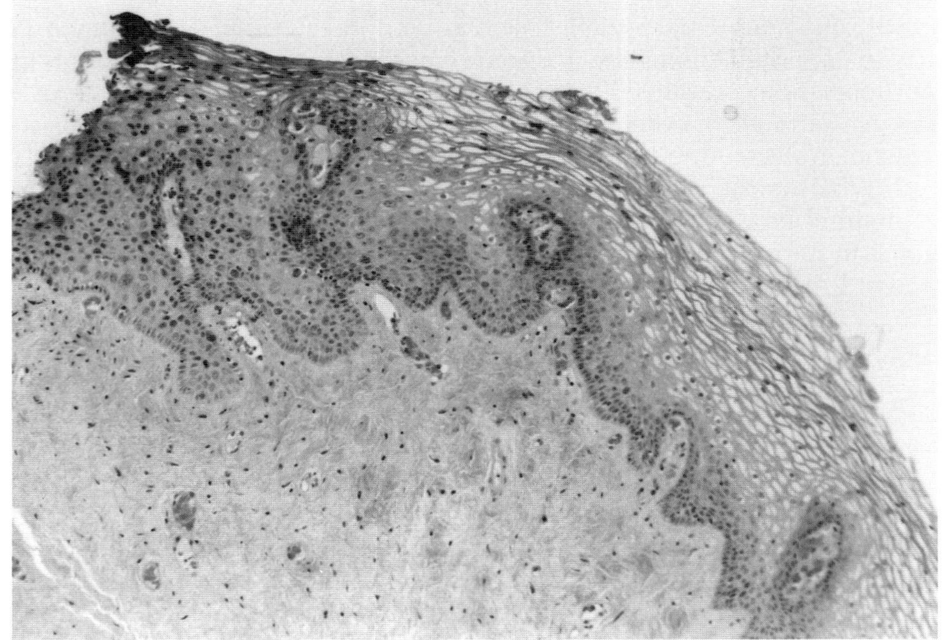

FIGURE 7.1. Low-grade VAIN. An abrupt transition from normal to atypical epithelium is present.

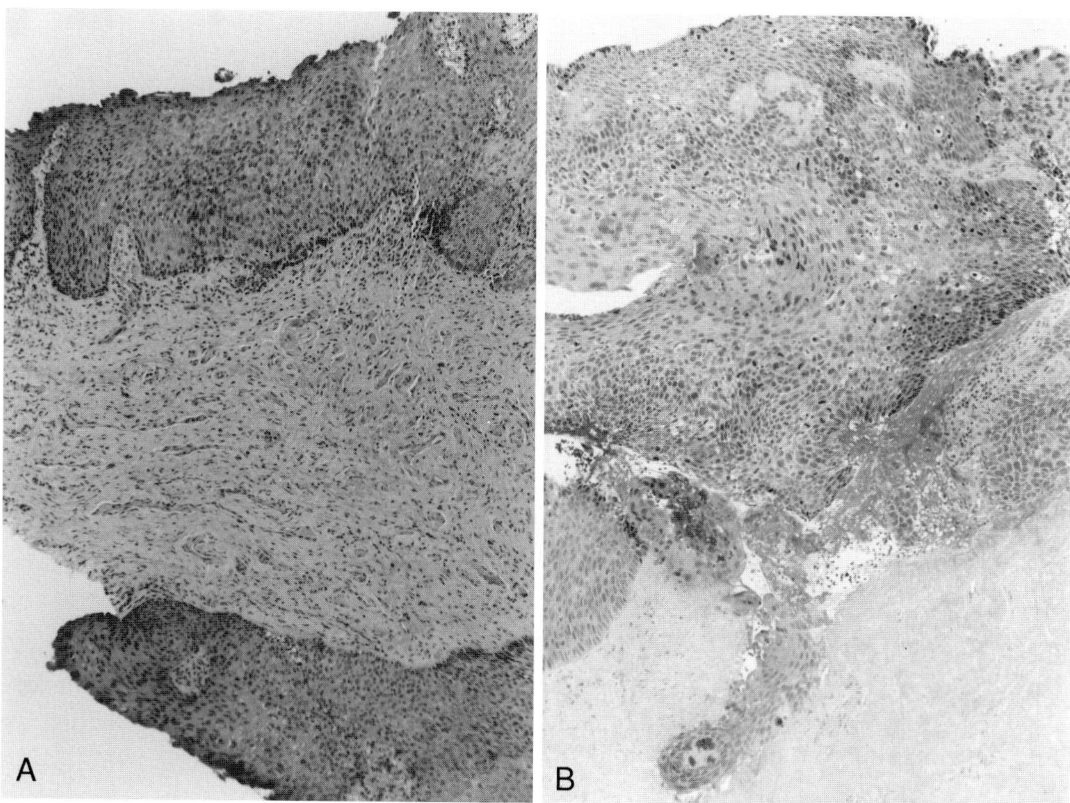

FIGURE 7.2.   High-grade VAIN. **A.** Full thickness maturation abnormality. **B.** Dysplastic epithelium is friable and specimens may not always have optimum orientation.

INVASIVE EPITHELIAL NEOPLASMS

Primary epithelial malignancies of the vagina are rare, representing 1–2% of gynecological malignancies (8). Extension from other carcinomas, particularly of the vulva and cervix, must first be ruled out. Some of the rarity of these lesions may actually be due to underreporting of the vagina as a primary site, caused by the strictness of the definition (Table 7.2). Environmental factors have been postulated to play a role in the development of vaginal carcinoma. These include human *Papillomavirus,* herpes simplex virus, in-utero exposure to diethystilbestrol, irritation secondary to pessary use, previous hysterectomy for benign disease, immunosuppression, cervical radiation therapy, and endometriosis (9).

Therapy for carcinomas of the vagina is individualized. Radiation therapy or surgical therapy alone or in combination are the usual primary therapies, depending on the stage of the disease. Palliative radiation alone or combined with chemotherapy has been used in advanced disease.

SQUAMOUS CELL CARCINOMA

Most invasive carcinomas of the vagina are squamous cell carcinomas. Of 53 women without DES exposure who had primary vaginal malignancies, 89% had squamous cell

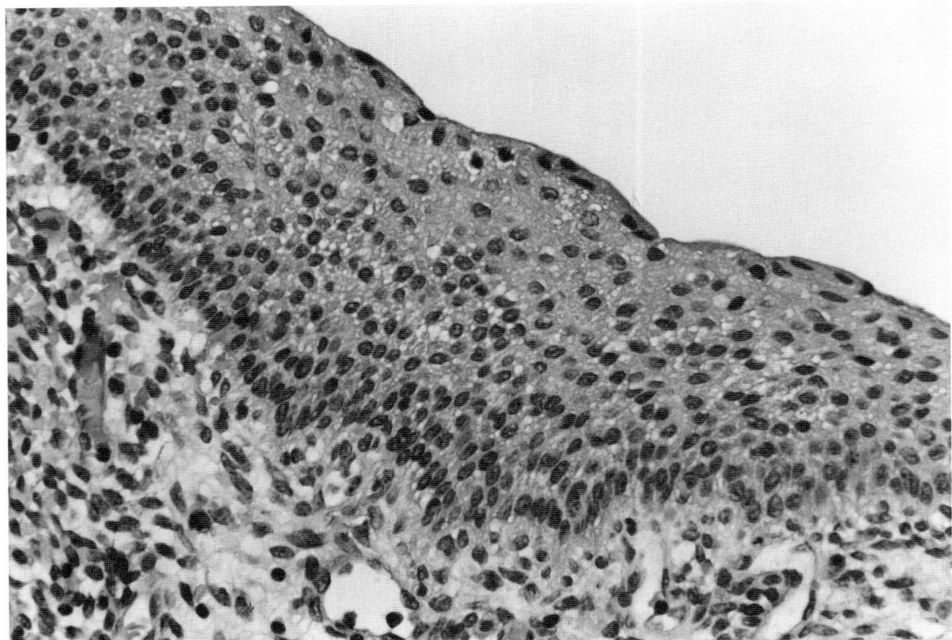

FIGURE 7.3. Repair. This epithelium is undergoing repair in an area of inflammation. Cells appear immature with less glycogen, but there is no nuclear pleomorphism. There is an open chromatin pattern with prominent nucleoli.

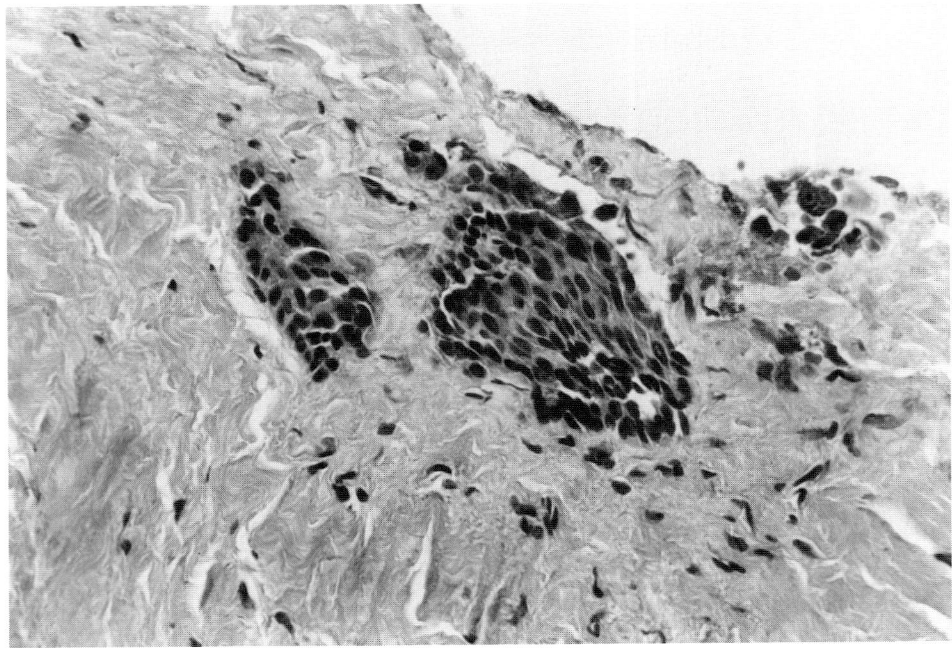

FIGURE 7.4. Atrophy. This fragment of atrophic vaginal epithelium may raise concern regarding a diagnosis of VAIN, but it lacks atypia or mitotic activity.

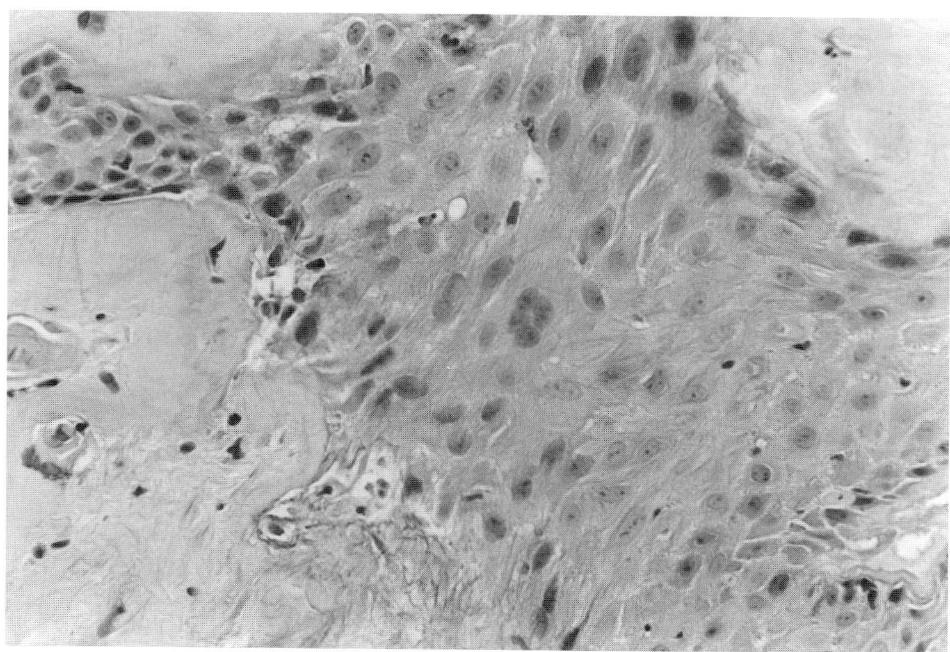

FIGURE 7.5.   Radiation. This radiated vaginal epithelium shows multinucleation and a few large nuclei. Chromatin is smudgy. There is no mitotic activity or hyperchromasia as in VAIN. Note the underlying fibrotic subepithelial tissue.

carcinomas and 11% had adenocarcinomas (10). Some of the lesions were detected during routine examination, by either abnormal cytology or detection of a lesion. For women with symptoms, bleeding was the most common, followed by discharge and urinary symptoms. Women who previously had hysterectomies had their cancers discovered later, after the onset of symptoms, and they had a worse outcome than women who had not had hysterectomies. The importance of continued gynecological care after hysterectomy was stressed. Many invasive vaginal squamous cell carcinomas have identifiable HPV DNA, usually type 16 (2).

Survival is related to disease stage, with reasonable 5-year survival for early stage disease (9) and extremely poor survival with more advanced disease (11). The FIGO staging of vaginal carcinoma can be seen in Table 7.3. No recognized category of microinvasive carcinoma in the vagina exists; however, lesions with less than 3-mm invasion and no lymphvascular space involvement have a low risk of metastases (12).

Grossly, vaginal squamous cell carcinomas may be exophytic or endophytic. Most cancers arise in the proximal third of the vagina (5). Histologically, the tumors may be well, moderately, or poorly differentiated (Figs. 7.6–7.8), and are identical histologically to squamous cell carcinomas arising elsewhere.

Verrucous Carcinoma

Verrucous carcinoma, a subtype of squamous cell carcinoma, is exceedingly rare in the vagina (8). Grossly and histologically, it is identical to the more common vulvar lesion (see Chapter 5). Pure verrucous carcinoma of the vagina may recur locally, but it rarely

TABLE 7.1. Rare Malignancies of the Vagina

Cloacogenic carcinoma
Verrucous carcinoma
Basal cell carcinoma
Endometrioid adenocarcinoma
Transitional cell carcinoma
Lymphoepithelioma-like carcinoma
Adenoid cystic carcinoma
Small cell carcinoma
Paravaginal mesonephric carcinoma
Malignant mixed mesodermal tumor
Malignant mixed tumor
Endometrioid stromal sarcoma
Carcinoid
Malignant schwannoma
Synovial-like sarcoma
Angiosarcoma
Malignant fibrous histiocytoma
Alveolar soft part sarcoma
Lymphoma
Endodermal sinus tumor
Gestational trophoblastic disease

TABLE 7.2. Criteria for Diagnosis of Primary Invasive Carcinoma of the Vagina

Tumor arises in the vagina
No clinical evidence of cervical or vulvar involvement
No histological evidence of cervical or vulvar involvement
No invasive carcinoma of the cervix within 5 years of diagnosis
No squamous intraepithelial lesion of the cervix within 2 years of diagnosis

Final two criteria adapted from Peters WA, Kumar NB, Morley GW. Carcinoma of the vagina: factors influencing treatment outcome. Cancer 1985;55:892–897.

TABLE 7.3. FIGO Staging of Primary Vaginal Cancer

0. Carcinoma-in-situ
I. Confined to vaginal wall
II. Subvaginal invasion but not to pelvic wall
III. Extension to pelvic wall
IV. Extension beyond the true pelvis or to bladder or rectal mucosa; bullous edema does not count as stage IV
    IVA. Adjacent organs and/or direct extension beyond true pelvis
    IVB. Distant spread

Adapted from Classification and staging of gynecologic malignancies: ACOG technical Bulletin #155, May 1991. Int J Gynecol Obstet 1992;38:319–323.

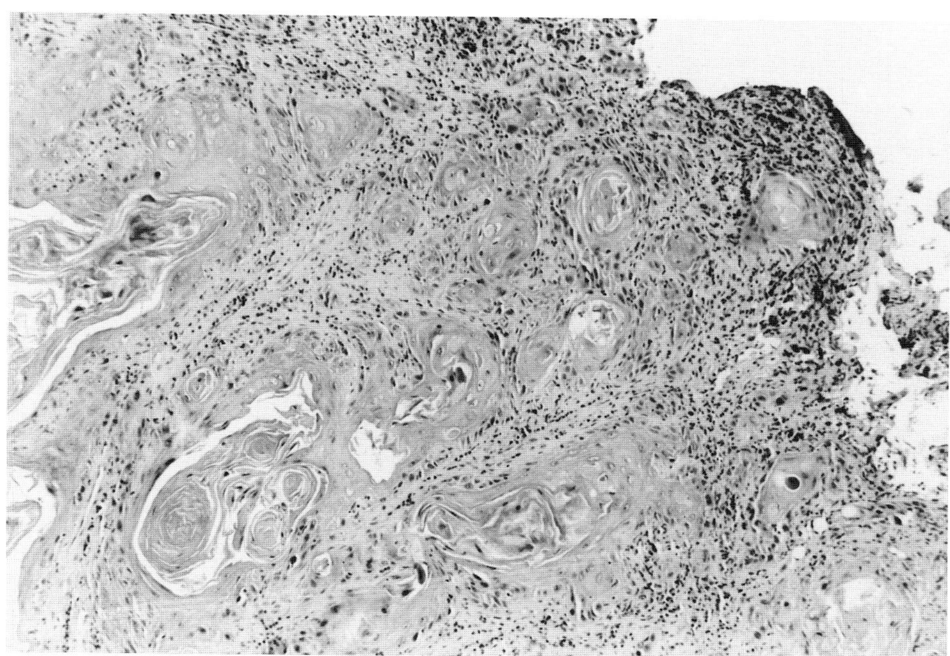

FIGURE 7.6.   Well-differentiated squamous cell carcinoma. The tumor is keratinized and maintains its resemblance to normal squamous epithelium.

metastasizes. If present along with usual squamous cell carcinoma, the more aggressive behavior of the squamous cell carcinoma predominates (5).

ADENOCARCINOMA OF THE VAGINA

Clear Cell Adenocarcinoma

The occurrence of clear cell adenocarcinoma of the vagina in the absence of intrauterine DES exposure is rare. This is in contradistinction to clear cell adenocarcinoma of the cervix, which occurs both with and without intrauterine DES exposure. In the United States, the highest likelihood of developing clear cell adenocarcinoma of the vagina or cervix after intrauterine diethylstilbestrol (DES) exposure was found for women between ages 14–22. The risk is quite small for DES progeny, at approximately 1 per 1000 exposed women (13). In one study (14), cytology only detected one-third of vaginal tumors; therefore, physical examination including colposcopy is important for women at risk. Reasons postulated for lack of cytological diagnosis in vaginal as opposed to cervical tumors were the failure to obtain a vaginal smear and the possibility that the major tumor bulk was growing under benign surface squamous metaplasia (14). Larger tumors may present with bleeding or discharge.

Both surgical and radiation therapy are methods for treatment. Surgery with or without adjuvant radiation is most common in early stage disease, with primary radiation used mostly in treating advanced disease (5). Follow-up must be prolonged due to the possibility of late recurrences (13). Stage and grade are the most important prognosticators (14). Overall, 5-year survivals have been good (5).

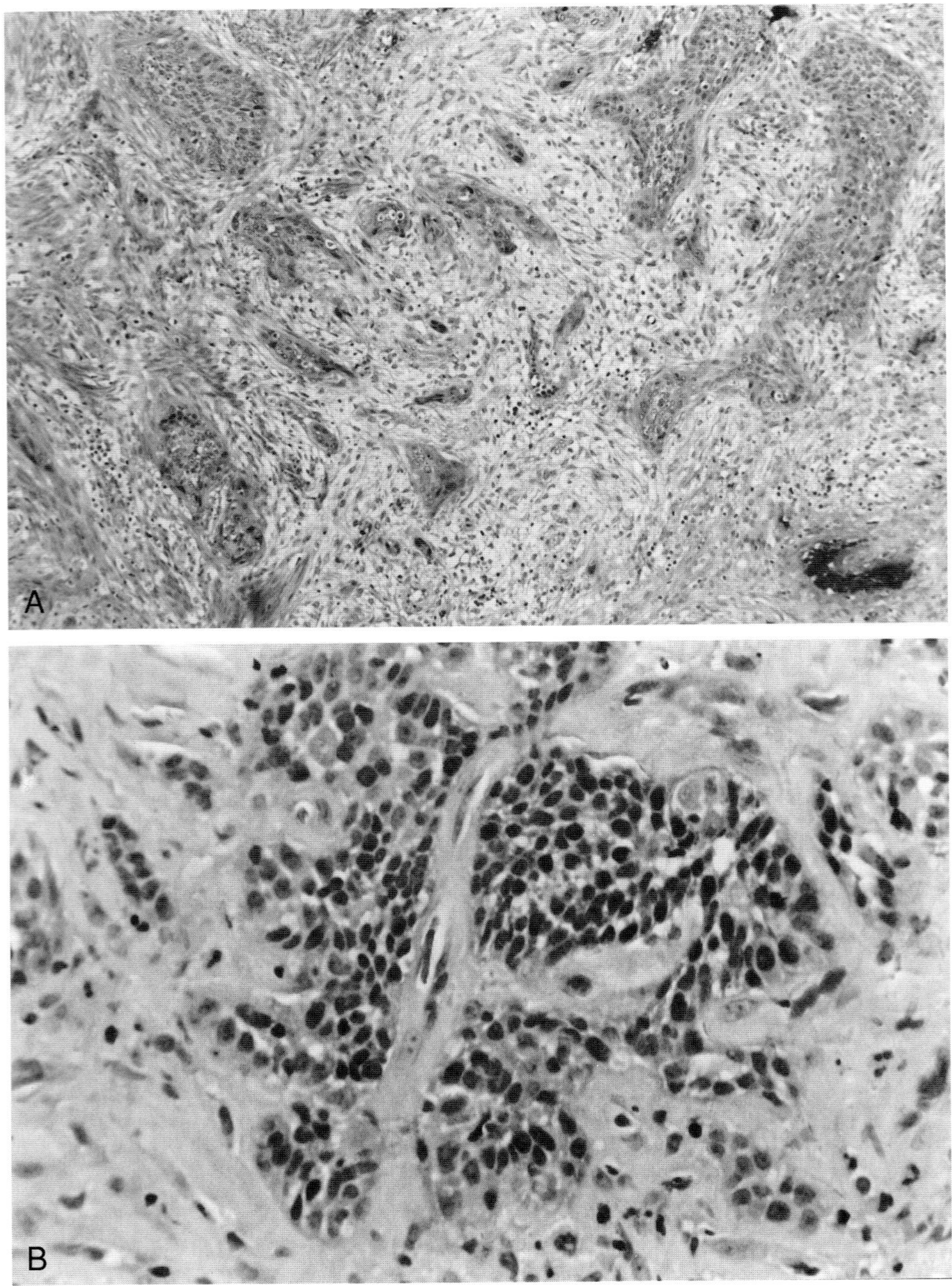

FIGURE 7.7. **A,B.** Moderately differentiated squamous cell carcinoma. With less differentiation, the resemblance to squamous epithelium decreases.

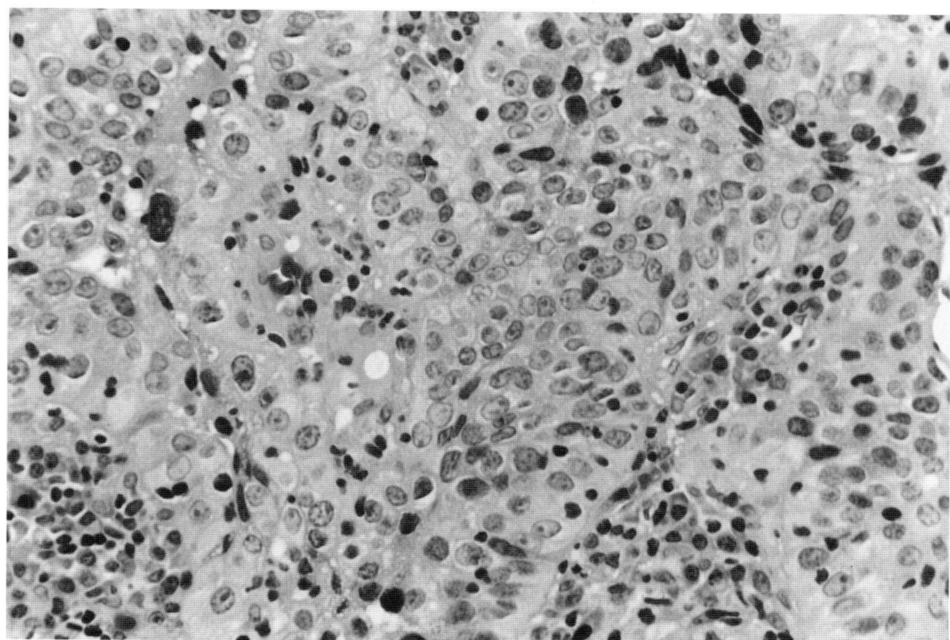

FIGURE 7.8.   Poorly differentiated squamous cell carcinoma no longer resembles squamous epithelium but is composed of sheets of undifferentiated malignant cells.

When grossly visible, lesions tend to be nodular. Histologically, clear cell adenocarcinoma is identical to clear cell carcinomas of the ovary and endometrium. Most commonly, the tumor may exhibit a solid clear cell pattern, with abundant cytoplasmic glycogen, or a tubulocystic pattern, with spaces lined by hobnail or flat cells (Fig. 7.9). Mixed patterns may also be seen.

Lesions that may be confused with clear cell adenocarcinoma include microglandular hyperplasia and the Arias-Stella reaction. Both of these are rare in the vagina. Microglandular hyperplasia is often associated with either pregnancy or the use of oral contraceptives. Careful searching usually reveals foci of mucinous epithelium, and there is no nuclear atypia. The Arias-Stella reaction is always associated with pregnancy and does not contain mitotic figures. Glands may be lined by hobnail cells, but they appear degenerative, and there are no areas of sheets of clear cells (15).

Endometrioid Adenocarcinoma

Vaginal adenocarcinoma with an endometrioid pattern is most often due to metastatic spread of a uterine primary; however, endometrioid carcinoma arising in vaginal endometriosis has been described (16).

OTHER EPITHELIAL MALIGNANCIES OF THE VAGINA

Small Cell Carcinoma

The diagnosis of small cell carcinoma of the vagina can be confusing because the terminology has been applied to poorly differentiated squamous cell carcinomas with small

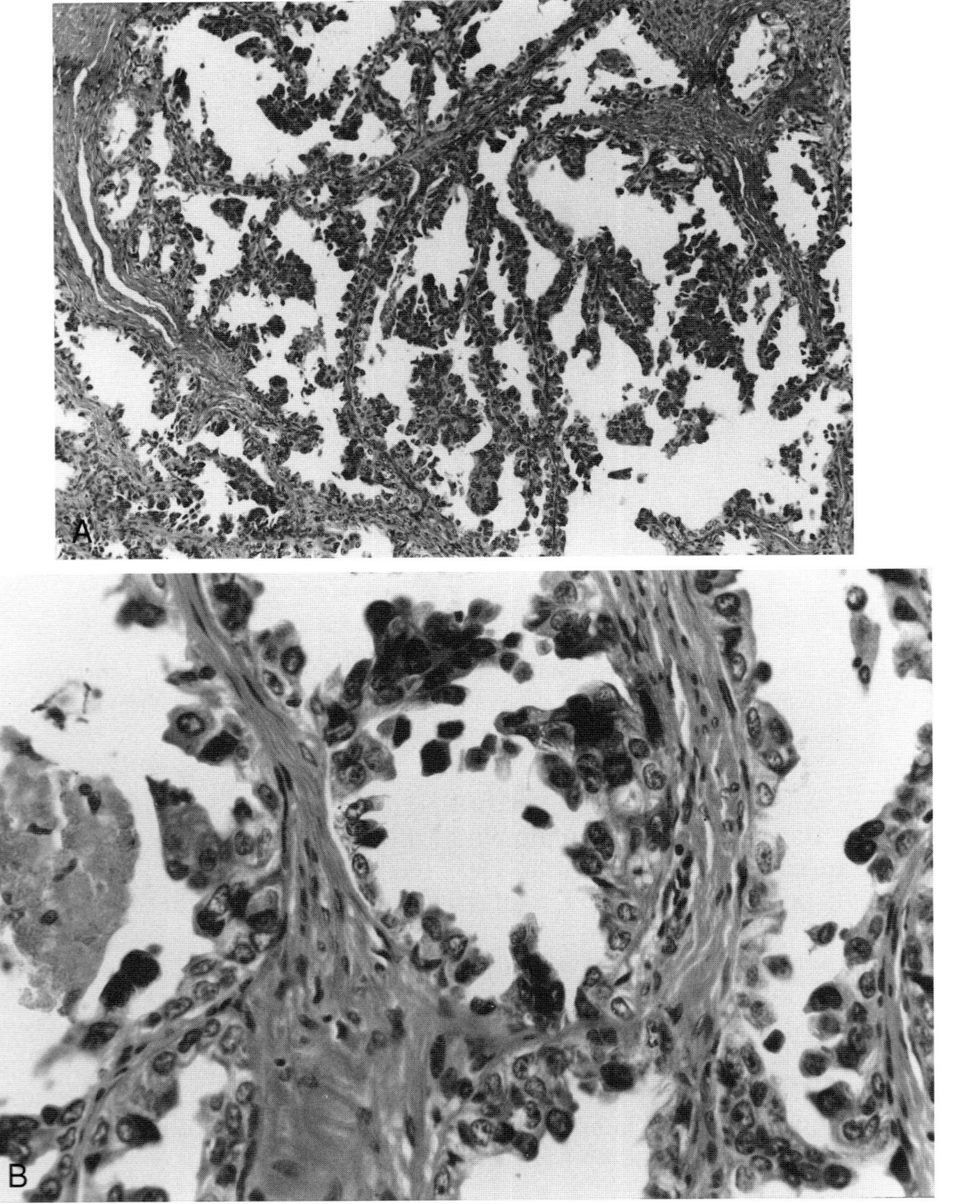

FIGURE 7.9.   Clear cell adenocarcinoma of the vagina. **A,B.** Tubulocystic pattern lined by hobnail cells.

cells as well as to tumors with neuroendocrine differentiation. Small cell carcinoma with neuroendocrine differentiation is extremely rare in the vagina, usually seen in older women, and reported cases have usually already spread beyond the vagina at the time of diagnosis. Immunohistochemistry and electron microscopy confirm the neuroendocrine differentiation in these tumors (2).

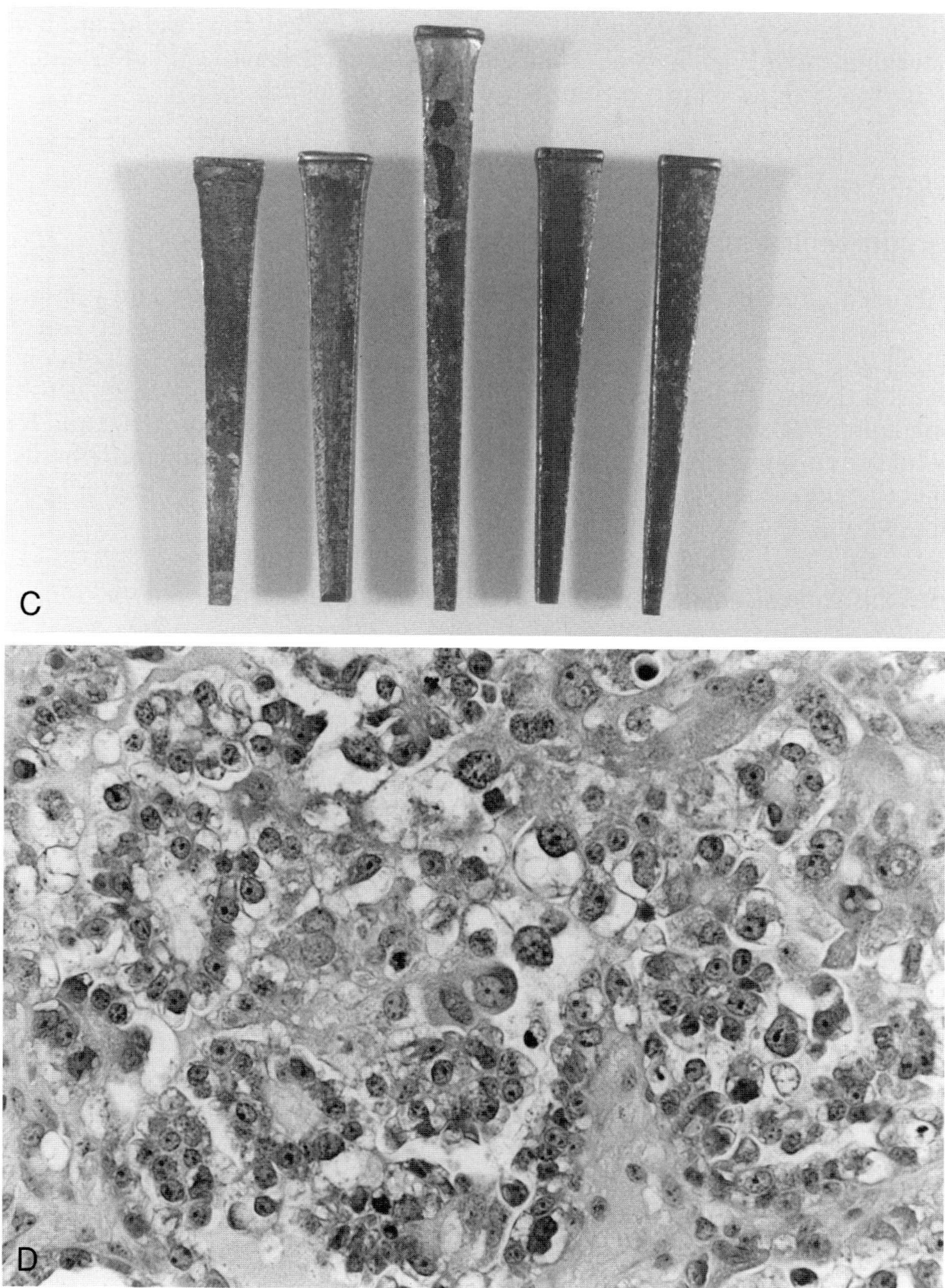

FIGURE 7.9.   (*continued*) **C.** Hobnails. **D.** The solid clear cell pattern, with abundant intracytoplasmic glycogen.

Carcinoma Arising in Neovaginas

Vaginal reconstruction with the creation of a neovagina performed after previous radical surgery for neoplasia or for congenital absence of the vagina may lead to an increased risk of vaginal neoplasia. As well as squamous cell carcinoma (17), adenocarcinoma arising in a neovagina constructed of bowel has been described (18).

OTHER PRIMARY VAGINAL MALIGNANCIES

Malignant Melnoma

Vaginal melanomas are extremely rare. Tumors occur in the elderly and present with bleeding, discharge, or mass. The prognosis is poor, with a 5–21% 5-year survival quoted in the literature (19). One study has correlated aggressive behavior with higher mitotic counts (20). Grossly, the tumors are usually pigmented, and the histology is the same as for melanomas elsewhere (Fig. 7.10). If the diagnosis is in question, S100 and HMB45 are useful immunohistochemical stains. The Chung and Breslow measurements used in vulvar melanoma are also applicable for vaginal melanomas (see Chapter 5). Due to the rarity of the lesion, therapeutic interventions have varied widely.

Sarcoma Botryoides (Embryonal Rhabdomyosarcoma)

This rare tumor is usually seen in children younger than age 5, with most patients around 2 years of age or younger (5). Most small tumors arise from the anterior vaginal wall. The most common symptom is a bloody discharge, followed by passage of tumor fragments. Gross polypoid tumor may protrude from the vagina (21).

Most of the patients in Hays' series (21) were treated with primary chemotherapy, or a combination of primary chemotherapy with radiation, often with secondary surgery, as opposed to initial excisional surgery. Therapy was aimed at avoiding exenteration and preserving the pelvic organs as much as possible. Most of the patients recovered well. Of the 28 patients with vaginal tumors, three deaths occurred, two from disease and one from a complication of therapy. Twenty-six of the patients had a localized tumor at diagnosis. Survival was good even with relapse and salvage therapy. Cytoreductive chemotherapy coupled with conservative surgery with or without radiation also led to excellent disease-free survival in a more recent series (22). Tumors were staged by a postsurgical classification in earlier studies (23), but more recent studies have used a clinical TNM staging system to compare various studies and to have staging before primary chemotherapeutic regimes (24).

Grossly, the tumors are usually polypoid (Fig. 7.11A); microscopically, the overlying epithelium is normal. The tumor consists of bland round to spindle cells in a loose myxoid or dense connective tissue stroma (Fig. 7.11B,C). Strap cells with cross-striations may be seen, but they can be absent. Tumor cells condense under the surface epithelium, forming the so-called "cambium layer." Immunohistochemical staining with muscle-specific actin, desmin, and myoglobin may be helpful. The tumor should not be confused with fibroepithelial papillomas, which do not have a cambium layer; mullerian papillomas in which the epithelium is the neoplastic (benign) element and there is an arborizing structure, or benign rhabdomyomas, which lack mitoses and atypia.

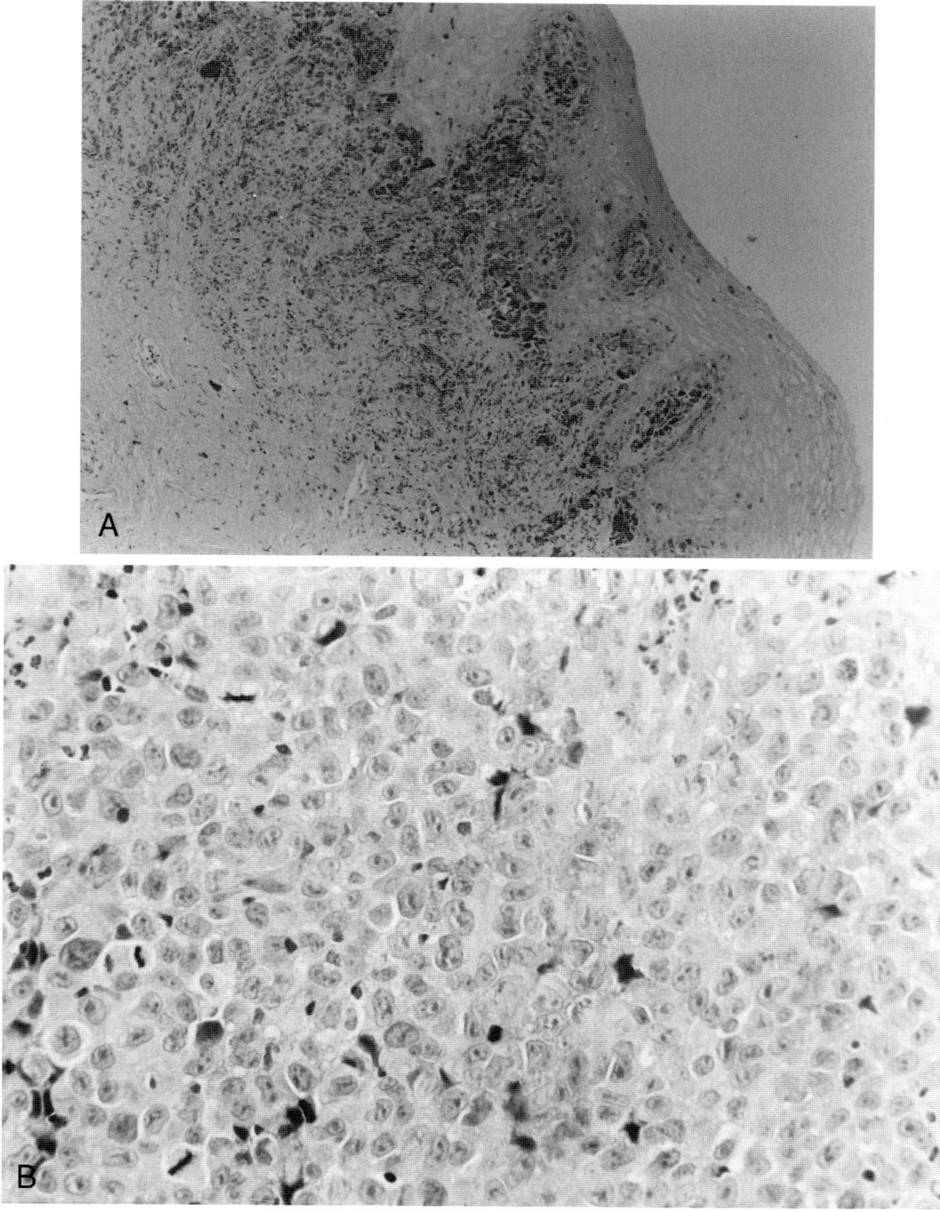

FIGURE 7.10.   Melanoma of the vagina. **A.** The lesion is pigmented. **B.** The tumor is composed of sheets of epithelioid cells with prominent nucleoli.

Leiomyosarcoma

Most vaginal smooth muscle neoplasms are either benign or only locally aggressive. If a vaginal smooth muscle neoplasm has 5 or more mitoses per 10 high-power fields and at least moderate atypia, it should be designated as a leiomyosarcoma (25). Prognosis has been correlated with degree of atypia, mitotic rate, and infiltrativeness of borders. Surgery is usually the primary therapy (5).

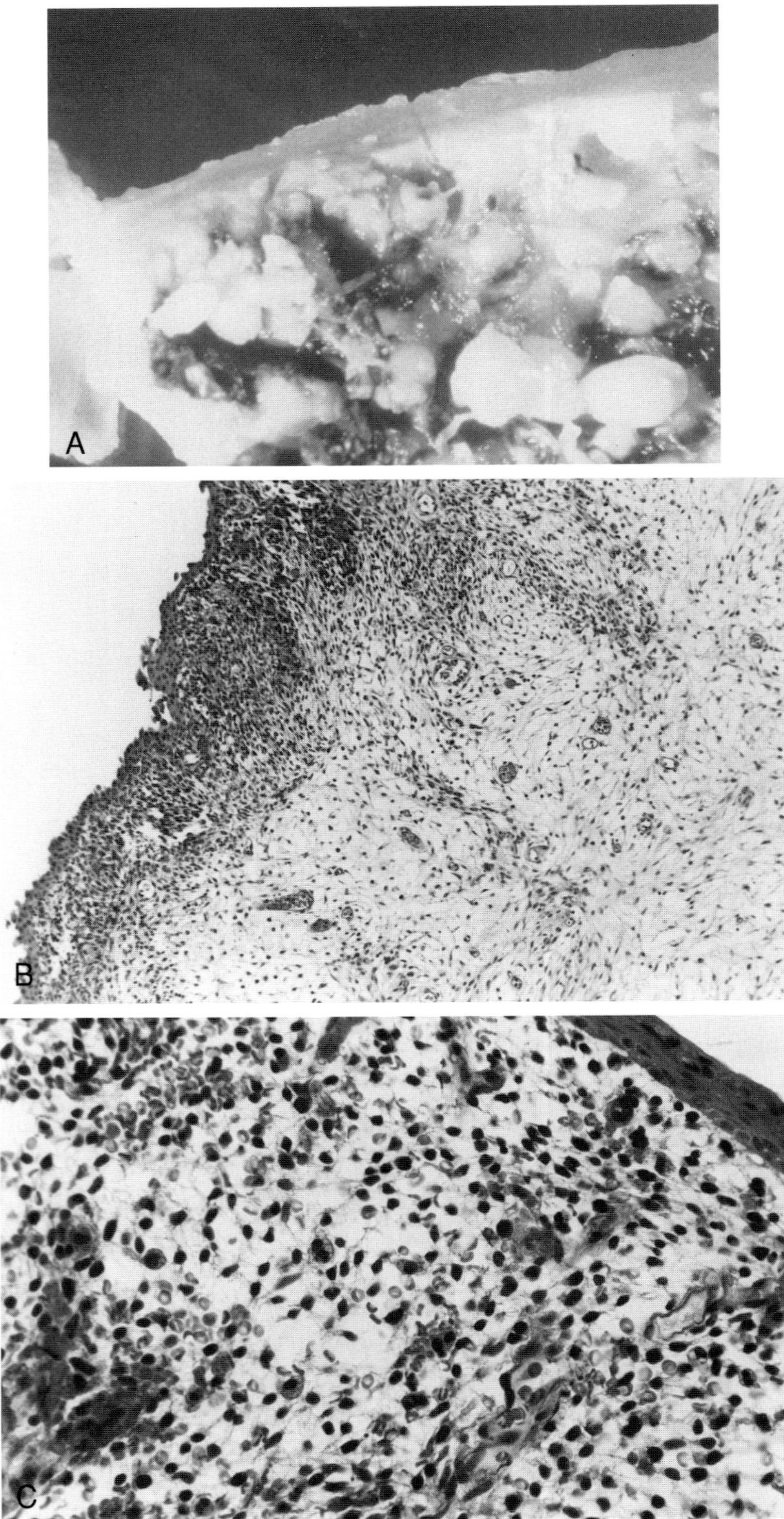

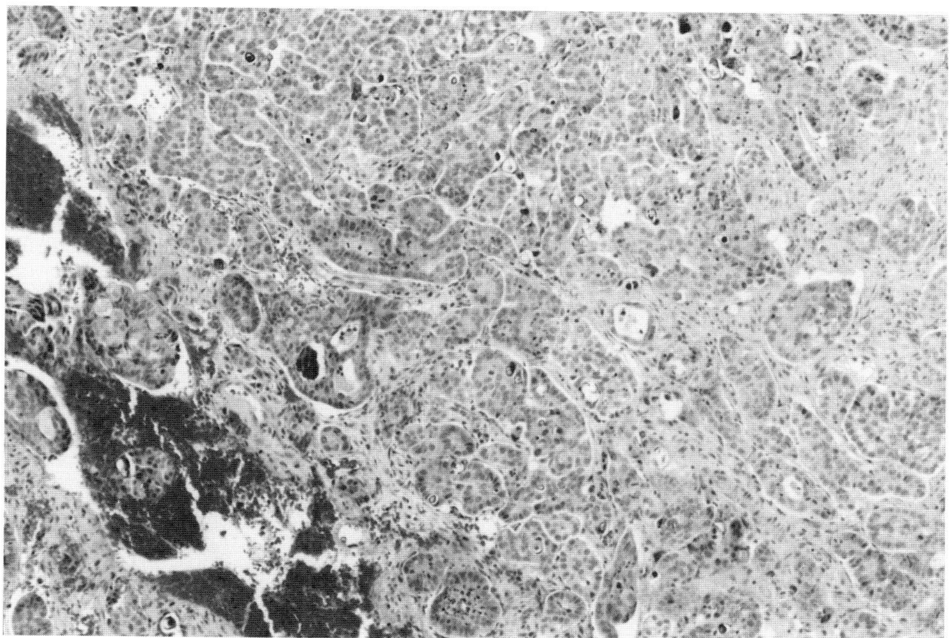

FIGURE 7.12.   Metastatic ovarian carcinoma to vaginal vault. The tumor is a papillary adenocarcinoma, consistent with this patient's previous history of papillary serous cystadenocarcinoma of the ovary.

Other Sarcomas

Vaginal sarcomas are extremely rare. A 20-year retrospective review at Memorial Sloan Kettering in New York City (26) yielded only 15 cases. Of these, there were eight leiomyosarcomas, two angiosarcomas, one adenosarcoma and four "others." Primary treatment consisted of surgery, with adjuvant chemotherapy for high-grade tumors. Grade was the most important predictor of outcome.

METASTATIC DISEASE

The vagina is a common site of metastases from both extragenital and genital primaries (27). The most common lesions metastasizing to the vagina originate in the cervix, endometrium, colon and rectum, ovary, vulva, and urinary tract (5) (Fig. 7.12).

FIGURE 7.11.   Sarcoma botryoides. **A.** This example of sarcoma botryoides, arising in the bladder, shows the polypoid nature of the lesion. **B.** Low-power view showing the cambium layer of tumor cells condensing under the surface epithelium. **C.** The tumor is composed of spindle cells in a loose stroma. Overlying squamous epithelium is unremarkable.

REFERENCES

1. Wright VC, Chapman W. Intraepithelial neoplasia of the lower female genital tract: etiology, investigation, and management. Semin Surg Oncol 1992;8:180–190.
2. Robboy SR, Welch WR. Selected topics in the pathology of the vagina. Hum Pathol 1991; 22:868–876.
3. Audet-Lapointe P, Body G, Vauclair R et al. Vaginal intraepithelial neoplasia [review] Gynecol Oncol 1990;36:232–239.
4. Aho M, Vesterinen E, Meyer B, et al. Natural history of vaginal intraepithelial neoplasia. Cancer 1991;68:195–197.
5. Zaino RJ, Robboy SJ, Bentley R, Kurman RJ. Diseases of the vagina. In: Kurman, RJ, ed. Blaustein's Pathology of the Female Genital Tract. 4th edition. New York: Springer-Verlag, 1994:131–183.
6. Clement PB, Benedet JL. Adenocarcinoma in situ of the vagina: a case report. Cancer 1979;43:2479–2485.
7. Cullimore JE, Leusley DM, Rollason TP, et al. A case of glandular intraepithelial neoplasia involving the cervix and vagina. Gynecol Oncol 1989;34:249–252.
8. Reinecke L, Thornley AL. Case report: radiotherapy–an effective treatment for vaginal verrucous carcinoma [review]. Br J Radiol 1993;66:375–378.
9. Merino MJ. Vaginal cancer: the role of infectious and environmental factors [review]. Am J Obstet Gynecol 1001;165(4pt2):1255–1262.
10. Manetta A, Gutrecht EL, Berman ML, et al. Primary invasive carcinoma of the vagina. Obstet Gynecol 1990;76:639–642.
11. Dixit S, Singhal S, Baboo HA. Squamous cell carcinoma of the vagina: a review of 70 cases. Gyncol Oncol 1993;48:80–87.
12. Peters WA, III, Kumar NB, Morley GW. Microinvasive carcinoma of the vagina: a distinct clinical entity? Am J Obstet Gynecol 1985;153:505–507.
13. Herbst AL, Anderson D. Clear cell adenocarcinoma of the vagina and cervix secondary to intrauterine exposure to diethylstilbestrol. Semin Surg Oncol 1990;6:343–346.
14. Hanselaar AG, Van Leusen ND, De Wilde PC, et al. Clear cell adenocarcinoma of the vagina and cervix: a report of the Central Netherlands Registry with emphasis on early detection and prognosis. Cancer 1991;67:1971–1978.
15. Robboy SJ, Scully RE, Welch WR et al. Intrauterine diethylstilbestrol exposure and its consequences. Pathologic characteristics of vaginal adenosis, clear cell adenocarcinoma, and related lesions. Arch Pathol Lab Med 1977;101:1–5.
16. Haskel S, Chen SS, Spiegel G. Vaginal endometrioid adenocarcinoma arising in vaginal endometriosis: a case report and literature review [review]. Gynecol Oncol 1989;34: 232–236.
17. Baltzer J, Zander J. Primary squamous cell carcinoma of the neovagina [review]. Gyncol Oncol 1989;35:99–103.
18. Ursic-Vrscaj M, Lindtner J, Lamovec J, et al. Adenocarcinoma in a sigmoid neovagina 22 years after Wertheim-Meigs operation. Case report. Eur J Gynaecol Oncol 1994;15;24–28.
19. Heller DS, Moomjy M, Koulos J, et al. Vulvar and vaginal melanoma. A clinicopathologic study. J Reprod Med 1994;39:945–948.
20. Borazjani G, Prem KA, Okagaki T, et al. Primary malignant melanoma of the vagina: a clinicopathological analysis of 10 cases. Gynecol Oncol 1990;37:264–267.
21. Hays DM, Shimada H, Raney RB Jr., et al. Clinical staging and treatment results in rhabdomyosarcoma of the female genital tract among children and adolescents [review]. Cancer 1988;61:1893–1903.
22. Andrassy RJ, Hays DM, Raney RB, et al. Conservative surgical management of vaginal and vulvar pediatric rhabdomyosarcoma: a report from The Intergroup Rhabdomyosarcoma Study III. J Ped Surg 1995;30:1034–1036.
23. Maurer HM, Moon T, Donaldson M, et al. The Intergroup Rhabdomyosarcoma Study: a preliminary report. Cancer 1977;40:2015–2026.

24. Rodary C, Flamant F, Donaldson SS. An attempt to use a common staging system in rhabdomyosarcoma: a report of an international workshop initiated by the International Society of Pediatric Oncologists (SIOP). Med Ped Oncol 1989;17:210–215.
25. Tavassoli FA, Norris HJ. Smooth muscle tumors of the vagina. Obstet Gynecol 1979;53: 689–693.
26. Curtin JP, Saigo P, Slucher B, et al. Soft tissue sarcoma of the vagina and vulva: a clinicopathological study. Obstet Gynecol 1995;86:269–272.
27. Mazur MT, Hsueh S, Gersell DJ. Metastases to the female genital tract. Analysis of 325 cases. Cancer 1984;53:1978–1984.

8

BENIGN DISEASES OF THE CERVIX

Debra S. Heller, MD

■

Normal Histology
Physiologic Changes of the Squamous Epithelium
Congenital Anomalies
Infections
Lesions That May Be Mistaken for Squamous Neoplasia
Lesions That May Be Mistaken for Glandular Neoplasia
Benign Tumors and Tumor-like Lesions

NORMAL HISTOLOGY

The cervix is an epithelial-lined structure with a fibromuscular stroma. The portion of the cervix protruding into the vagina is called the ectocervix, or portio vaginalis. The central opening, the external os, is small and round in the nulliparous woman, but becomes larger and slit-shaped in the parous one. The ectocervix is lined in continuity with the vagina by stratified squamous epithelium, which is nonkeratinized under normal circumstances. The endocervical canal is lined by endocervical mucosa, a single layer of mucinous columnar epithelium. The endocervical mucosa invaginates into the cervical stroma where it is arranged in complex crypts and folds appearing as glandular structures on histological sections. The point where the squamous mucosa meets the glandular mucosa is the squamocolumnar junction (SCJ). The SCJ shifts over the course of a woman's life. The original squamocolumnar junction is often located on the portio vaginalis. This leads to endocervical mucosa, which is red and granular in appearance, being visible to the examining eye. This has been mistakenly called cervical erosion although ectropion is a more accurate term.

During the course of reproductive life, the new squamocolumnar junction migrates up the endocervical canal and is often well up the canal by the time a woman reaches menopause. This shifting of the SCJ is secondary to cervical repair by squamous metaplasia, which is usually present in the area between the original squamocolumnar junction and the new squamocolumnar junction. This zone between the original and new squamocolumnar junctions, lying between the mature squamous epithelium of the ectocervix and the endocervical mucosa, is called the transformation zone or T-zone (Fig. 8.1).

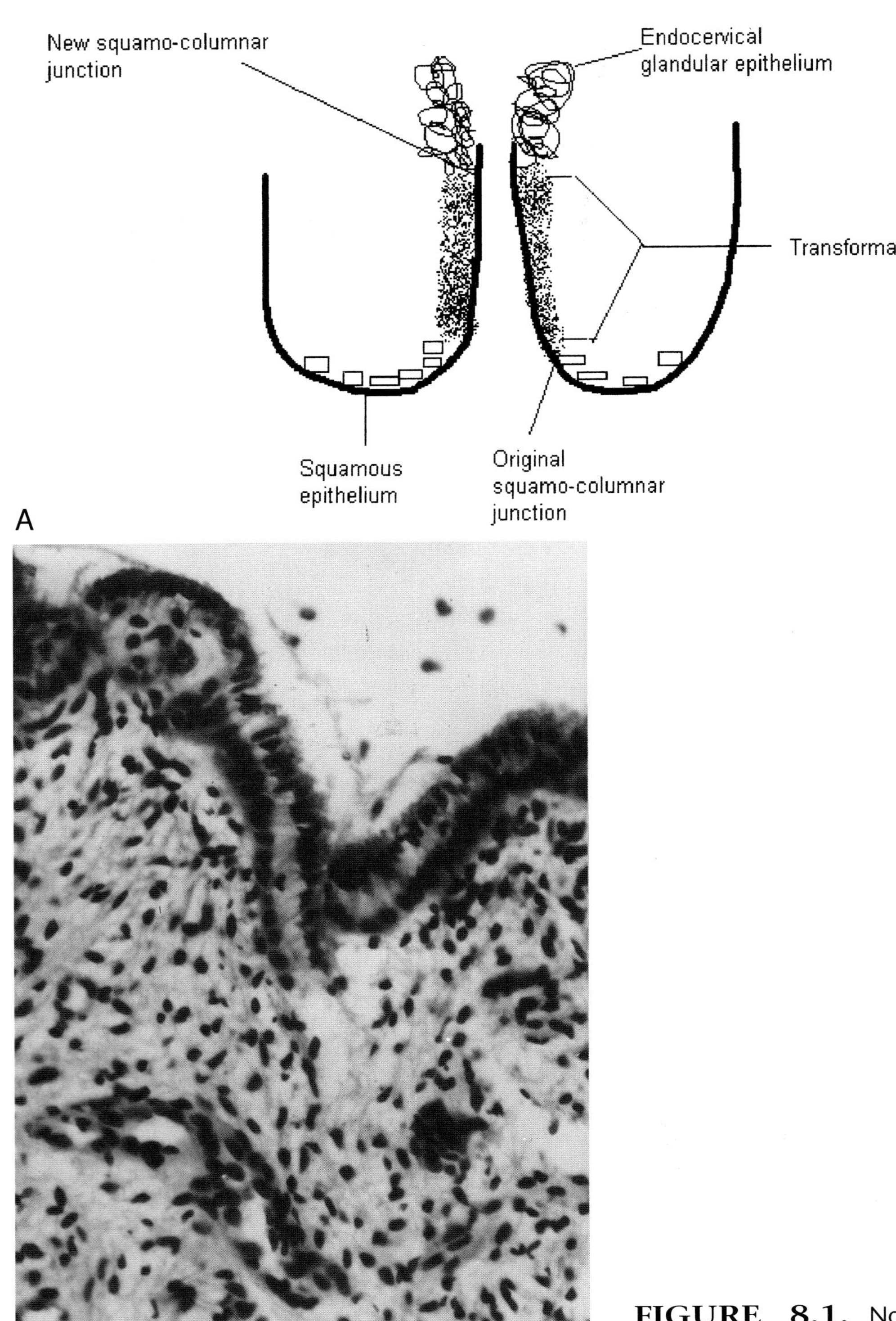

FIGURE 8.1. Normal cervix. **A.** Transformation zone. **B.** Reserve cell hyperplasia.

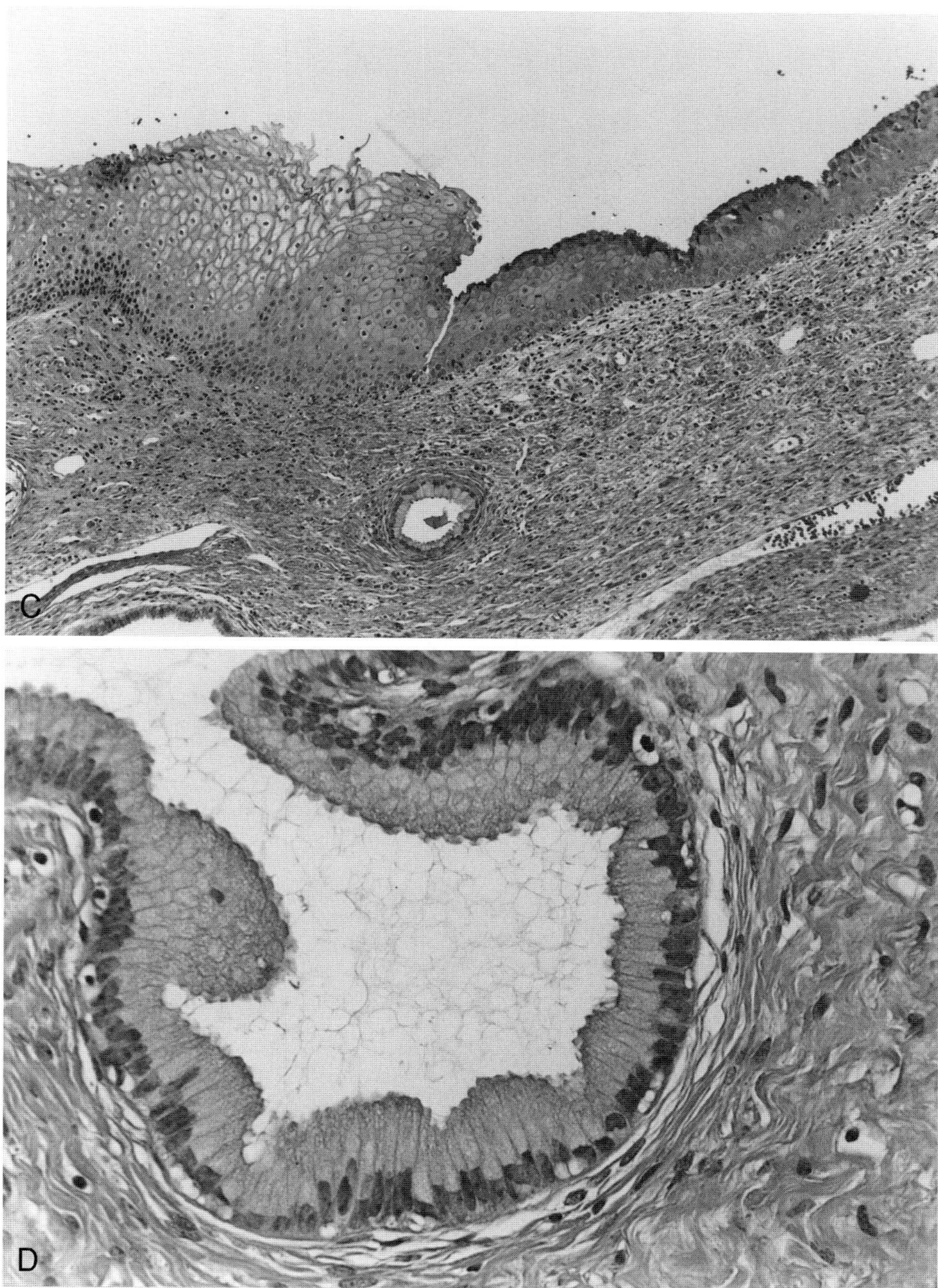

FIGURE 8.1. *(continued)* **C.** Transformation zone. Mature squamous epithelium meets metaplastic squamous epithelium at the site of the original squamocolumnar junction. **D.** normal endocervical gland, lined by single layer of mucinous epithelium. *(figure continues)*

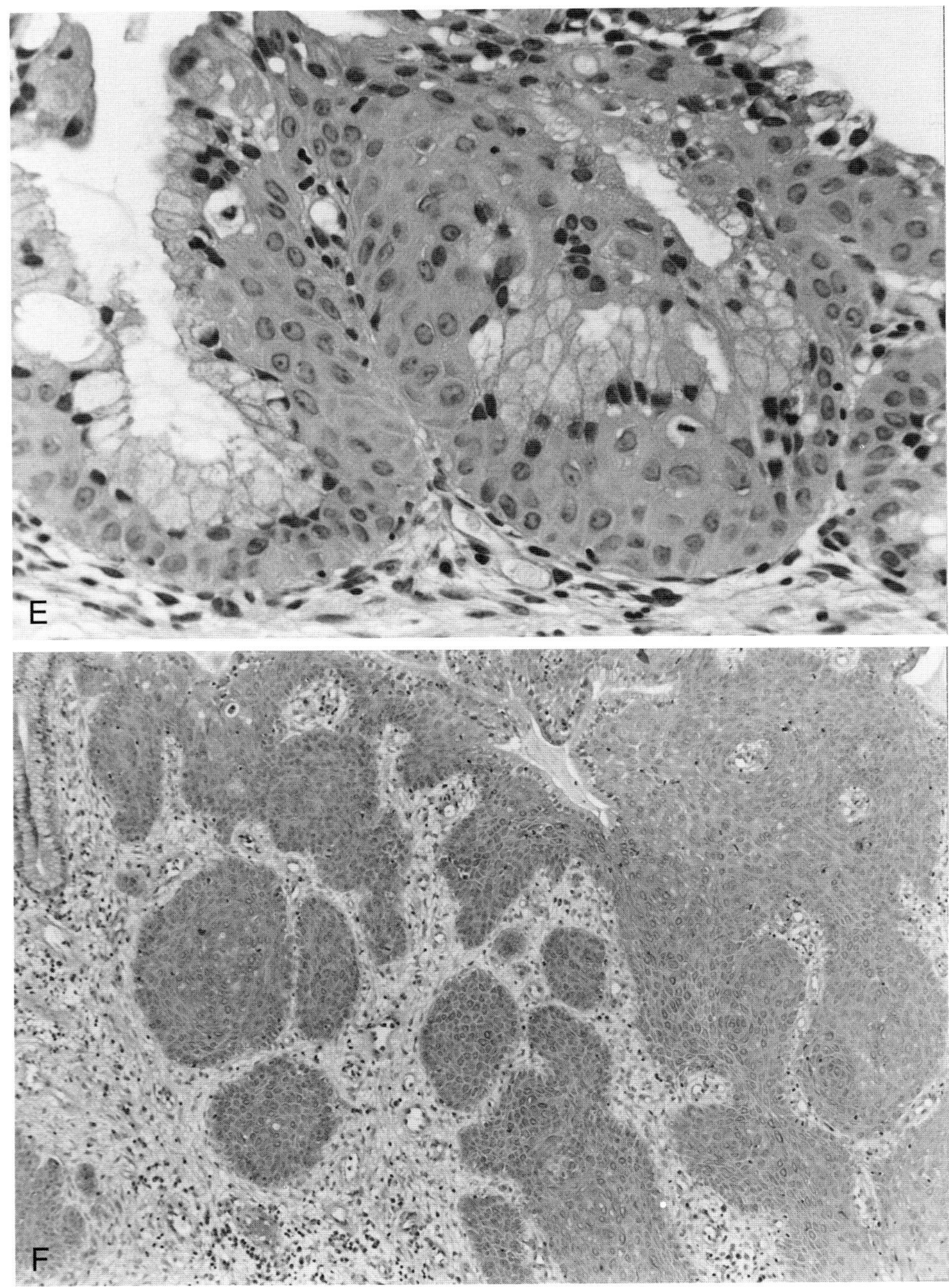

FIGURE 8.1. *(continued)* **E.** Squamous metaplasia of endocervical glands in the transformation zone. **F.** Florid squamous metaplasia of endocervical glands.

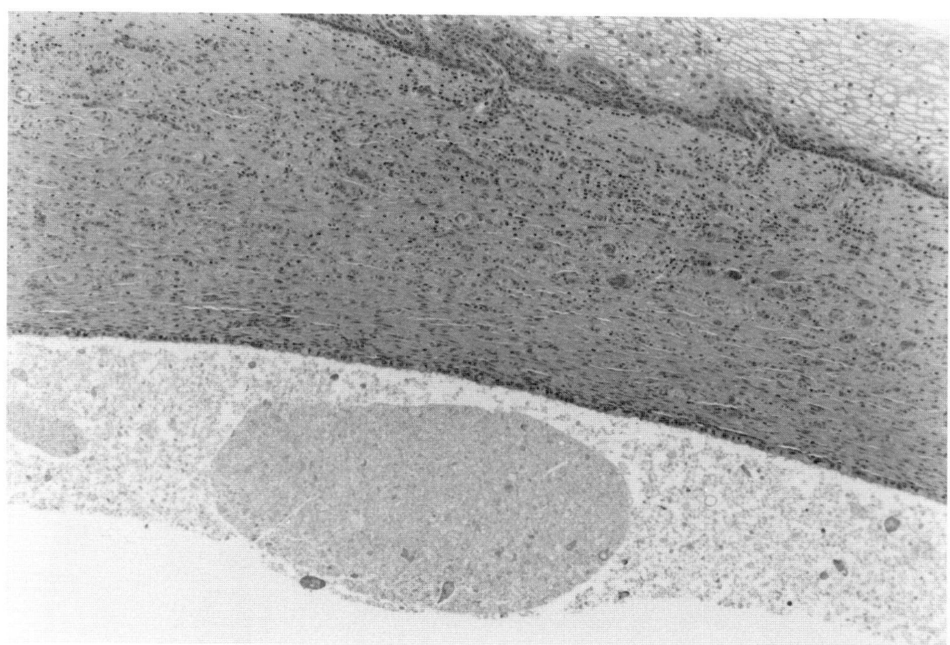

FIGURE 8.2. Nabothian cyst. Inspissated secretions are present in a cystically dilated endocervical gland lined by cuboidal epithelium.

This region is important because most squamous neoplasms arise there. In clinical practice, the transformation zone must be visualized during colposcopy for the examination to be considered adequate. If a cervical biopsy does not include the T-zone, meaning no metaplastic squamous epithelium or endocervical epithelium is present, even if the biopsy is negative, one cannot conclude that no lesion is present in the T-zone. Squamous metaplasia undergoes stages of maturation, beginning with reserve cell hyperplasia (Fig. 8.1B), progressing through immature metaplasia (Fig. 8.1C), and finally reaching mature squamous metaplasia. Reserve cell hyperplasia consists of a single layer of cuboidal epithelium under the endocervical epithelium. Immature squamous metaplasia shows well-demarcated cell borders, and the cells contain abundant eosinophilic cytoplasm. Glycogen is minimal, and residual endocervical mucinous cells may be present. Mature squamous metaplasia histologically is identical to ectocervical squamous epithelium. When endocervical glands become blocked as a result of the upward-growing squamous metaplasia, Nabothian cysts (Fig. 8.2) can occur. Lined by a flattened endocervical epithelium, these cysts contain inspissated secretions. The metaplastic epithelium covers the surface of the endocervical canal as it migrates and also replaces the columnar mucinous epithelium of the endocervical glands, leaving round aggregates of metaplastic squamous epithelium in its place (Fig. 8.1F). When squamous intraepithelial lesions (SIL) involve these endocervical glands replaced by squamous metaplastic epithelium, the round contour and lack of stromal reaction helps distinguish the process from an invasive one.

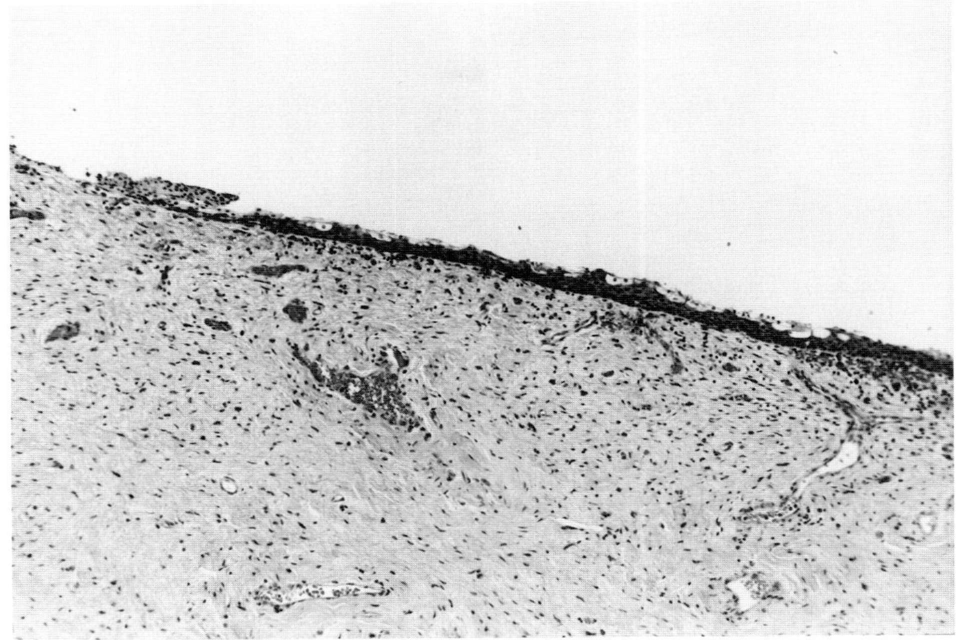

FIGURE 8.3. Atrophy. Lack of maturation is present, but the cell arrangement is orderly and there is lack of mitotic activity and atypia.

PHYSIOLOGIC CHANGES OF THE SQUAMOUS EPITHELIUM

The normal squamous epithelium of the cervix during reproductive life is well glycogenated, and it matures toward the surface in distinctive layers, the parabasal, intermediate, and superficial layers, which are best appreciated on cytology. In menopause, the absence of hormonal stimulation often leads to atrophy (Fig. 8.3), in which a monotonous population of small cells with no maturation exists. This should not be confused with SIL, which shows disorderly cell arrangements and nuclear atypia not seen in atrophy.

Chronic irritation of the cervix, as in prolapse, can lead to epithelial hyperplasia, hyperkeratosis, and parakeratosis.

CONGENITAL ANOMALIES

Cervical duplication or atresia may occur in conjunction with other anomalies of the mullerian system. Intrauterine DES exposure has led to a variety of structural anomalies of the cervix, including hypoplastic cervix, pseudopolyps, cervical coxcomb, ridge, or hood.

INFECTIONS
SEXUALLY TRANSMITTED DISEASES

In a study by Kiviat and colleagues of mucopurulent cervicitis associated with known infection with *Chlamydia*, herpes, *Trichomonas,* or gonorrhea, the histologic findings included intraepithelial and luminal polymorphonuclear leukocytes, reactive endocervical cells, edema, subepithelial inflammation, granulation tissue, necrotic ulceration, focal loss of surface columnar cells, and spongiosis (1). Although no finding was entirely specific for a given infection, certain trends were found in this study. Follicular cervicitis (Fig. 8.4) was seen in 67% of cases of documented *Chlamydia* infection. Herpes infection

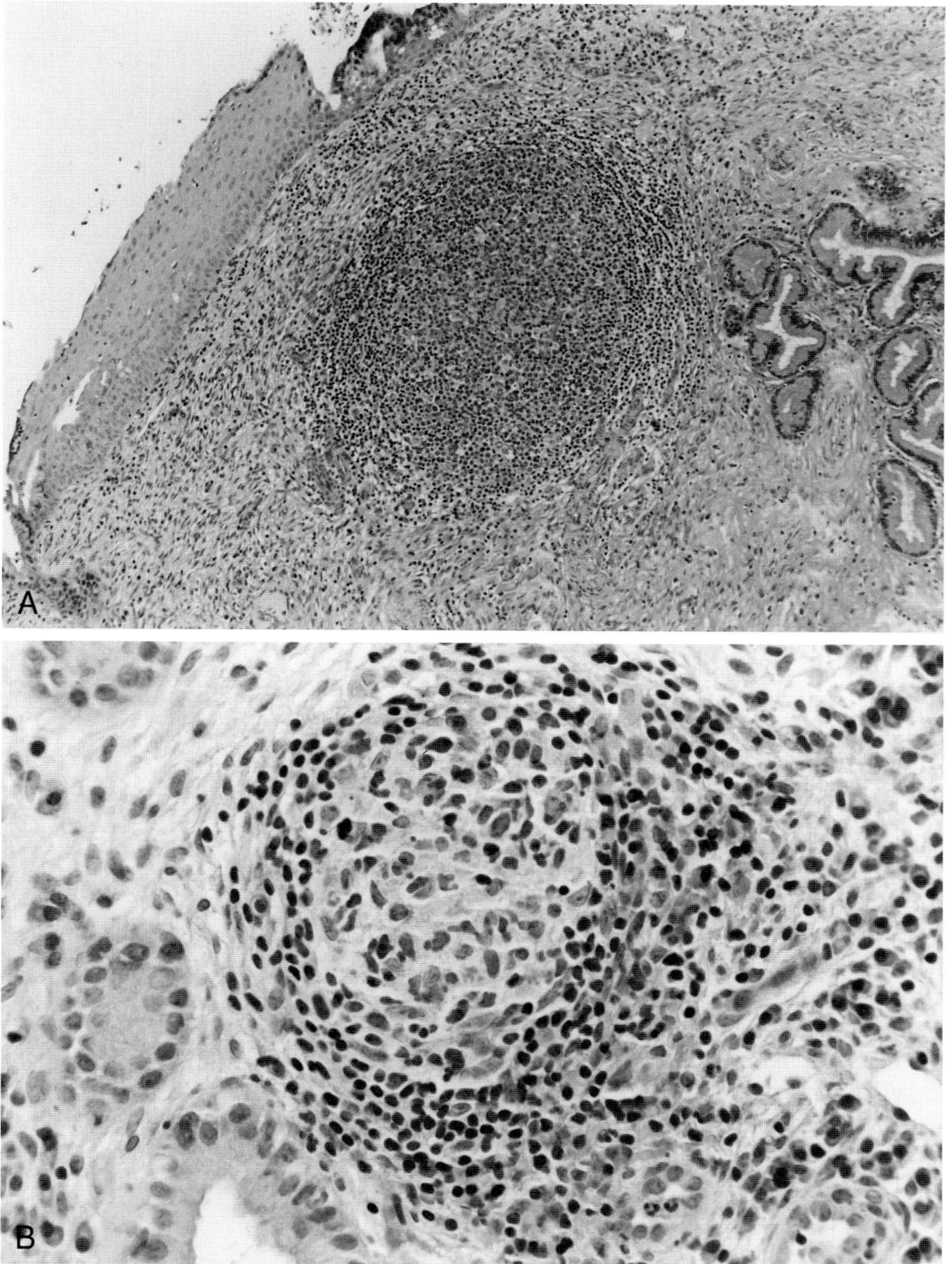

FIGURE 8.4 **A,B.** Follicular cervicitis. A well-developed follicle with a germinal center is present.

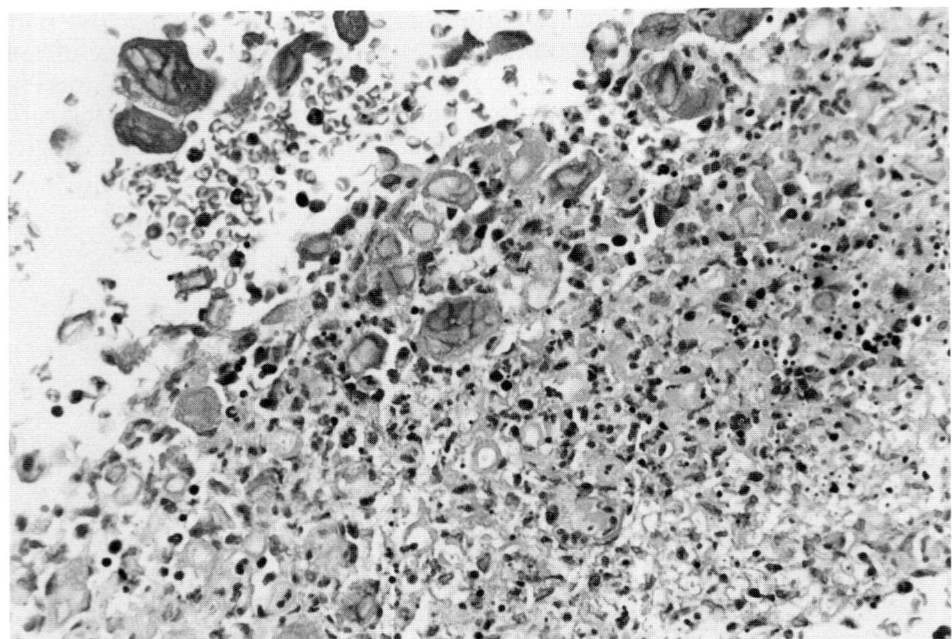

FIGURE 8.5.   Herpetic cervicitis. Characteristic viral inclusions are seen in this necrotic lesion.

was associated with necrotic ulcers with a lymphohistiocytic infiltrate, but the finding was nonspecific. Characteristic viral inclusions are sometimes seen in herpetic cervicitis (Fig. 8.5). Gonorrheal cervicitis was not associated with marked inflammatory changes but with focal loss of surface epithelium. Spongiosis was seen in some cases of *Trichomonas* infection. The authors recommend suspecting *Chlamydia* in cases of well-developed germinal centers, dense plasma cell infiltrate in the subepithelial zone, and undisturbed architecture; on the other hand, a disturbed architecture, necrotic ulcers, and a lymphohistocytic infiltrate suggest herpes infection.

OTHER INFECTIONS OF THE CERVIX

Actinomyces may colonize the cervix, and the typical sulphur granules may be seen on a Pap smear or endocervical curettage (Fig. 8.6A). Most of these women are intrauterine contraceptive device users. Genital tuberculosis may affect the cervix (Fig. 8.6B,C), but this is rare in the United States. Cervical involvement is common in endemic areas of schistosomiasis (Fig. 8.6D,E). Although some older studies have suggested an association with cervical carcinoma, not all studies support this conclusion (2).

LESIONS THAT MAY BE MISTAKEN FOR SQUAMOUS NEOPLASIA

ATROPHY

Although lack of maturation may suggest SIL, the disorderly cell arrangement, atypia, and mitotic activity of SIL is lacking in atrophy (Fig. 8.3).

POSTMENOPAUSAL SQUAMOUS ATYPIA

Jovanovic and colleagues (3) describe a lesion they call postmenopausal squamous atypia (PSA), which may be confused with koilocytosis due to perinuclear halos, nuclear hyperchromasia, nuclear size variability, and multinucleation. No HPV was detected in the 30 biopsies they analyzed. Distinction from koilocytosis may be made by noting less variation in nuclear size and staining intensity and finer, more evenly distributed chromatin. Perinuclear halos are also more uniform in PSA (Fig. 8.7).

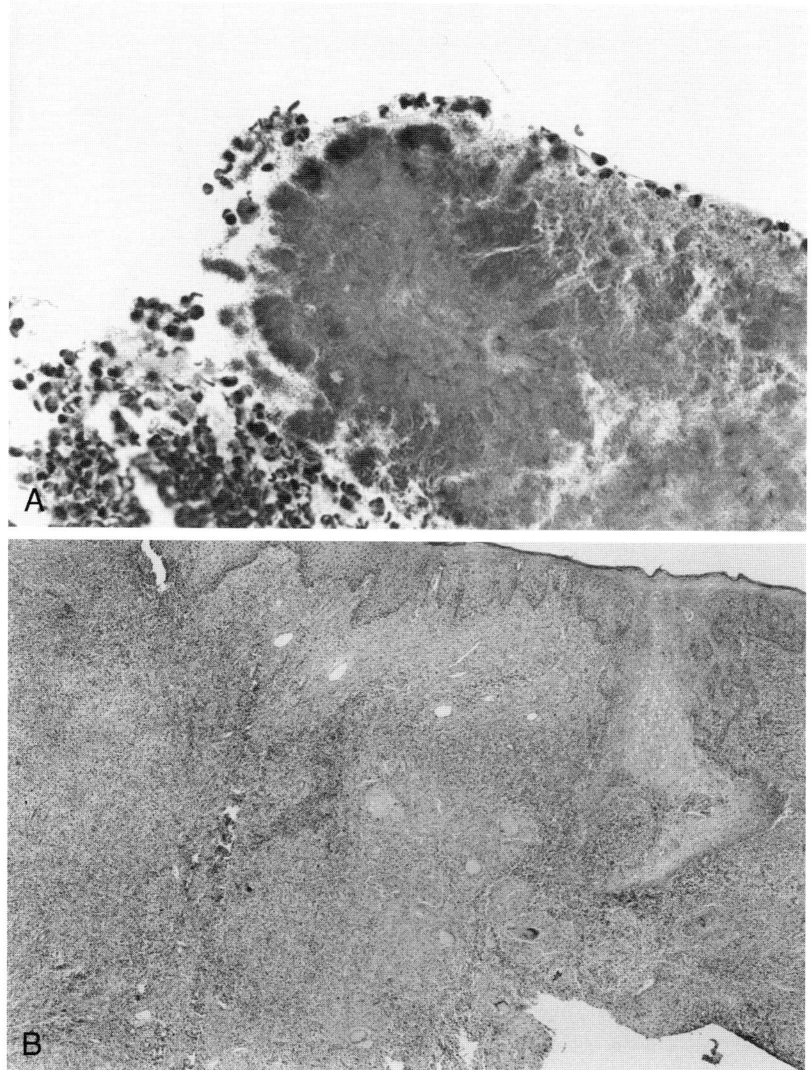

FIGURE 8.6.   **A.** Actinomyces colonization of the cervix. A typical colony of organisms, the sulphur granule, is present in this endocervical curettage specimen. **B,C.** Tuberculosis of the cervix. Granulomatous cervicitis secondary to genital tuberculosis is seen. **D,E.** Schistosomiasis. The organism elicits a granulomatous response. *(figure continues)*

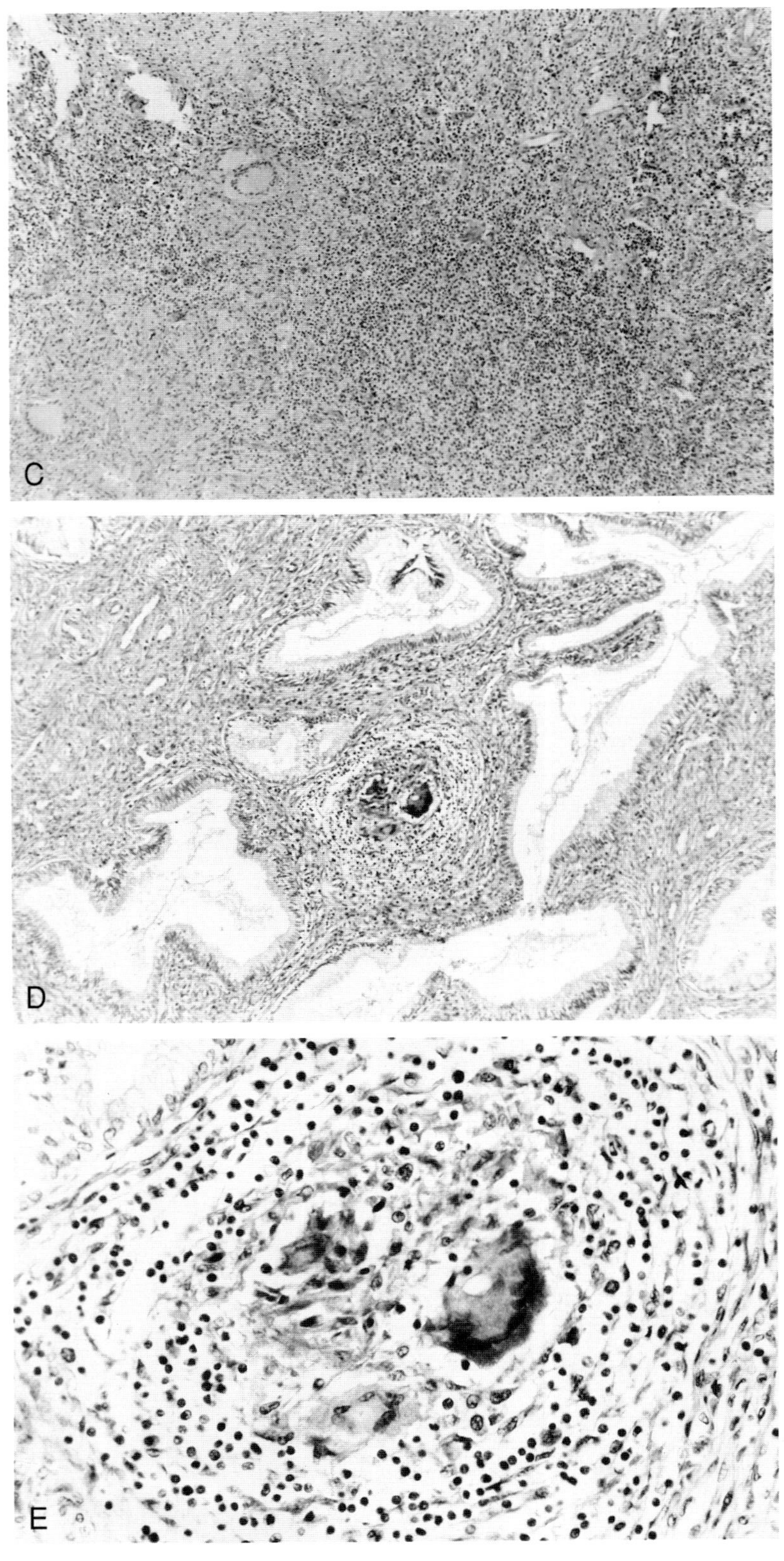

FIGURE 8.6 *(continued)*

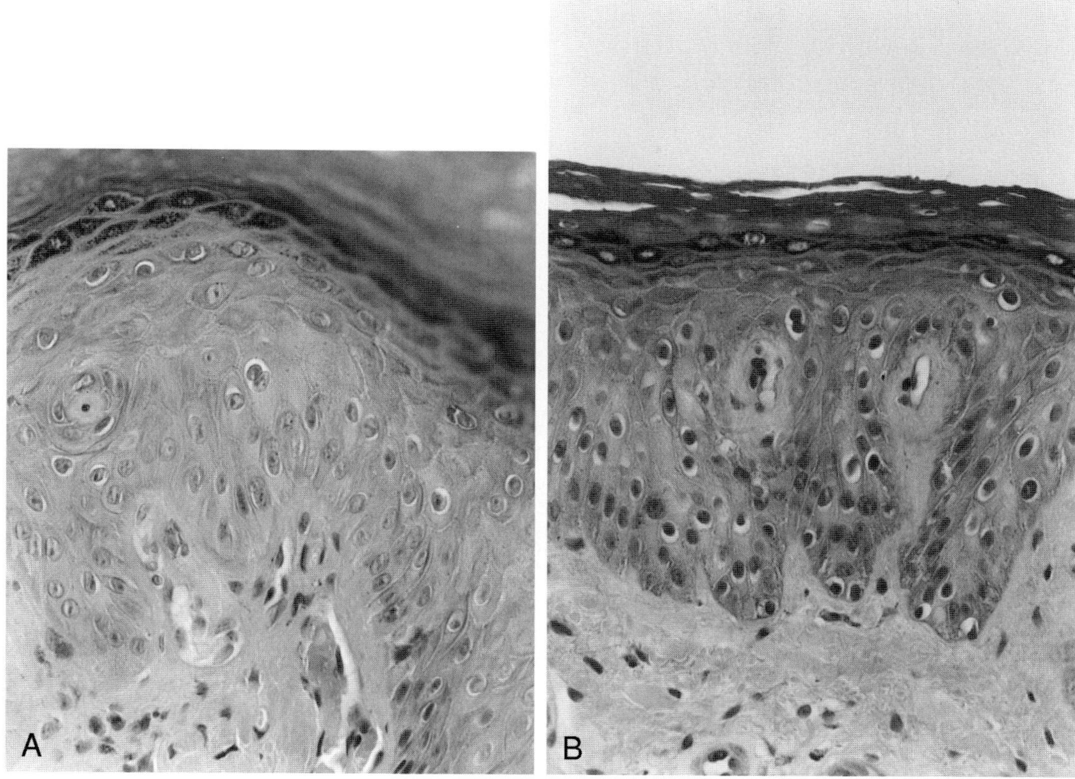

FIGURE 8.7.   Postmenopausal squamous atypia. **A,B.** Occasional multinucleated cells and perinuclear halos are seen. The atypia of koilocytosis is absent.

PSEUDOINVASION

McLachlin and colleagues (4) describe a case in which lymphvascular space involvement was mimicked after dysplastic squamous epithelium was pushed into vascular spaces with the needle used for local anesthetic administration.

SQUAMOUS METAPLASIA

Although extensive squamous metaplasia (Fig. 8.1f) may be associated with inflammatory cells, the lack of infiltration and atypia should distinguish the finding from a malignancy.

ATYPICAL SQUAMOUS METAPLASIA/REPAIR

Atypical squamous metaplasia has a low mitotic count; mitotic activity is usually confined to the lower third of the epithelium, and only occasionaly is superficial atypia or multinucleation present. Atypical squamous metaplasia can be distinguished from SIL

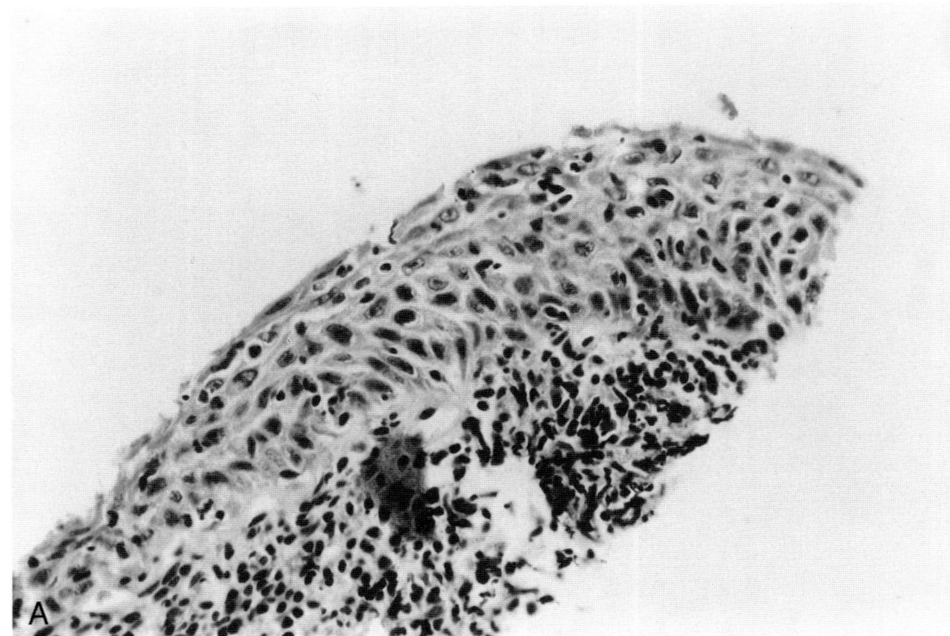

FIGURE 8.8. Repair. **A,B,C.** Examples of reparative atypia, with a marked chronic inflammatory background.

(squamous intraepithelial lesions) by its monotonous cell population, uniformity, minimal nuclear atypia, and scant mitotic activity (Fig. 8.8) (5).

TRANSITIONAL METAPLASIA

Transitional metaplasia is a not uncommon finding that may be mistaken for SIL. The cells of transitional metaplasia frequently contain the grooved nuclei seen in transitional epithelium but lack the atypia and mitotic activity of SIL.

PLACENTAL SITE NODULE

More often seen in the uterus, these lesions may occur in the cervix, and they are considered to be a subinvoluted implantation site. Eosinophilic nodules containing scattered atypical cells, which are intermediate trophoblasts, may be confused with a keratinizing squamous cell carcinoma. In a difficult case, positivity of human placental lactogen and placental alkaline phosphatase will confirm the trophoblastic nature of the placental site nodule (Fig. 8.9).

LESIONS THAT MAY BE MISTAKEN FOR GLANDULAR NEOPLASIA

PAPILLARY ENDOCERVICITIS

Papillary endocervicitis has a micropapillary configuration, which may lead it to be confused with the villoglandular variant of endocervical adenocarcinoma. The epithe-

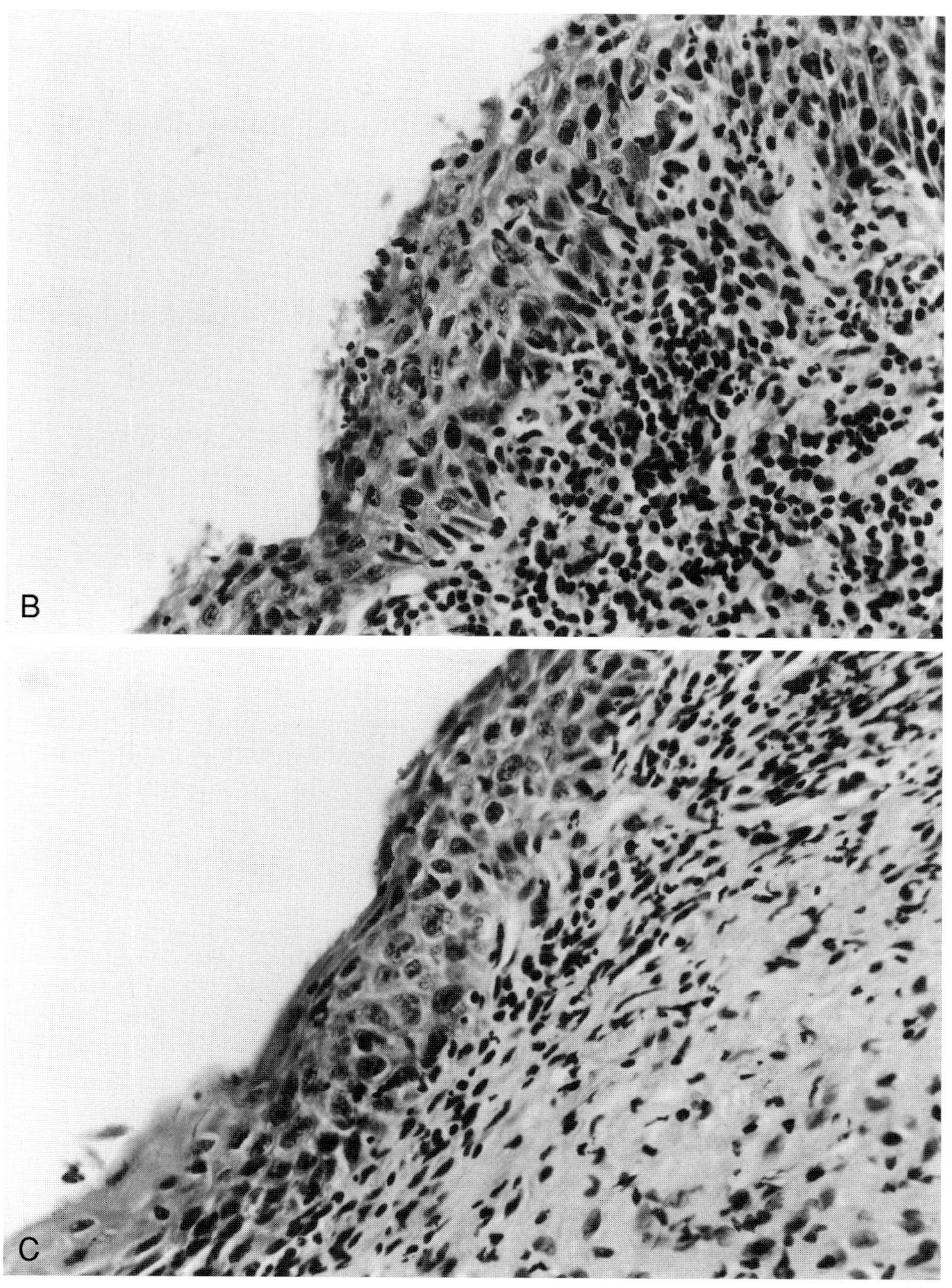

FIGURE 8.8. *(continued)*

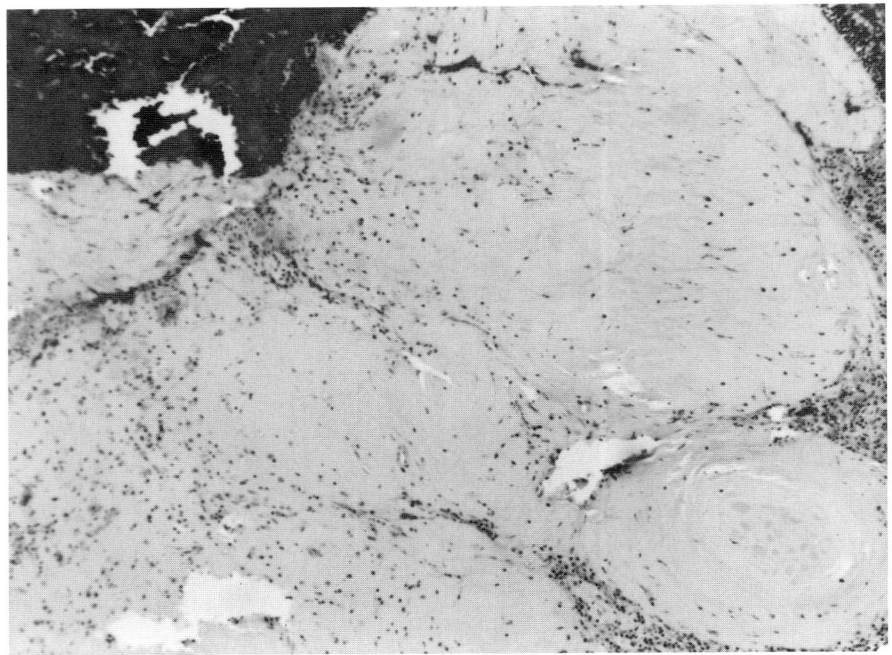

FIGURE 8.9. Placental site nodule. Hyalinized paucicellular nodules represent subinvoluted implantation sites.

lium in papillary endocervicitis is a single layer of benign endocervical epithelium, as opposed to the stratification and cytological atypia seen in villoglandular carcinoma. The underlying stroma of papillary endocervicitis contains chronic inflammatory cells (Fig. 8.10) (6).

TUNNEL CLUSTERS

Endocervical tunnel clusters are common incidental findings that may raise concern of malignancy when detected deep in the cervical stroma. The lesion is composed of clusters of tubular structures that may be cystically dilated and are lined by a flat-to-cuboidal epithelium (Fig. 8.11). Although mild cytologic atypia and occasional mitoses may be present, no infiltrating pattern nor desmoplastic response in tunnel clusters exists, thus distinguishing them from adenoma malignum (6). CEA may be focally positive on the lumenal surface of tunnel clusters but not staining the cytoplasm—as in some cases of AIS and invasive endocervical adenocarcinoma (7).

DEEP ENDOCERVICAL GLANDS

Endocervical glands and nabothian cysts may be found deep in the endocervical stroma, leading to a possible misdiagnosis of adenoma malignum. These deep glands do not exhibit the irregularities of size and shape, nor the infiltrative, atypical, or desmoplastic features seen at least focally in adenoma malignum (8). Daya and colleagues (9) found CEA was negative in two cases of deep endocervical glands.

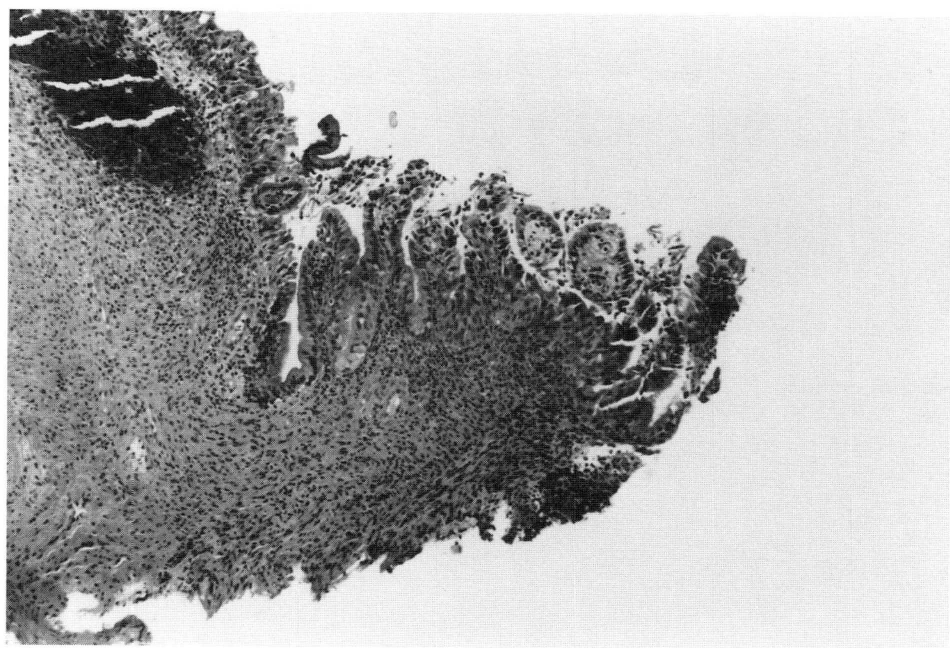

FIGURE 8.10.   Papillary endocervicitis. There is a papillary architecture and chronic inflammation. The lining is a single layer of normal endocervical cells.

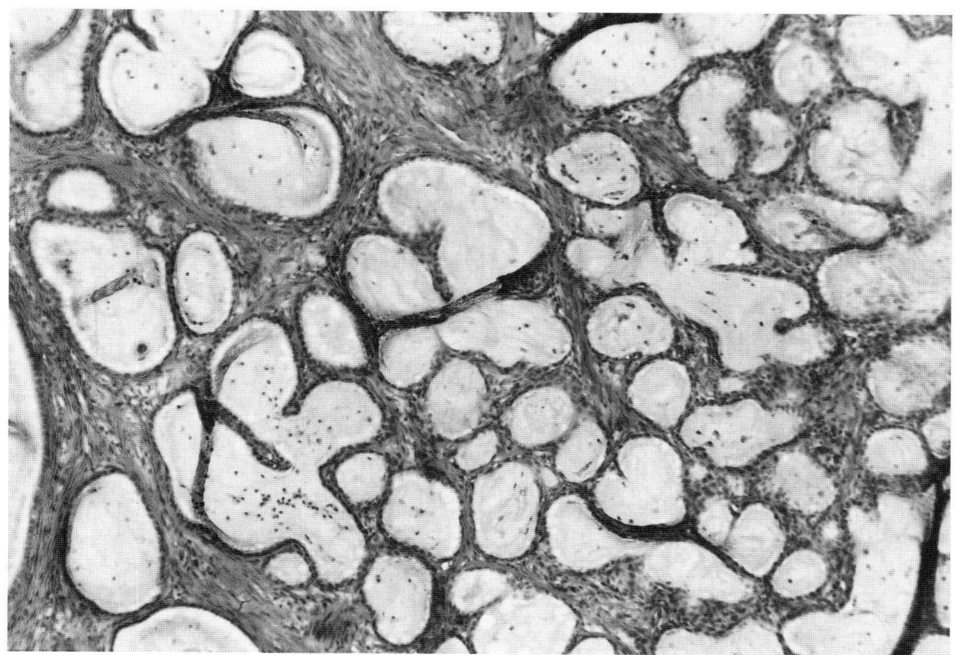

FIGURE 8.11.   Tunnel clusters. A cluster of dilated tubules lined by flattened epithelium and containing inspissated secretions is present.

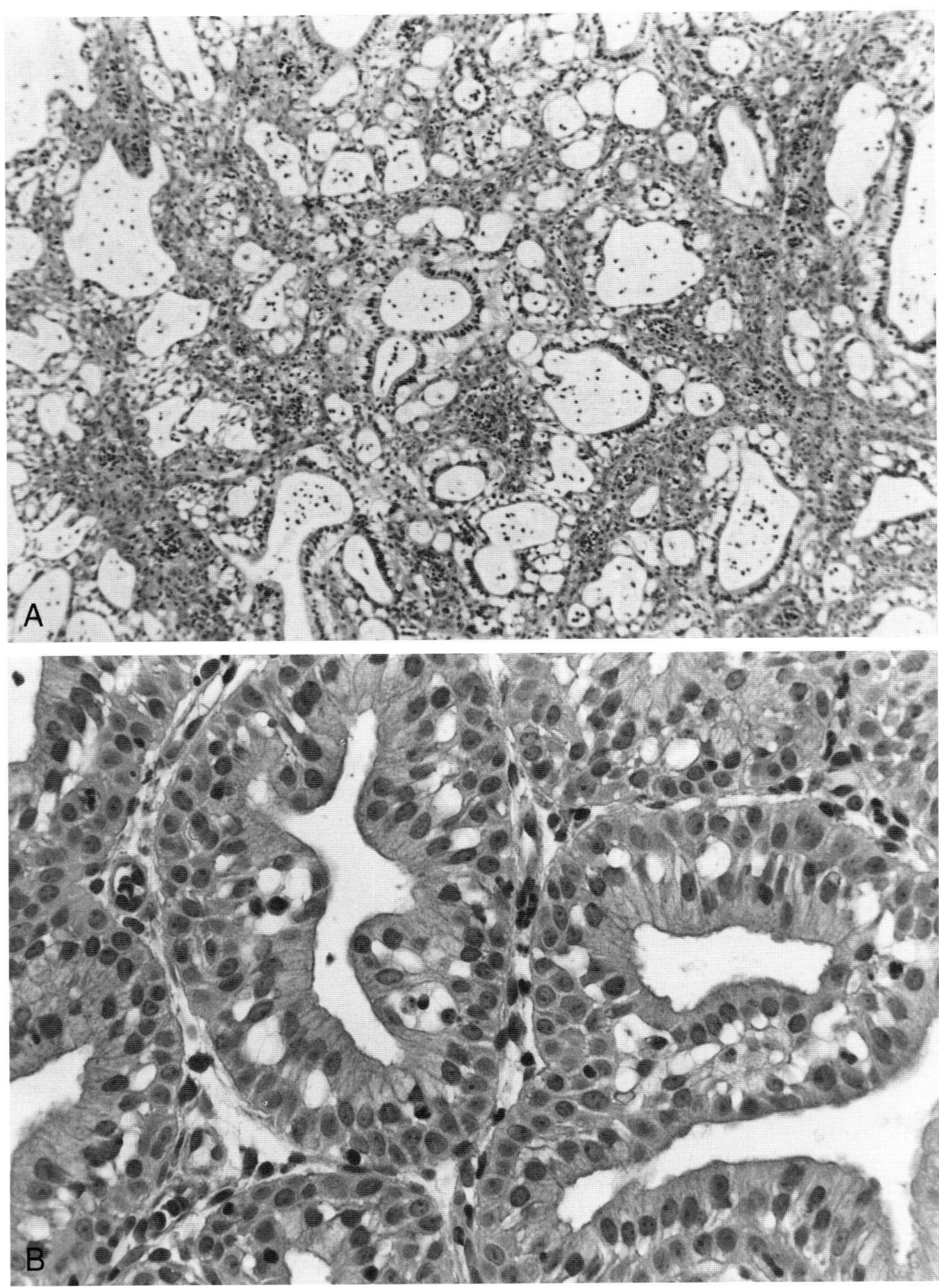

FIGURE 8.12. Microglandular hyperplasia. **A.** Crowded clusters of glands. **B.** Areas of clear cytoplasm should not be mistaken for clear cell carcinoma.

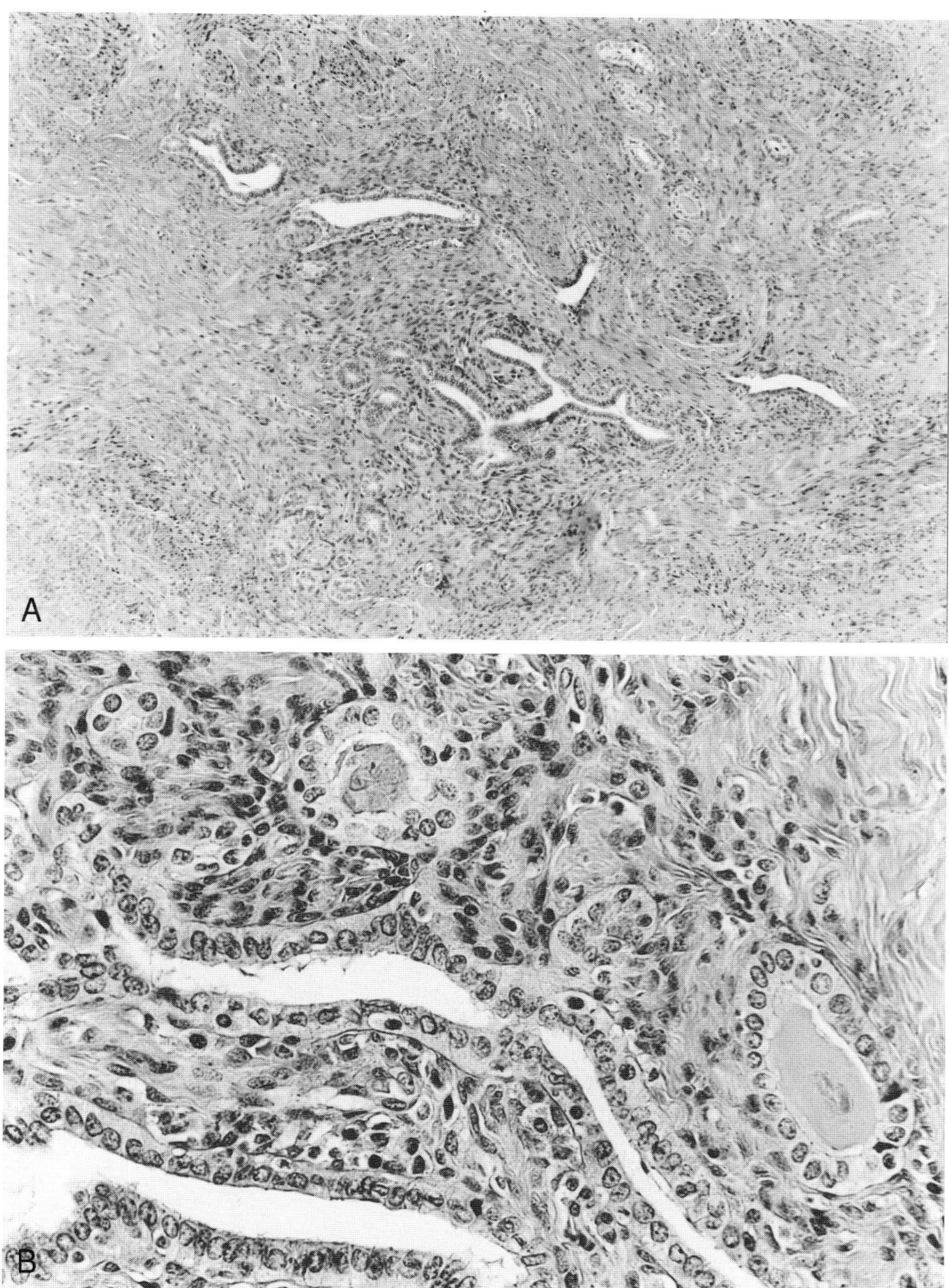

FIGURE 8.13. Mesothelial remnants. **A.** Remnants of the mesothelial duct and tubules are not uncommon. **B.** Mesothelial remnants lined by cuboidal epithelium. Tubules contain bright eosinophilic material.

MICROGLANDULAR HYPERPLASIA

Although it may be associated with bleeding or discharge, microglandular hyperplasia is often an incidental finding. The condition may be associated with progesterone exposure, particularly with oral contraceptive usage, and in some cases with pregnancy (Fig. 8.12). Histologically, the appearance of crowded glands may lead to a diagnosis of adenocarcinoma; however, the cells usually lack atypia, and mitotic activity is minimal or absent. Carcinoembryonic antigen is usually absent in microglandular hyperplasia and may be present in mucinous endocervical adenocarcinoma, but caution must be exercised here due to lack of consistency in these findings (6).

The most common type of cervical adenocarcinoma confused with microglandular hyperplasia is clear cell adenocarcinoma. This is due to the subnuclear vacuoles seen in microglandular hyperplasia. These vacuoles contain mucin, rather than glycogen, and no papillary areas are present in microglandular hyperplasia.

Uncommon atypical forms of microglandular hyperplasia may also be confused with carcinoma, but more typical areas should be searched for. Features of these atypical variants of microglandular hyperplasia include solid areas, pseudoinfiltration, stromal hyalinization, signet or hobnail cells, moderate atypia, and occasional mitoses (10).

MESONEPHRIC REMNANTS AND HYPERPLASIA

A not infrequent finding on hysterectomy specimens is mesonephric remnants, consisting of a main duct surrounded by dilated tubules lined by cuboidal or columnar epithelium, and often containing brightly staining PAS-positive eosinophilic material (Fig. 8.13). Less commonly seen is mesonephric hyperplasia (Fig. 8.14), which may be lobu-

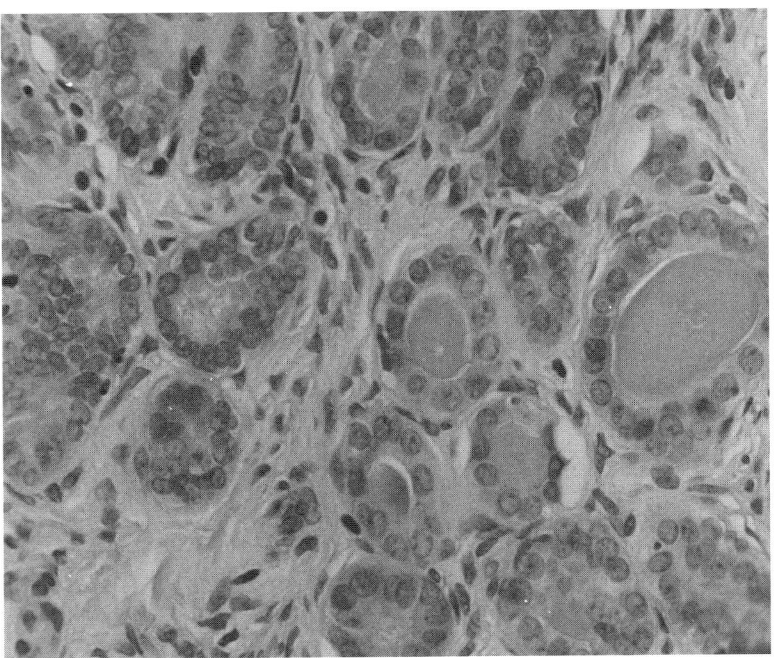

FIGURE 8.14. Mesothelial hyperplasia. An increased number of tubules exists, but intervening stroma is present.

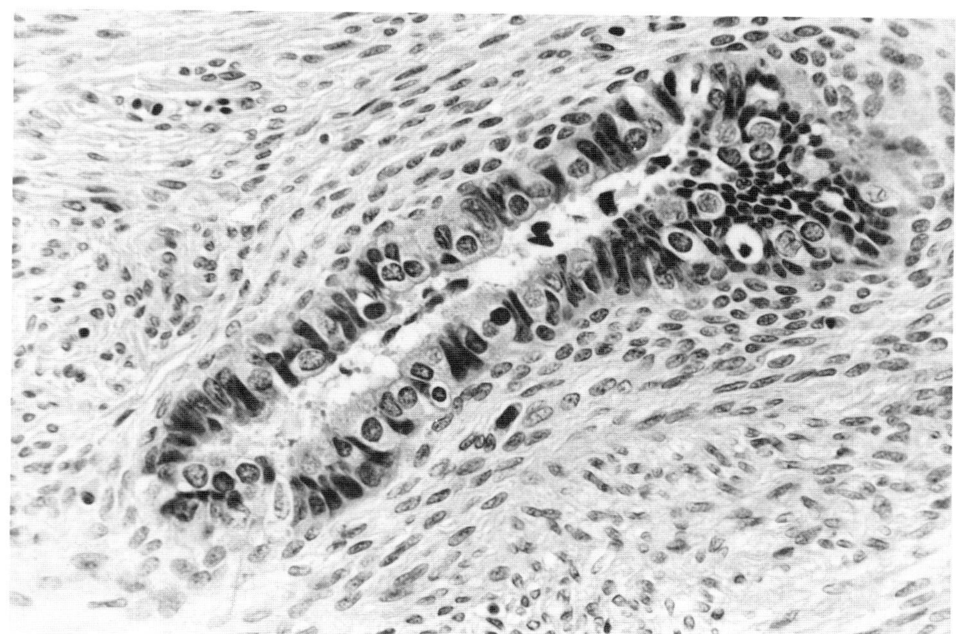

FIGURE 8.15. Tubal metaplasia of the endocervix. Cells resembling the lining of the fallopian tube are present.

lar, diffuse, or ductal. In cases of lobular mesonephric hyperplasia, larger lobules with less organization and more irregular shapes are present. Diffuse mesonephric hyperplasia consists of a diffuse proliferation of tubules. Mesonephric ductal hyperplasia shows papillary tufting within the duct. True mesonephric carcinomas are rare. Mesonephric hyperplasia lacks the back-to-back tubules, atypia, and invasiveness of a mesonephric carcinoma (11).

Although mild atypia and occasional mitoses may be present in mesonephric hyperplasia, there is not as much as in most clear cell carcinomas, with which the lesion may also be confused. In addition, clear cell carcinomas have cells with clear cytoplasm or a hobnail configuration. Mesonephric hyperplasia may be distinguished from adenoma malignum by the lack of gland irregularity in size and shape, absence of tall mucinous cells, and the lack of stromal reaction (6).

DIFFUSE LAMINAR ENDOCERVICAL GLANDULAR HYPERPLASIA

In this lesion, crowding of the endocervical glands confined to a band-like pattern in the upper third of the endocervical stroma occurs. Mild atypia and occasional mitoses may be present, and inflammation is frequent; however, no desmoplastic response exists as in adenoma malignum (12).

GLANDULAR HYPERPLASIA NOS (NOT OTHERWISE SPECIFIED)

Young and Clement (6) describe the occurrence of endocervical glandular hyperplasia that does not extend deep into the endocervical stroma and occurs in a lobular arrangement. The lack of stromal reaction and atypia distinguish this condition from adenocarcinoma.

TUBAL METAPLASIA

A common finding in the endocervical glands is tubal metaplasia (Fig. 8.15), which can be mistaken for endocervical dysplasia or adenocarcinoma in situ. The glandular architecture in tubal metaplasia is normal, and the epithelium consists of ciliated and nonciliated columnar and intercalary cells. Atypia and mitotic activity are absent, and CEA is negative in these areas (6).

LESS COMMON METAPLASIAS THAT MAY MIMIC GLANDULAR NEOPLASIA

Endometrioid metaplasia, usually admixed with tubal metaplasia, or ectopic endometrial glands may be seen in the cervical stroma. Intestinal metaplasia with goblet and argentaffin cells may be seen in association with cervical neoplasms, but this is an uncommon independent finding (6).

ENDOMETRIOSIS

Cervical endometriosis (Fig. 8.16) can be superficial or deep. A history of previous cervical surgery may or may not exist. Histologically, the presence of glands and stroma

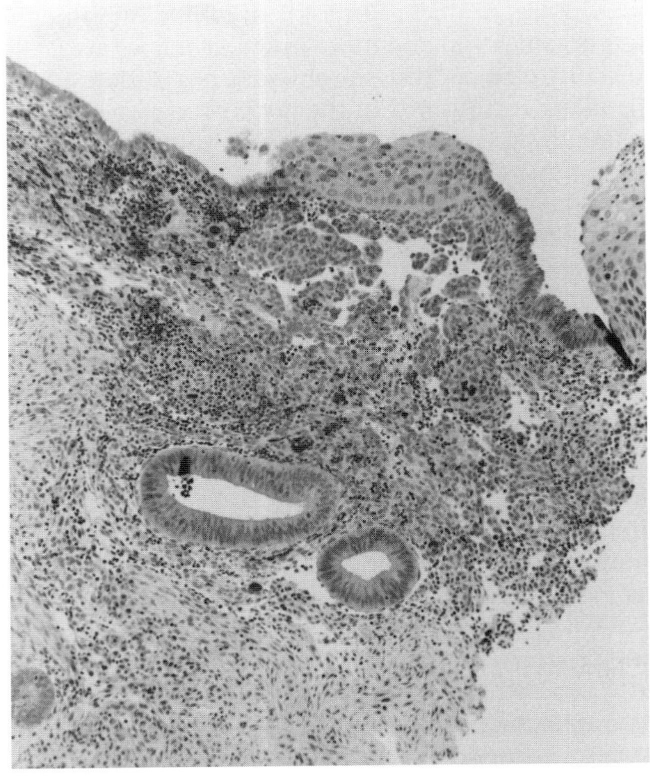

FIGURE 8.16. Endometriosis. Endometriosis is present, consisting of both glands and stroma, in this cervical biopsy. The overlying epithelium showed low-grade SIL in this case.

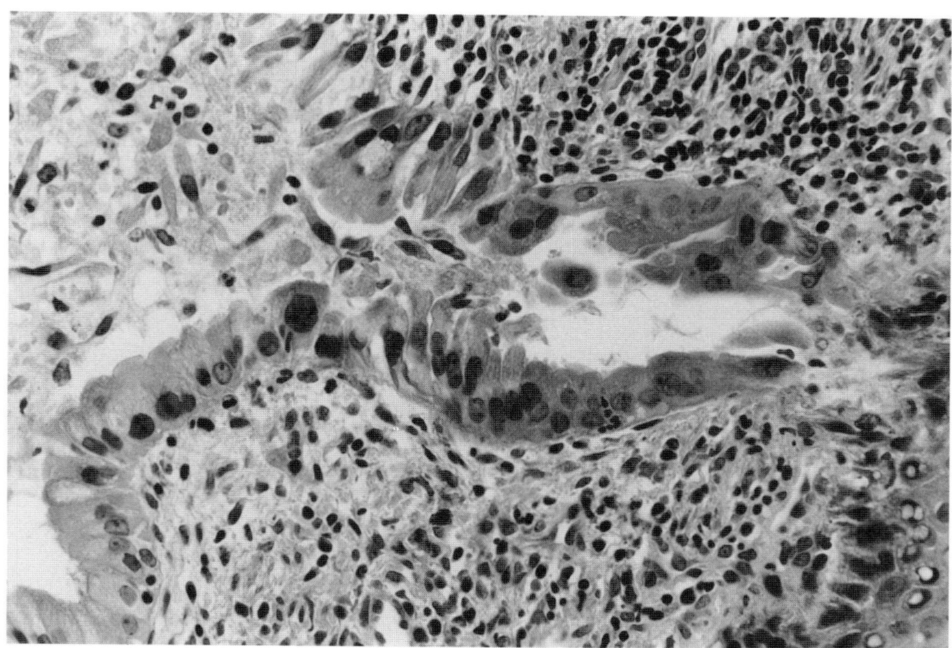

FIGURE 8.17.   Endocervical repair. Smudgy nuclei and scattered multinucleation is seen.

make the distinction relatively simple in most cases; however, cytologic interpretation may be a problem.

ARIAS-STELLA REACTION (ASR)

Although this pregnancy-related change is most often seen in the endometrium, it is not rare in the cervix. The cervical lesion is usually focal and does not cause a mass. The cells in ASR may be atypical, but minimal or no mitotic activity occurs. There is also no cellular stratification and a low nucleus-to-cytoplasmic (n/c) ratio in ASR. The finding of adjacent decidua may be helpful. This is in distinction to clear cell adenocarcinoma, the most likely lesion in the differential, where there are the additional findings of invasiveness, stratification, high n/c ratio as well as papillary, solid, and tubular patterns to help make the distinction. Also, in the absence of a history of in utero DES exposure, clear cell carcinoma of the cervix is less likely. Adenocarcinoma in situ (AIS) can be distinguished from ASR by its more consistent atypia and greater numbers of mitoses. AIS also lacks major cytoplasmic vacuolization, hobnail cells, and optically clear nuclei, which may be seen in ASR. ASR must be considered before diagnosing cervical adenocarcinoma in a pregnant patient (6).

RUPTURED ENDOCERVICAL GLAND

The tissue reaction provoked by a ruptured endocervical gland should not be confused with stromal response to an invasive adenocarcinoma.

CYTOMEGALOVIRUS INFECTION

The cytologic atypia may raise the concern of malignancy; however, single cell involvement in CMV infection exists, with characteristic inclusions (6).

RADIATION EFFECT

Radiation may lead to marked cytologic atypia, which can be confused with adenocarcinoma. In addition to lack of mitotic activity in radiation change, vascular and stromal changes may also be seen in areas treated with radiation.

REACTIVE ATYPIA

Reactive inflammatory atypia may also be present in endocervical glands. Smudgy enlarged single nuclei and multinucleation can be seen (Fig. 8.17).

BENIGN TUMORS AND TUMOR-LIKE LESIONS

A variety of benign tumors and tumor-like lesions (Fig. 8.18) can arise from the cervix, and they are histologically identical to these lesions arising elsewhere (Table 8.1).

ENDOCERVICAL POLYPS

Endocervical polyps are the most common polypoid lesion projecting from the cervix, and these represent hyperplasia rather than neoplasia. They may be asymptomatic, or

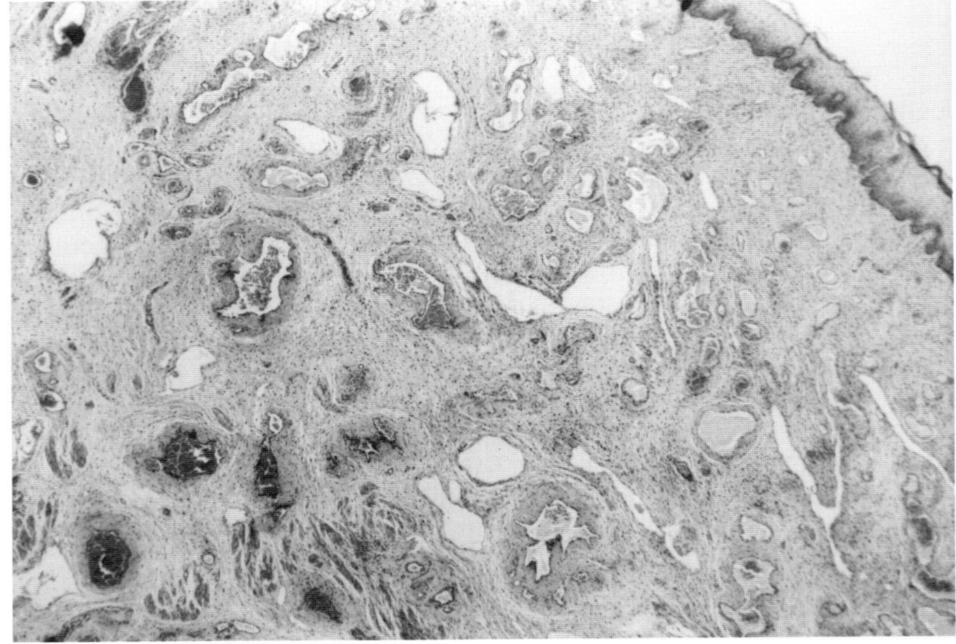

FIGURE 8.18. Hemangioma of the cervix, which grossly appeared as a purple lesion.

TABLE 8.1.   Uncommon Benign Neoplasms
and Tumor-like Lesions of the Cervix

Leiomyoma
Mullerian papilloma
Rhabdomyoma
Papillary adenofibroma
Adenomyoma of endocervical type
Hemangioma
Lipoma
Schwannoma
Ganglioneuroma
Neurofibroma
Granular cell tumor
Squamous papilloma
Blue nevus
Mature teratoma
Pseudosarcoma botryoides

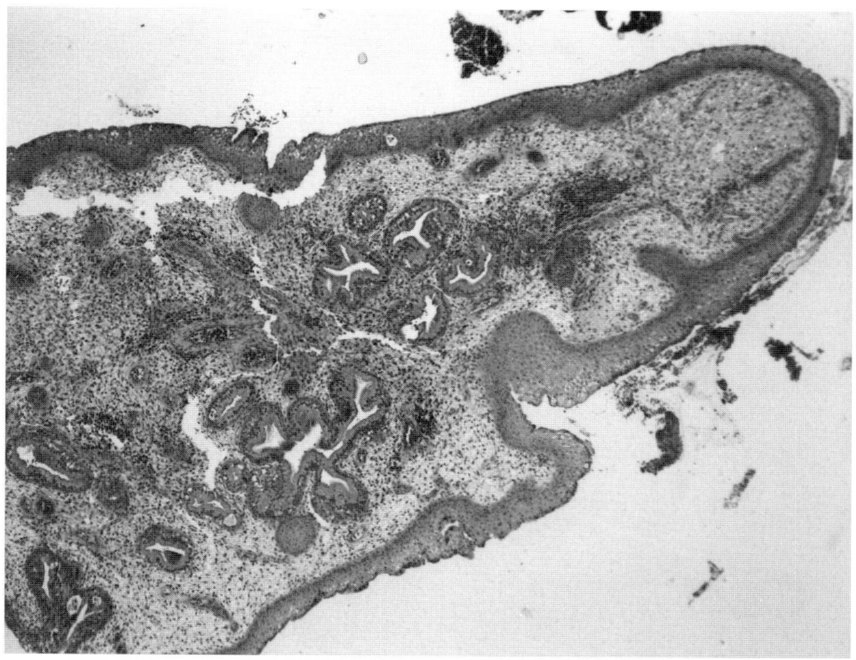

FIGURE 8.19.   Endocervical polyp containing endocervical glands and lined by metaplastic squamous epithelium.

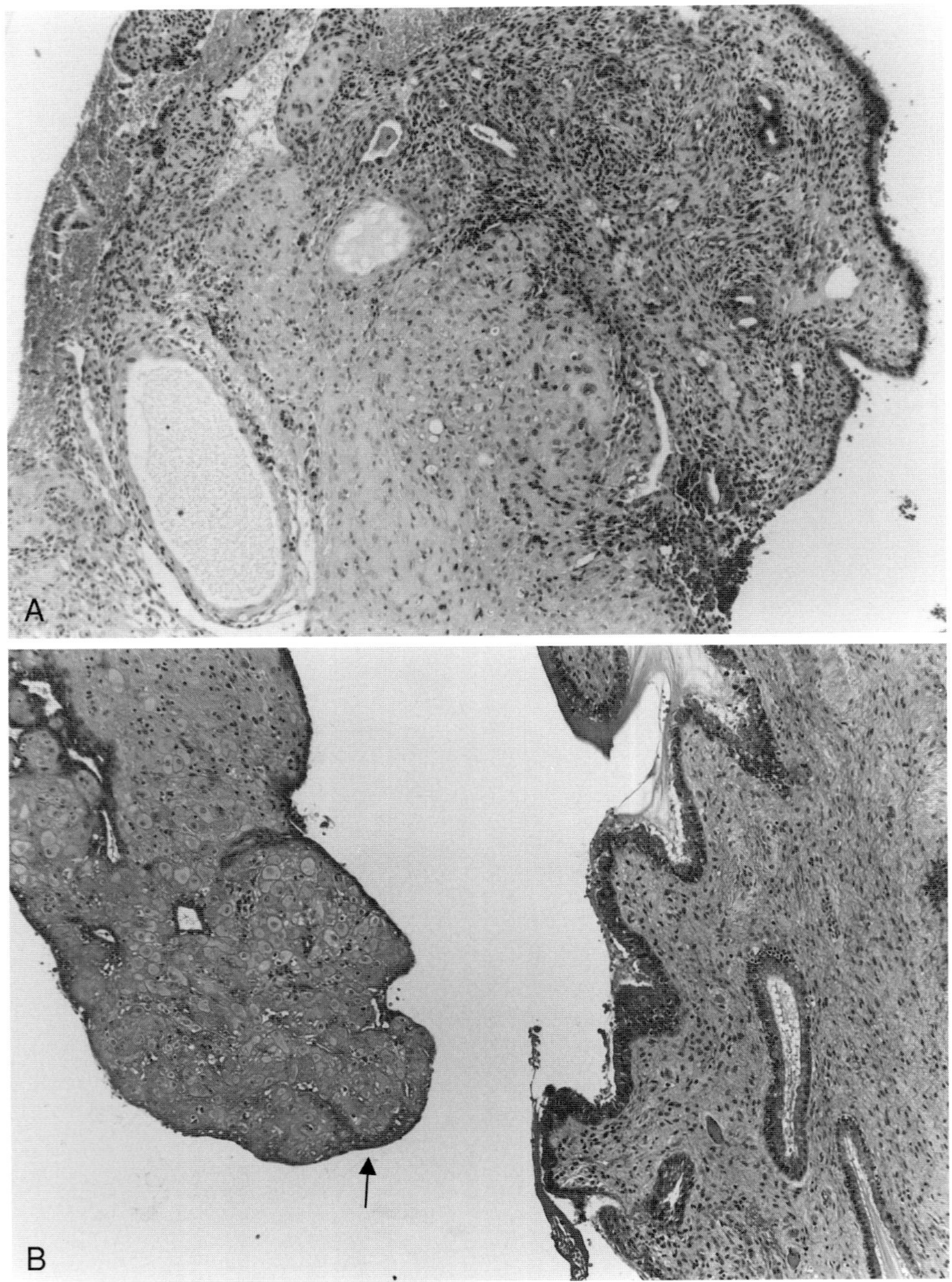

FIGURE 8.20. Decidualization. **A.** Focal decidualization of the cervix. **B.** Decidual polyp.

they may present with mucoid vaginal discharge or vaginal bleeding, usually of minimal amount. Histologically, the most common pattern (Fig. 8.19) is one of endocervical glands, often with exuberant squamous metaplasia in a fibrovascular stroma. Severe inflammation, ulceration, and granulation tissue often exist. Other polyps may have a predominance of vascular or fibrous tissue, or there may be a mixture of endometrial and endocervical glands. In pregnancy, the cervix may become focally decidualized (Fig. 8.20A), and at times a polypoid projection of this tissue occurs (Fig. 8.20B). The pseudosarcomatous polyp previously described in the vulva and vagina can also occur in the cervix, and this should not be mistaken for a true sarcoma botryoides, which can also arise from the cervix. Other polypoid lesions of the cervix, including aborting submucosal leiomyoma, squamous papilloma, adenofibroma, and cervical malignancies should be distinguishable by histology.

ADENOMYOMAS OF ENDOCERVICAL TYPE

Gilks and colleagues (13) described ten cases of adenomyomas of endocervical type, which can be distinguished from adenoma malignum by their gross circumscription, polypoid shape, lobular arrangement of glands, and lack of stromal response.

LEIOMYOMA

Leiomyomas histologically identical to those of the uterine corpus may arise in the cervix (Fig. 8.21). Aborting fundal submucous leiomyomas may present as a polypoid protrusion from the cervical os.

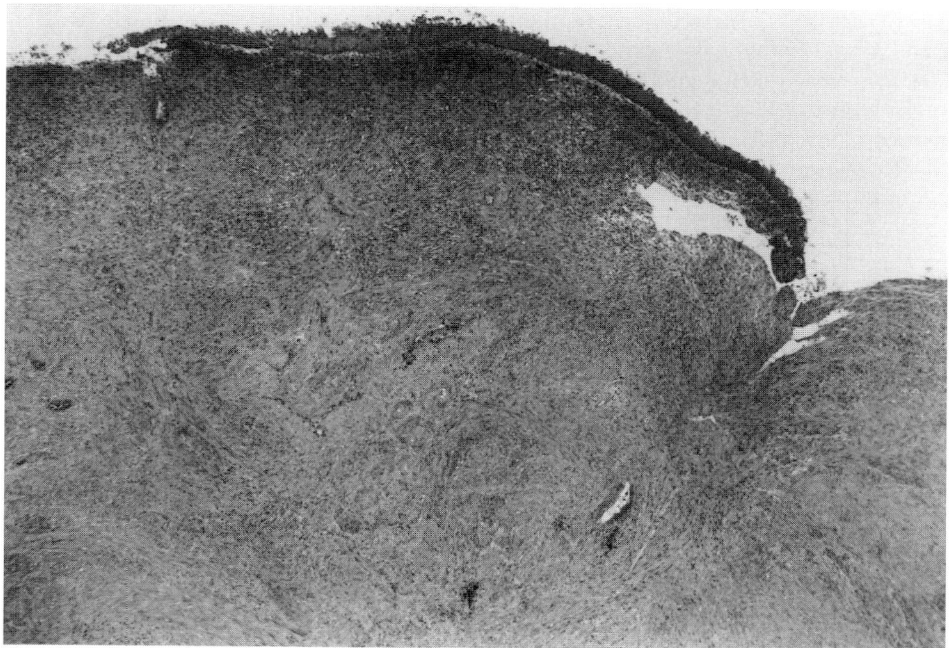

FIGURE 8.21.   Cervical leiomyoma, lined by squamous epithelium.

REFERENCES

1. Kiviat NB, Paavonen JA, Wolner-Hanssen P, et al. Histopathology of endocervical infection caused by Chlamydia trachomatis, herpes simplex virus, Trichomonas vaginalis, and Neisseria gonorrhoea. Hum Pathol 1990;21:831–837.
2. Moubayed P, Lepere JF, Mwakyoma H, et al. Carcinoma of the uterine cervix and schistosomiasis. Int J Gynaecol Obstet 1994;45:133–139.
3. Jovanovic AS, McLachlin CM, Shen L, et al. Postmenopausal squamous atypia: a spectrum including pseudo-koilocytosis. Mod Pathol 1995;8:408–412.
4. McLachlin C, Devine P, Muto M, et al. Pseudoinvasion of vascular spaces: report of an artifact caused by cervical lidocaine injection prior to loop diathermy. Hum Pathol 1994; 25:208–211.
5. Fu YS, Reagan JW. Benign and malignant epithelial lesions of the uterine cervix. In: Fu YS, Regan JW. Pathology of the Uterine Cervix, Vulva, and Vagina. Philadelphia: WB Saunders, 1989:225–335.
6. Young RH, Clement PB. Pseudoneoplastic glandular lesions of the uterine cervix [review]. Semin Diagn Pathol 1991;8:234–249
7. Sickel JZ. Surgical pathology of the uterine cervix. Diagnostic problems and controversies [review]. Clin Lab Med 1995;15:493–516.
8. Clement PB, Young RH. Deep nabothian cysts of the uterine cervix. A possible source of confusion with minimal-deviation adenocarcinoma (adenoma malignum). Int J Gynecol Pathol 1989;8:340–348.
9. Daya D, Young RH. Florid deep glands of the uterine cervix. Another mimic of adenoma malignum. Am J Clin Pathol 1995;103:614–617.
10. Young RH, Scully RE. Atypical forms of microglandular hyperplasia of the cervix simulating carcinoma. A report of 5 cases and review of the literature [review]. Am J Surg Pathol 1989;13:50–56.
11. Ferry JA, Scully RE. Mesonephric remnants, hyperplasia, and neoplasia in the uterine cervix. A study of 49 cases. Am J Surg Pathol 1990;14:1100–1111.
12. Jones MA, Young RH, Scully RE. Diffuse laminar endocervical glandular hyperplasia. A benign lesion often confused with adenoma malignum (minimal deviation adenocarcinoma) Am J Surg Pathol 1991;15:1123–1129.
13. Gilks CB, Young RH, Clement PB, et al. Benign endocervical adenomyomas and adenoma malignum. Mod Pathol 1996;9:220–224.

MALIGNANT DISEASES OF THE CERVIX

Debra S. Heller, MD

■

Intraepithelial Lesions of the Uterine Cervix
Microinvasive Squamous Cell Carcinoma
Invasive Squamous Cell Carcinoma
Adenocarcinoma of the Uterine Cervix
Adenosquamous Carcinoma
Other Primary Malignancies of the Uterine Cervix
Metastatic Tumors to the Uterine Cervix

INTRAEPITHELIAL LESIONS OF THE UTERINE CERVIX
SQUAMOUS INTRAEPITHELIAL LESIONS

In the 1960s, Richart developed the concept of a spectrum of invasive squamous changes of increasing severity in the cervix, and called the lesions cervical intraepithelial neoplasia (CIN) (1). With our expanding knowledge of the role of human *Papillomavirus* in the development of cervical carcinoma, it appears that cervical preinvasive lesions have two different clinically significant potential outcomes: those that will progress and those that will not. Nuovo and colleagues (2) have demonstrated that while wide heterogeneity exists in the types of HPV seen in low-grade CIN lesions, high-grade CIN lesions usually contain intermediate to high-risk types of HPV DNA. Considering the pathobiology of the disease as well as treatment planning, diagnosing squamous lesions of the cervix using a two-tiered system (3) is more practical as it provides better correlation with Bethesda system cytological diagnoses. In the two-tiered system, lesions previously diagnosed as CIN 1 are classified as low-grade cervical intraepithelial neoplasia or low-grade squamous intraepithelial lesions (SIL), and lesions formerly diagnosed as either CIN 2 or 3 are classified as high-grade cervical intraepithelial neoplasia or high-grade SIL. Although commercial kits for HPV typing are available, their clinical usefulness is controversial, and they have not yet come to play a major role in the management of patients with SIL; however, using these tests in the management of atypical (ASCUS) pap smears may prove beneficial. In the presence of a negative endocervical curettage, following an adequate colposcopic examination, the approach to low-grade SIL varies from observation to resection/ablation whereas high-grade lesions are generally treated more aggressively with one of the resection/ablative techniques. However, in women with SIL—particularly high-grade—if the colposcopic examination is unsatisfactory due to nonvisualization of the upper end of the transformation zone or lesion, or if a positive endocervical curettage exists, the presence of preinvasive or invasive disease high up in the endocervical canal must be determined. A loop electroexcisional procedure (LEEP) conization using an endoloop to obtain an endocervical specimen or a cold knife conization may be performed in these cases.

Low-grade Squamous Intraepithelial Lesions (LOSIL)

Low-grade SIL (CIN 1) is characterized histologically by abnormal maturation confined to the lower one-third of the squamous epithelium. Basal cell proliferation, mild nuclear atypia, and mitotic activity occurs, usually in the lower third. The cytopathic effects of HPV, including koilocytosis and multinucleation, are often seen (Fig. 9.1). Koilocytotic atypia may be pronounced in the upper epithelium; however, with maturation present, this should not be mistaken for a higher grade of SIL. To diagnose koilocytosis, nuclear atypia must be present, as well as perinuclear halos, and care should be taken not to overdiagnose low-grade SIL.

High-grade Squamous Intraepithelial Lesions (HISIL)

High-grade SIL (CIN 2 and CIN 3) is characterized by a more profound derangement of maturation than low-grade SIL, extending beyond the lower third of the squamous

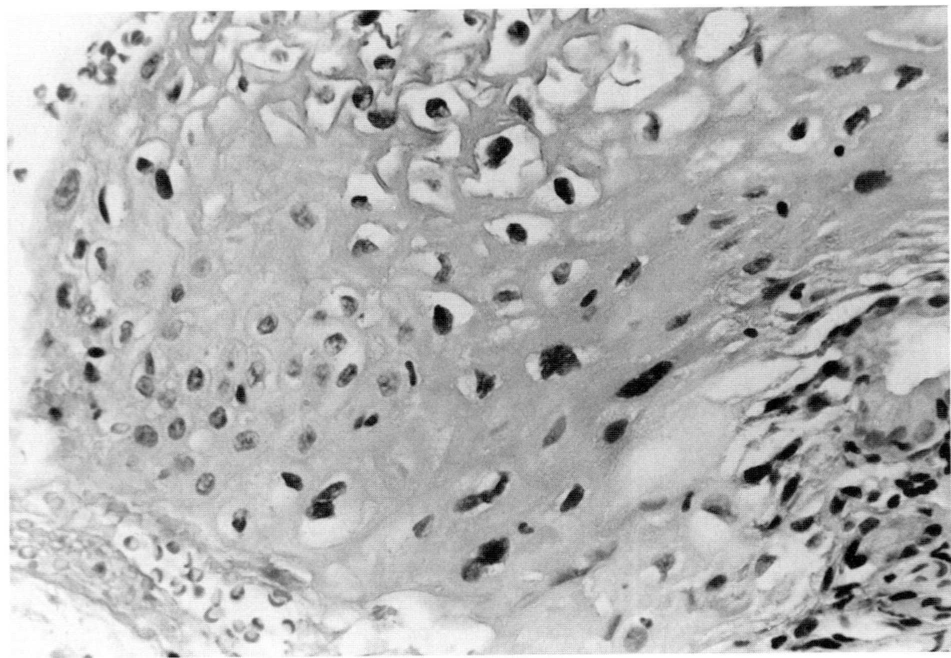

FIGURE 9.1. Low-grade squamous intraepithelial lesion. Koilocytotic atypia is present, but there is maturation.

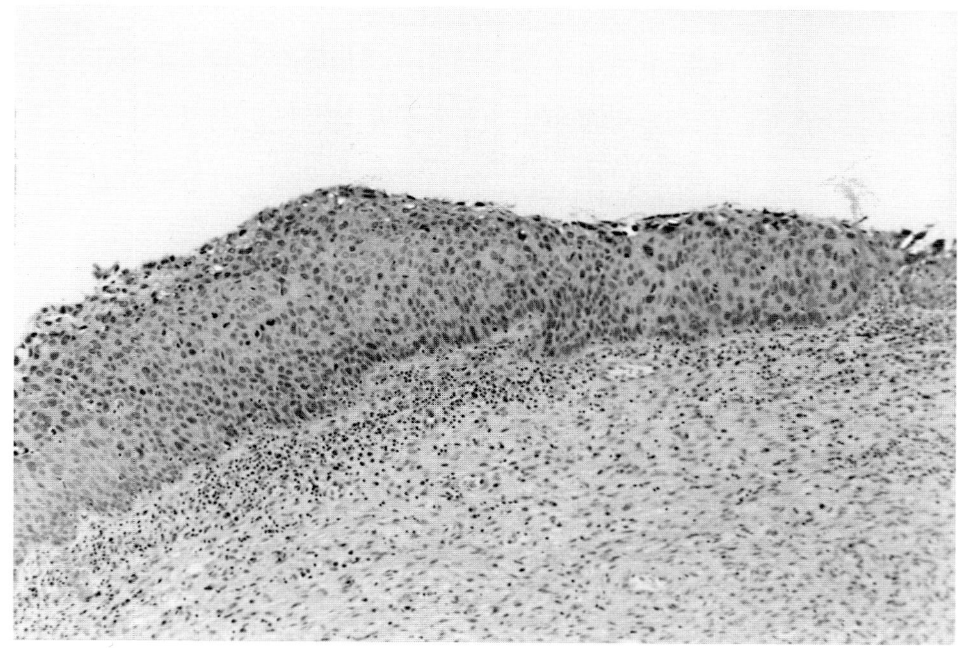

FIGURE 9.2.   High-grade squamous intraepithelial lesion. There is atypia and lack of maturation throughout the entire epithelial thickness.

epithelium (Fig. 9.2). Koilocytosis is less pronounced than in low-grade SIL, and mitoses, including atypical mitotic figures, are more frequent.

Lesions that may be confused with high-grade SIL include immature squamous metaplasia, atrophy, and transitional cell metaplasia (Figs. 9.3 and 9.4). Squamous metaplasia is much more orderly, lacks significant atypia and atypical mitoses, and residual mucinous epithelium may be seen. Atrophic epithelium is thin, with no maturation and a high nuclear-to-cytoplasmic ratio; however, no nuclear atypia or mitotic activity exist. In cases in which distinguishing atrophy from a high-grade squamous lesion is difficult, a short course of estrogen will mature atrophic epithelium but will not eliminate SIL. Transitional metaplasia resembles transitional epithelium, having frequent grooved nuclei. The lack of atypia and significant mitotic activity separates transitional metaplasia from SIL.

A variety of histological factors have been suggested to predict invasive disease in the unsampled cervix in patients with high-grade SIL. Tidbury and colleagues (4) noted that CIN 3 lesions associated with microinvasion were larger than those without invasive foci. Leung and colleagues (5) noted that invasion may be missed if biopsies are not deep enough and suggested suspecting invasion if two or more of the following features are present: giant bizarre cells, large keratinizing cells, keratin pearls, necrosis, or neovascariziation. Al-Nafussi and colleagues (6) found an increased frequency of invasive carcinoma in high-grade intraepithelial lesions with extensive surface and endocervical gland involvement, luminal necrosis, frequent mitoses, greater nuclear atypia, apoptosis, and pericryptal concentric fibrosis and inflammation.

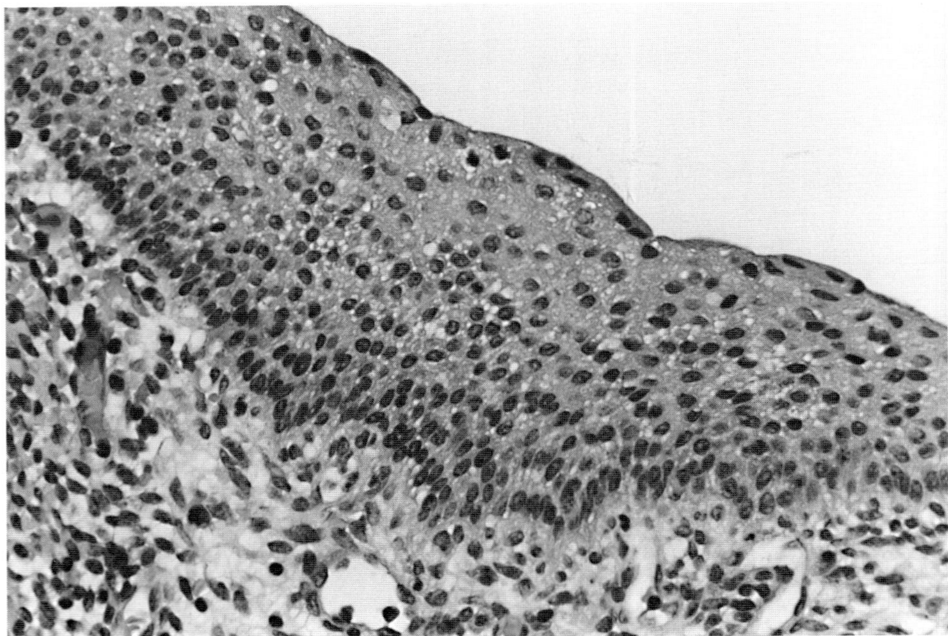

FIGURE 9.3. Immature metaplasia. The nuclear atypia of SIL is absent, and there is epithelial maturation.

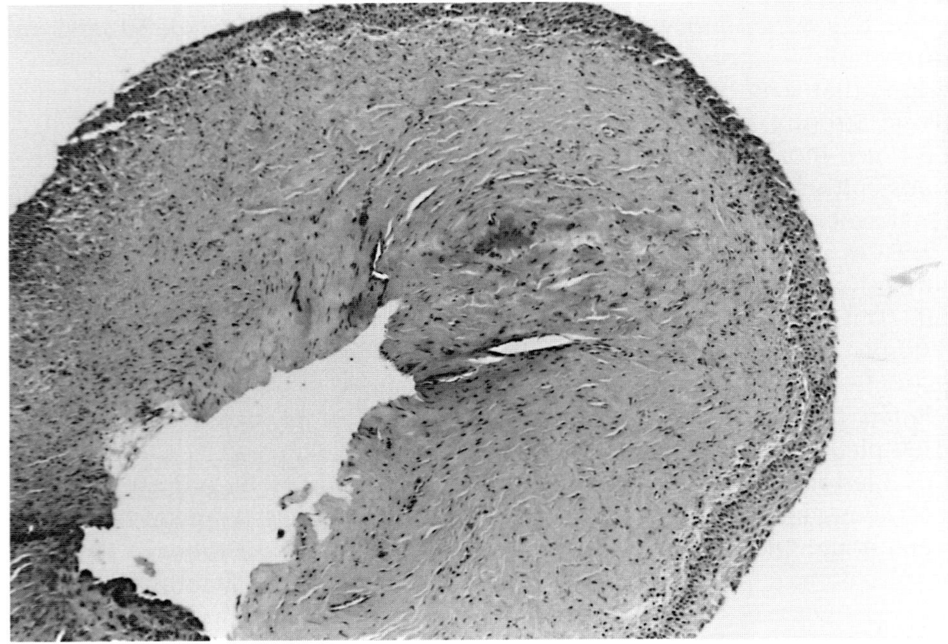

FIGURE 9.4. Atrophy. Maturation is absent, but the atypia and mitotic activity seen with SIL is not seen.

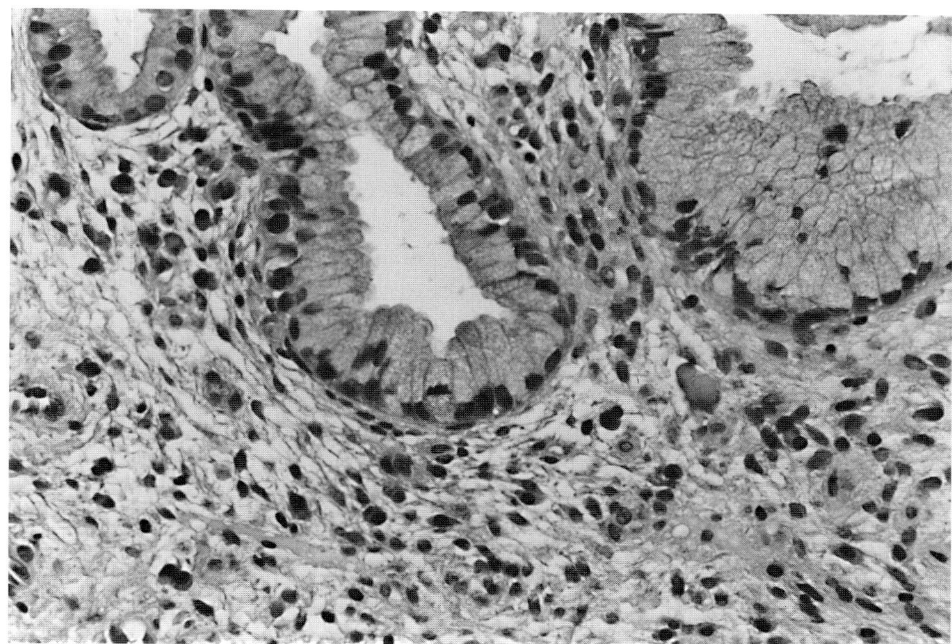

FIGURE 9.5. Endocervical glandular dysplasia. Mild atypia of endocervical epithelium with the occasional mitosis falls short of the criteria of AIS. The clinical significance of this lesion is unclear.

GLANDULAR INTRAEPITHELIAL LESIONS OF THE UTERINE CERVIX

Endocervical Dysplasia

Atypical endocervical lesions that are not severe enough to classify as adenocarcinoma-in-situ (AIS) are classified as endocervical dysplasia. These lesions may consist of only a few glands exhibiting mild nuclear atypia, stratification, and occasional mitoses (Fig. 9.5). The biology of these lesions and the criteria for distinguishing them from AIS is not as well established as with squamous lesions.

Adenocarcinoma-in-Situ

Most adenocarcinoma-in-situ of the endocervix is of the endocervical type. Endometrioid and intestinal patterns also occur. Endocervical-type AIS is composed of mucin-containing cells that exhibit stratification, atypia, and mitotic activity (Fig. 9.6). AIS may show a complex architecture, with outpouching and cribriforming of glands. The features distinguishing AIS from frankly invasive adenocarcinoma include lack of penetration beyond the normal endocervical crypt depth, a mixture of normal and neoplastic glands, and a lack of stromal reaction. At times the distinction may be difficult, and frankly invasive adenocarcinoma cannot be ruled out on a punch biopsy specimen.

AIS is frequently associated with HPV type 18, and there is also a frequent association of AIS with squamous intraepithelial lesions (7). Lesions that should be distinguished from AIS include microglandular hyperplasia, tubal metaplasia, endometriosis, Arias-Stella reaction, cervicitis, and inspissated endocervical glands with rupture and inflam-

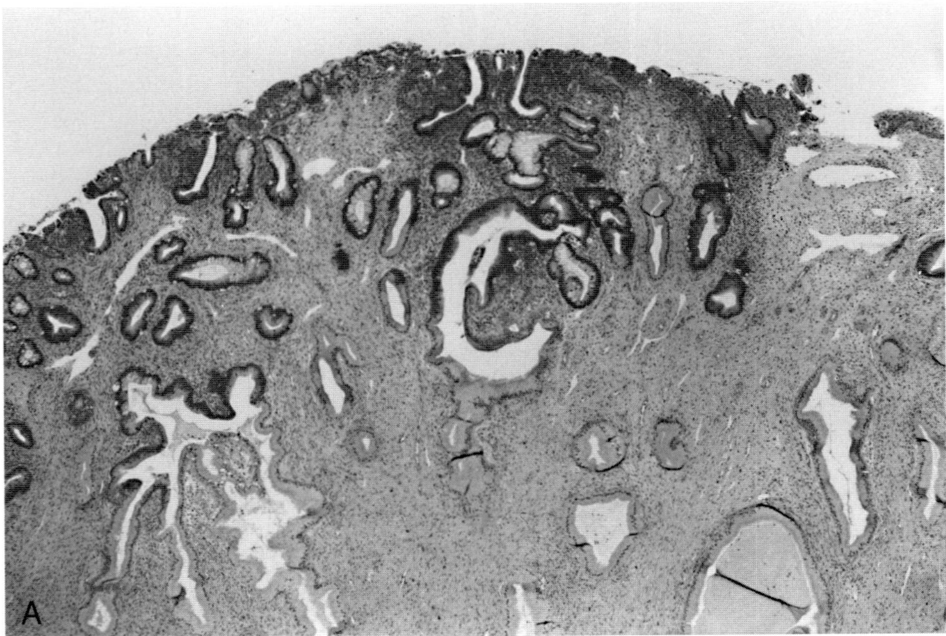

FIGURE 9.6. Adenocarcinoma-in-situ (AIS), endocervical-type. **A.** The neoplastic glands do not invade beyond the normal crypt depth and are admixed with normal glands.

mation (see Chapter 8) (8). Immunohistochemical staining for carcinoembryonic antigen (CEA) may be positive in AIS, but this is of limited diagnostic use (8).

ENDOCERVICAL CURETTAGE (ECC) SPECIMENS

Abnormal Squamous Fragments in an ECC

A positive endocervical curettage after colposcopy suggests disease extending up into the endocervical canal, and thus requires further investigation. A LEEP conization or cold knife conization may be used in these cases. A positive ECC at the time of cone biopsy with high-grade SIL is an important predictor of residual SIL and invasive carcinoma. Some investigators recommend repeating the cone proceedure in women 50 years and older or for whom fertility is not an issue who have high-grade SIL on cone biopsy, a negative cone margin, and a positive ECC to rule out invasion. For women concerned about fertility, they suggest close follow-up (9). A potential diagnostic difficulty is that strips of neoplastic squamous epithelium on an ECC do not always reflect disease up in the endocervical canal. Fragmentation of neoplastic epithelium on the exocervix can occur, even if the ECC is performed before biopsies, contaminating the ECC specimen. Abundant strips of neoplastic squamous epithelium, dysplastic changes within metaplastic squamous epithelium, or the presence of attached mucinous or metaplastic squamous epithelium suggests a true endocervical lesion (Fig. 9.7). If one or two detached neoplastic fragments are present in an otherwise normal ECC, we report this as such and allow the clinician to determine the significance.

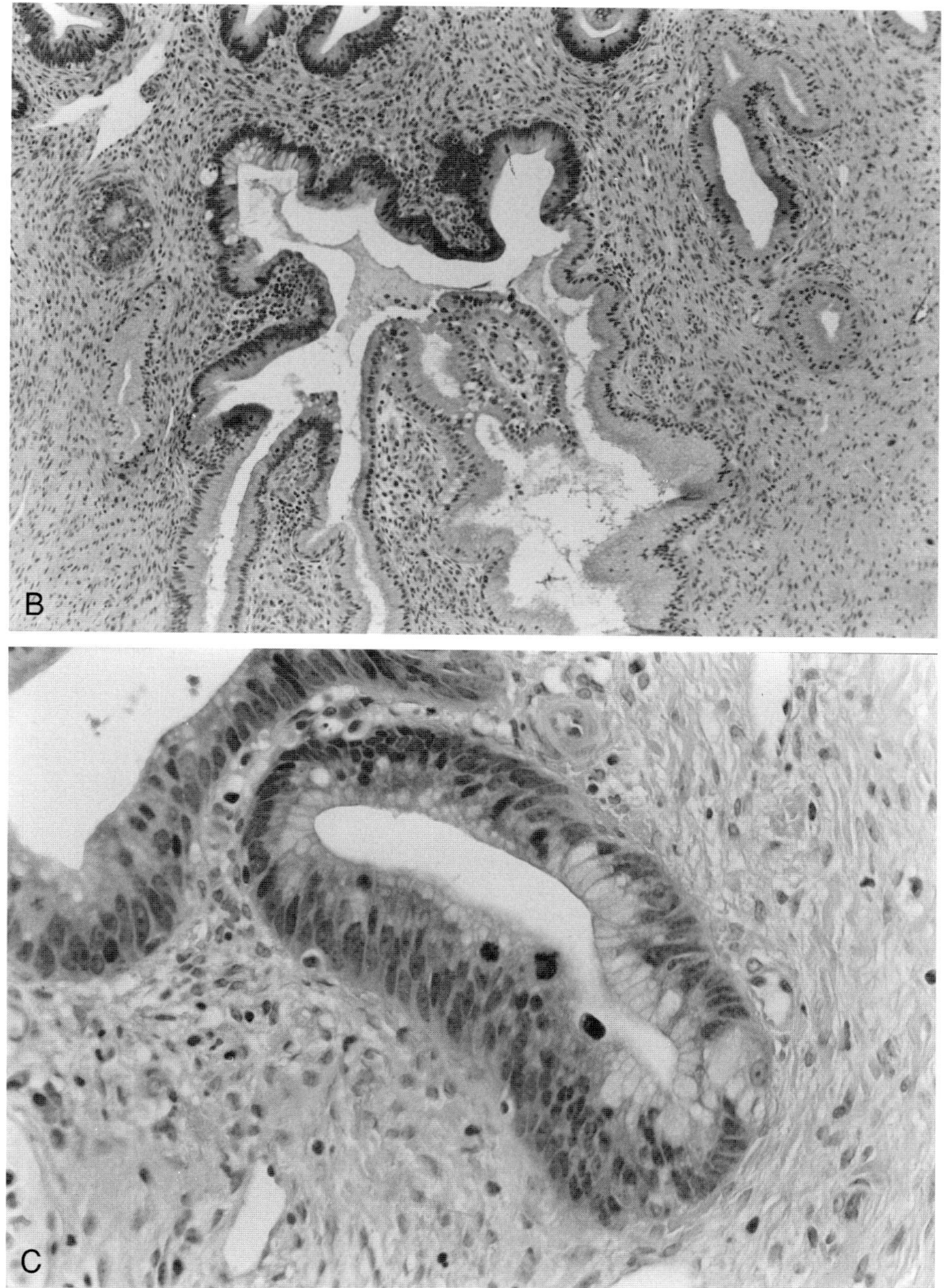

FIGURE 9.6.   *(continued)* **B.** An endocervical gland partially replaced by AIS. **C.** Glands show nuclear stratification, atypia, and mitotic activity.

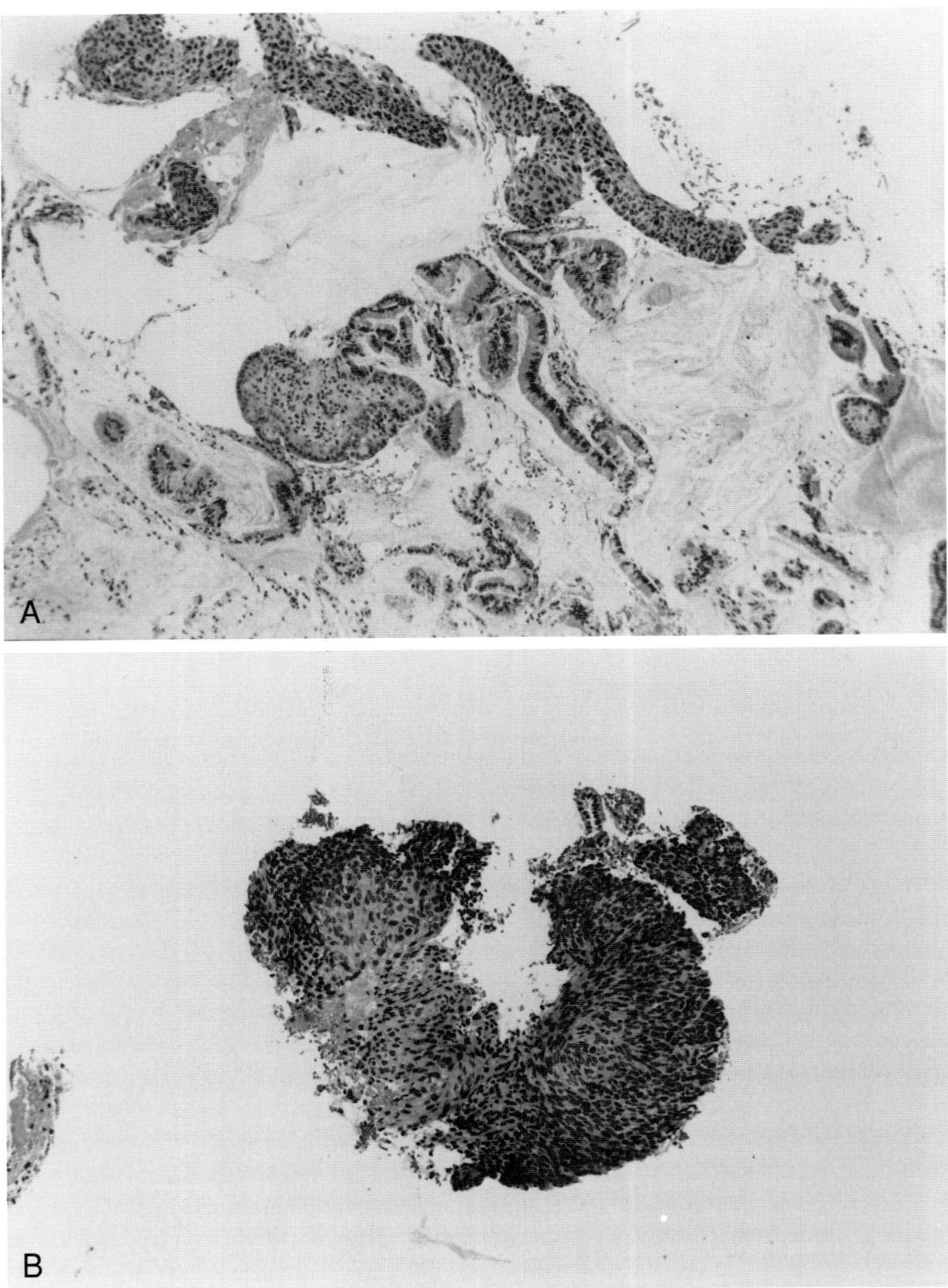

FIGURE 9.7. Endocervical curettings. **A.** Abundant strips of neoplastic squamous epithelium. **B.** Neoplastic squamous epithelium in the shape of an endocervical gland replaced by SIL.

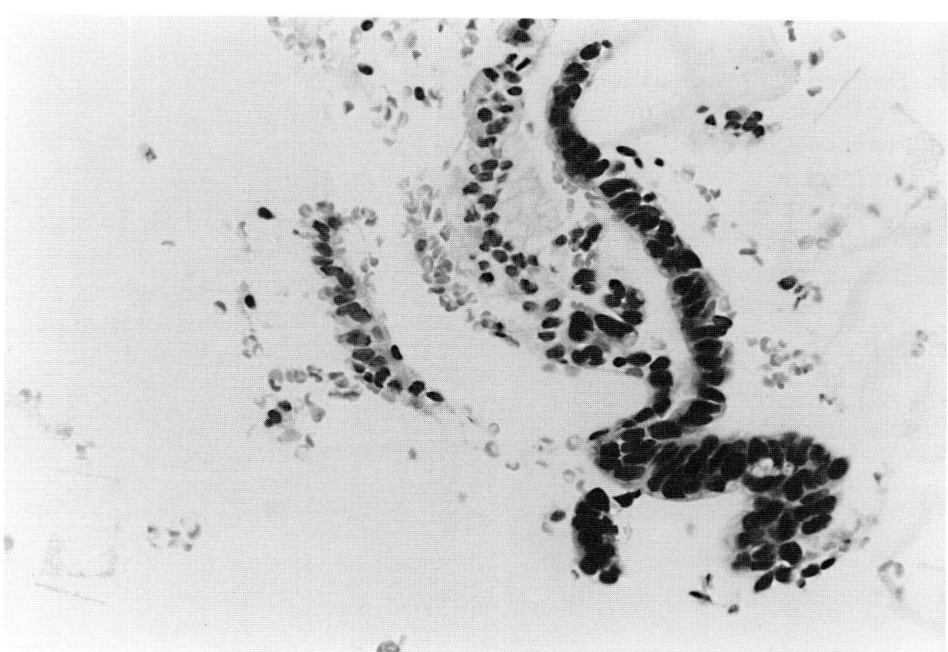

FIGURE 9.8.   Endocervical curettings. Strips of atypical glandular fragments admixed with normal endocervix. The severity of the lesion cannot be assessed from this specimen.

Abnormal Glandular Fragments in an ECC

The presence of abnormal glandular fragments in an ECC requires further investigation because the severity of a glandular lesion cannot be ascertained from an ECC (Fig. 9.8).

LEEP SPECIMENS

Most pathology laboratories are now receiving LEEP specimens. It may be difficult to determine the margins on a LEEP due to problems of orientation, fragmentation, and cautery artifact. An additional problem seen on LEEPs and occasionally on cold knife cone biopsies is a squamous or glandular lesion approaching the deep margin of resection (Fig. 9.9). Even if this depth is less than the accepted definition of microinvasion, a microinvasive squamous lesion, or an AIS in the case of glandular neoplasia cannot be diagnosed. It can only be stated that the lesion reaches the deep margin, and a measurement can be given. The clinician then needs to evaluate the patient for residual disease.

COLD KNIFE CONE BIOPSIES

For squamous intraepithelial lesions, most studies show less residual disease in patients with negative cone biopsy endocervical margins than with positive ones; nonetheless, some risk of residual disease with negative margins does exist. Positive cone margins do correlate with a greater risk of harboring or developing invasive cancer. Regardless of margin status, all patients need continuous follow-up. Jansen and colleagues (10)

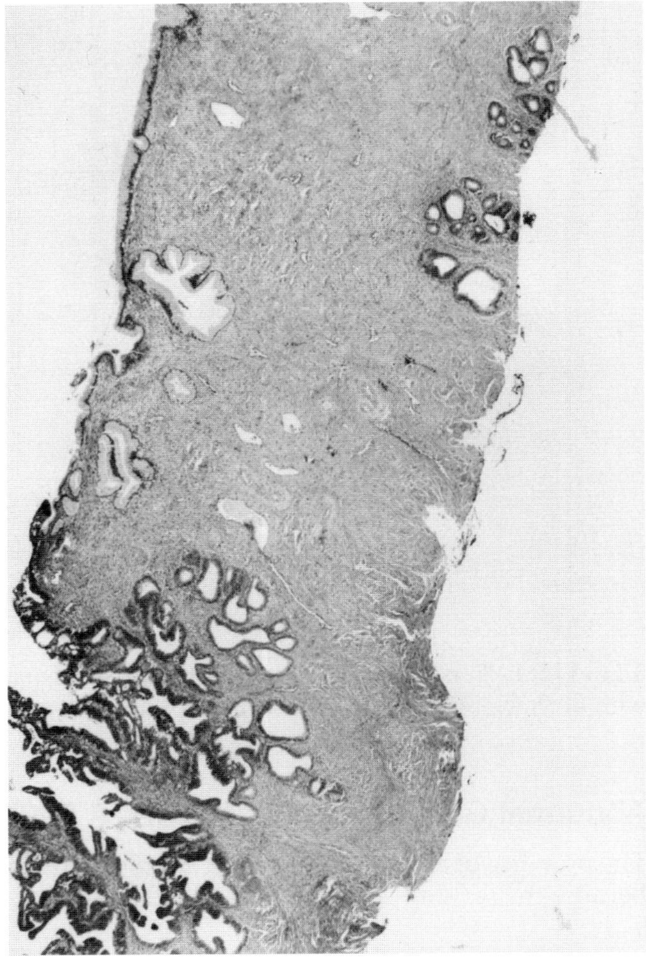

FIGURE 9.9. Positive LEEP margin. Endocervical neoplasia is present at the deep margin of this LEEP. Even though the entire thickness of the specimen in this case measured 3mm, no distinction between AIS and invasive adenocarcinoma (nor between microinvasive and invasive squamous cell carcinoma in the case of a squamous lesion) can be made from this type of specimen.

feel that low-grade SIL at a cone margin is not clinically significant, but that high-grade SIL at the endocervical margin of a cone is, and that cytology is a reliable way to follow up patients who have positive endocervical margins. Repeat colposcopies, ECCS, repeat conization, and hysterectomy are other therapeutic options. Therapy is individualized, taking into consideration the patient's age and reproductive plans.

The risk appears to be higher for glandular intraepithelial neoplasia. Although some authors feel that a negative cone biopsy endocervical margin on a young patient with AIS permits clinical follow-up, residual disease, both AIS and invasive adenocarcinoma, may be present after both a positive and negative cone margin (11).

MICROINVASIVE SQUAMOUS CELL CARCINOMA

The definition of microinvasion has varied over the years in an attempt to separate out those minimally invasive neoplasms with essentially no metastatic potential, and which may require less aggressive therapy. Up until recently, the definition by the Society of Gynecologic Oncologists (SGO) of microinvasion was significantly more stringent than the FIGO staging; however, recently FIGO has amended its staging system so that it now more closely resembles the SGO definition (12). The SGO (13) defines microinvasive lesions as lesions that invade 3 mm or less below the basement membrane in one or more foci, in the absence of lymphvascular space involvement. The current FIGO staging of cervical cancer can be seen in Table 9.1. Up to 10% of patients with lesions invading over 3mm but not exceeding 5mm have lymph node metastases (14) . Lesions over 1 mm but not exceeding 3 mm in invasion have a low but not absent risk of metastatic disease (15). Because of the variability of classification and therapy in these cases, it is important to report the measured depth of invasion and greatest tumor width. Multifocality, confluency, and lymphvascular space involvement (Fig. 9.10) should be described when present. The clinician can then decide whether cone biopsy alone, total hysterectomy, or in cases determined to be of high risk for metastatic spread, radical hysterectomy with pelvic lymphadenectomy is indicated. In a radical hysterectomy, the parametria are removed with the uterus (Fig. 9.11), and should be examined separately, as should the vaginal resection margin. There is increased morbidity after a radical hysterectomy as opposed to a total hysterectomy, and the procedure is usually performed by gynecological oncologists.

Histologically, microinvasion is characterized by paradoxically more mature appearing tongues of squamous epithelium invading the stroma. These tongues may arise from the surface or from an endocervical gland replaced by SIL. The invasive focus provokes an inflammatory or desmoplastic stromal reaction (Fig. 9.12). It is important to adequately sample a cone biopsy or hysterectomy to reach the final diagnosis of microinvasion. To this end, levels may be a necessary part of the evaluation. A frankly invasive carcinoma cannot be excluded on the basis of a cervical punch biopsy showing microinvasion.

TABLE 9.1.   FIGO Staging for Cervical Cancer (12)

  IA. Preclinical carcinomas
     IA1. Depth of invasion no greater than 3 mm; tumor width does not exceed 7 mm
     IA2. Depth of invasion over 3 mm but not over 5 mm; tumor width does not exceed 7 mm
  IB. Clinically evident lesions, and preclinical lesions greater than IA
     IB1. Clinical lesions no greater than 4 cm in size
     IB2. Clinical lesions over 4 cm in size
  II. Tumor spread beyond cervix but not to pelvic wall; vaginal involvement, but not lower third
     IIA. No obvious parametrial involvement; upper 2/3 vagina involved
     IIB. Obvious parametrial involvement, but not to sidewall
  III. Spread to pelvic sidewall or lower third of vagina; all cases of hydronephrosis, unless of known other etiology
     IIIA. No extension to pelvic sidewall, tumor involves lower third of vagina
     IIIB. Extension to sidewall; hydronephrosis or nonfunctioning kidney
  IV. Extension beyond true pelvis, or involving bladder or rectal mucosa (bullous edema of bladder does not permit assignment of stage IV)
     IVA. Adjacent organs
     IVB. Distant spread

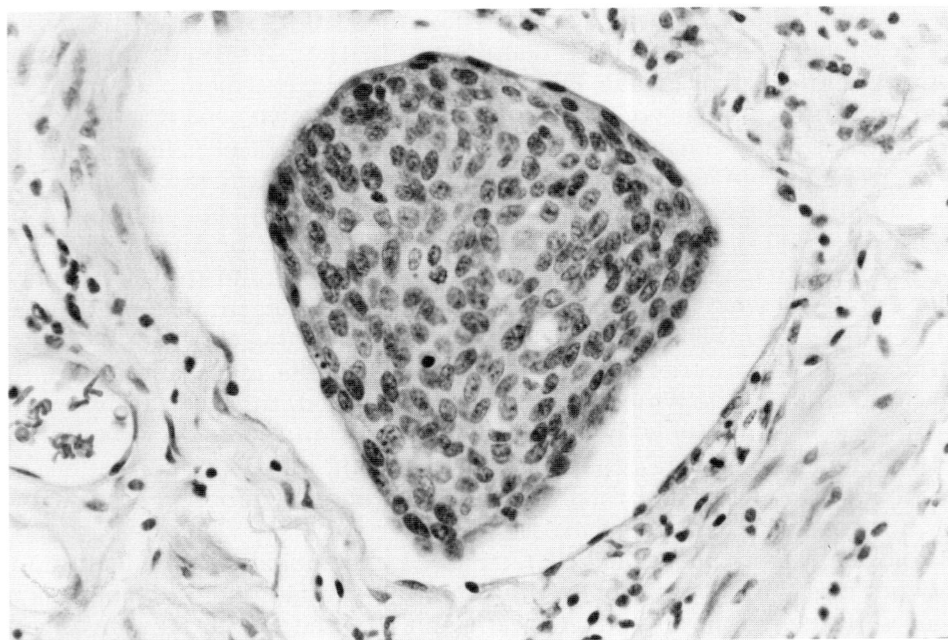

FIGURE 9.10. Lymphvascular space involvement. A true lymphvascular space, lined by endothelial cells, containing squamous cell carcinoma. It may not be possible to distinguish a lymphatic vessel from a capillary in the absence of erythrocytes.

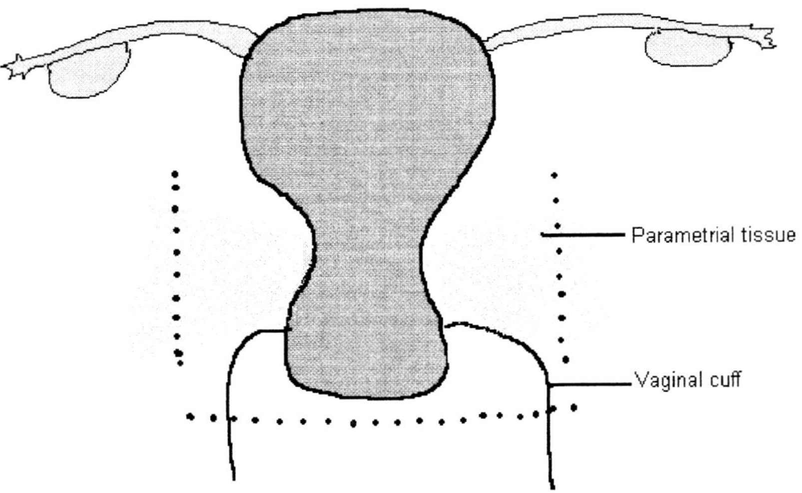

FIGURE 9.11. Radical hysterectomy. In a total abdominal hysterectomy (TAH), the uterus, with or without adnexa, is removed. In a radical hysterectomy, parametrial tissue and a vaginal cuff are removed (dotted lines). Pelvic lymphadenectomy is performed as part of the procedure.

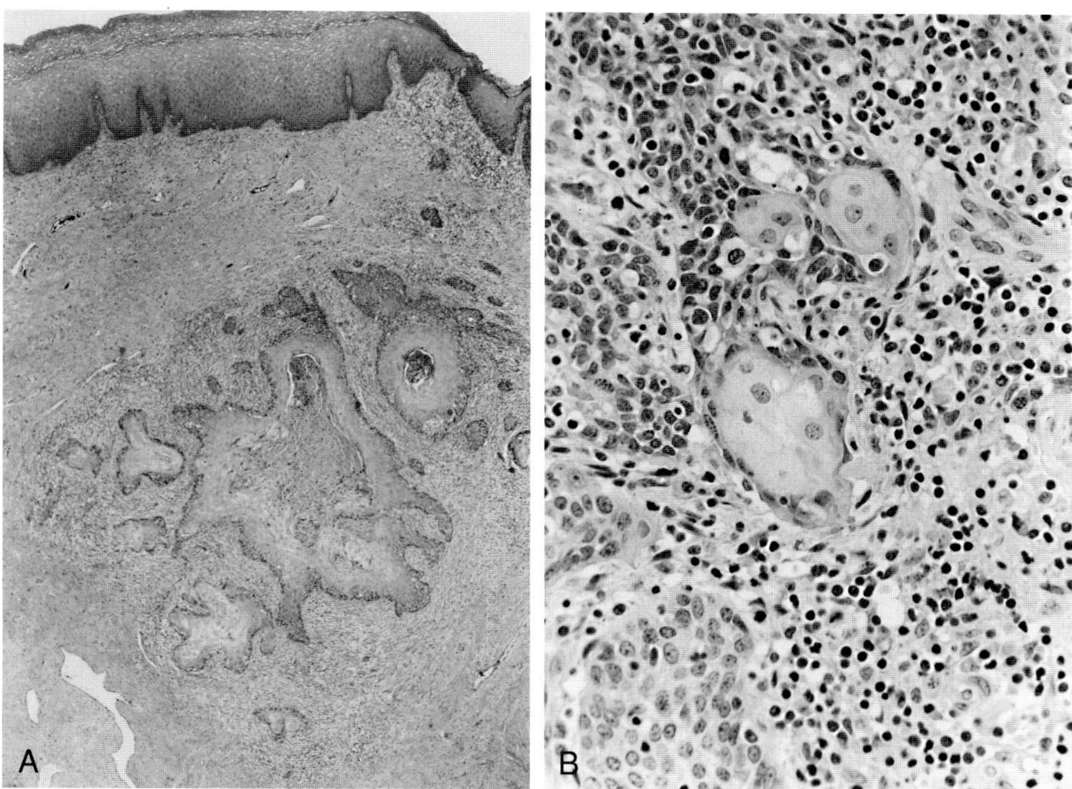

FIGURE 9.12. Microinvasion. **A.** This microinvasive lesion showed a confluent pattern, invaded to a depth of 3.0 mm and measured 2.5 mm in greatest width. **B.** Microinvasive tongues of tumor appear paradoxically mature. A stromal reaction is present.

Microinvasion must be distinguished from high-grade SIL with endocervical gland involvement. Endocervical glands replaced by SIL are rounded and uniform as opposed to the irregular outline of invasive foci. While inflammation may surround an endocervical gland involved with SIL, no desmoplasia exists. SIL does not show the paradoxical maturation of the cells with abundant eosinophilic cytoplasm as is seen with microinvasion.

It is important to distinguish tangential sectioning and healing biopsy sites from true microinvasion. A rare problem, pseudoinvasion of vascular spaces after local anesthesia has also been described (16).

No established criteria is universally accepted for an equivalent form of early invasion for adenocarcinoma of the cervix.

MEASURING DEPTH OF INVASION

The measurement of the depth of invasion of squamous cell lesions can be difficult. Traditionally, the depth of invasion is measured from the epithelial-stromal junction of either the adjacent surface epithelium or the gland from which the focus arises to

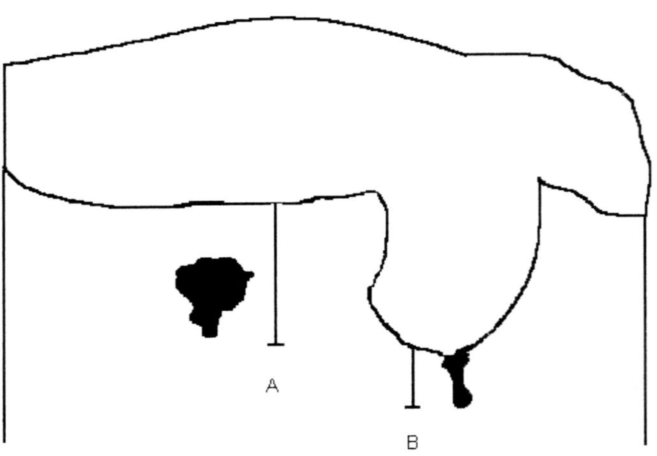

FIGURE 9.13. Depth of invasion. Invasion is measured from the basement membrane of the surface epithelium **(A)**, or endocervical gland **(B)**, from which the invasive focus arises, to the deepest point of invasion.

the deepest point of invasion (Fig. 9.13). Factors that can make this measurement problematic include surface ulceration, tissue fragmentation, the healing of a previous biopsy site, and inability to determine from where an invasive focus arises.

INVASIVE SQUAMOUS CELL CARCINOMA

Traditionally, squamous cell carcinomas of the cervix have been classified as large cell keratinizing, large cell nonkeratinizing, and small cell nonkeratinizing in an attempt to predict outcome (17). In later studies, some of the tumors classified as small cell nonkeratinizing were actually found to be tumors with neuroendocrine differentiation or adenoid basal carcinomas. While some authors have suggested that large cell nonkeratinizing tumors have the best prognosis, large cell keratinizing the second best, and small cell nonkeratinizing the worst (18), not all studies support a prognostic difference to either cell type or tumor grade (15, 19), and not all pathologists report the cell type. Grading, based on a modification of the Broder's classification (20), while of unclear usefulness, should be reported. Depth of invasion and the presence of lymphvascular space invasion should also be reported, as they may affect subsequent treatment planning. A majority of invasive squamous cell carcinomas are positive for human *Papillomavirus* (HPV), depending on the testing method, and most contain intermediate-risk to high-risk HPV types, including types 16 and 18.

WELL-DIFFERENTIATED SQUAMOUS CELL CARCINOMA (GRADE 1)

Well-differentiated (grade 1) squamous cell carcinomas resemble squamous epithelium, showing keratinization at least focally, often with keratin pearls, and intracellular bridges. Mitotic activity and atypia are usually minimal (Fig. 9.14). Most large cell keratinizing carcinomas can be included in this category.

Young and colleagues (21) described a hyalinizing variant of squamous cell carcinoma that can be mistaken for a placental site trophoblastic tumor, but which has a different clinical presentation, does not exhibit the muscle splitting of PSTT, and is negative for human placental lactogen.

A warty (condylomatous) variant of squamous cell carcinoma similar to the vulvar

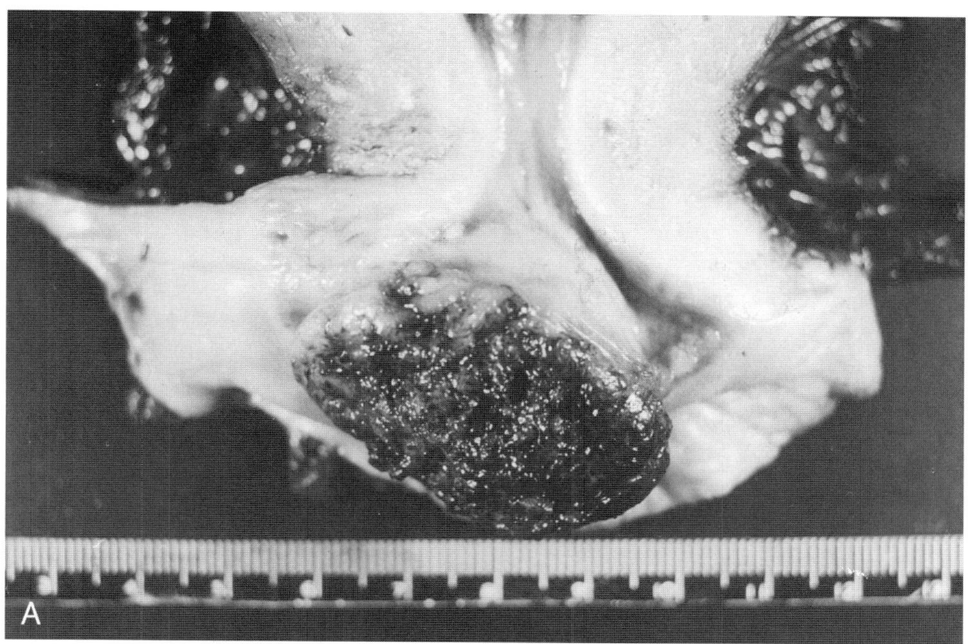

FIGURE 9.14. Well-differentiated squamous cell carcinoma. **A.** Exophytic cervical tumor. *(figure continues)*

lesion can occur, and it can be distinguished from verrucous carcinomas by its aggressively invasive rather than pushing margins.

MODERATELY DIFFERENTIATED SQUAMOUS CELL CARCINOMA (GRADE 2)

Moderately differentiated (grade 2) squamous cell carcinoma may show individual cell keratinization, but is more atypical and mitotically active than grade 1 tumors (Fig. 9.15). Most large cell nonkeratinizing carcinomas fall into this category.

POORLY DIFFERENTIATED SQUAMOUS CELL CARCINOMA (GRADE 3)

Poorly differentiated squamous cell carcinomas (grade 3) barely resemble squamous epithelium. Most small cell nonkeratinizing carcinomas can be classified in this grade. Cells are immature with scant cytoplasm, little or no keratinization, marked pleomorphism, and abundant mitotic activity (Fig. 9.16). The lesions should be distinguished from small cell undifferentiated carcinomas (neuroendocrine carcinomas) and adenoid basal carcinomas of the cervix. A rare variant, spindle cell squamous cell carcinoma, similar to that described in the vulva, must be distinguished from sarcomas and melanomas.

PROGNOSTIC FACTORS

Stage, lymphatic and vascular invasion, lymph node status, volume of tumor, and stromal depth of invasion provide important prognostic information. Pelvic node involve-

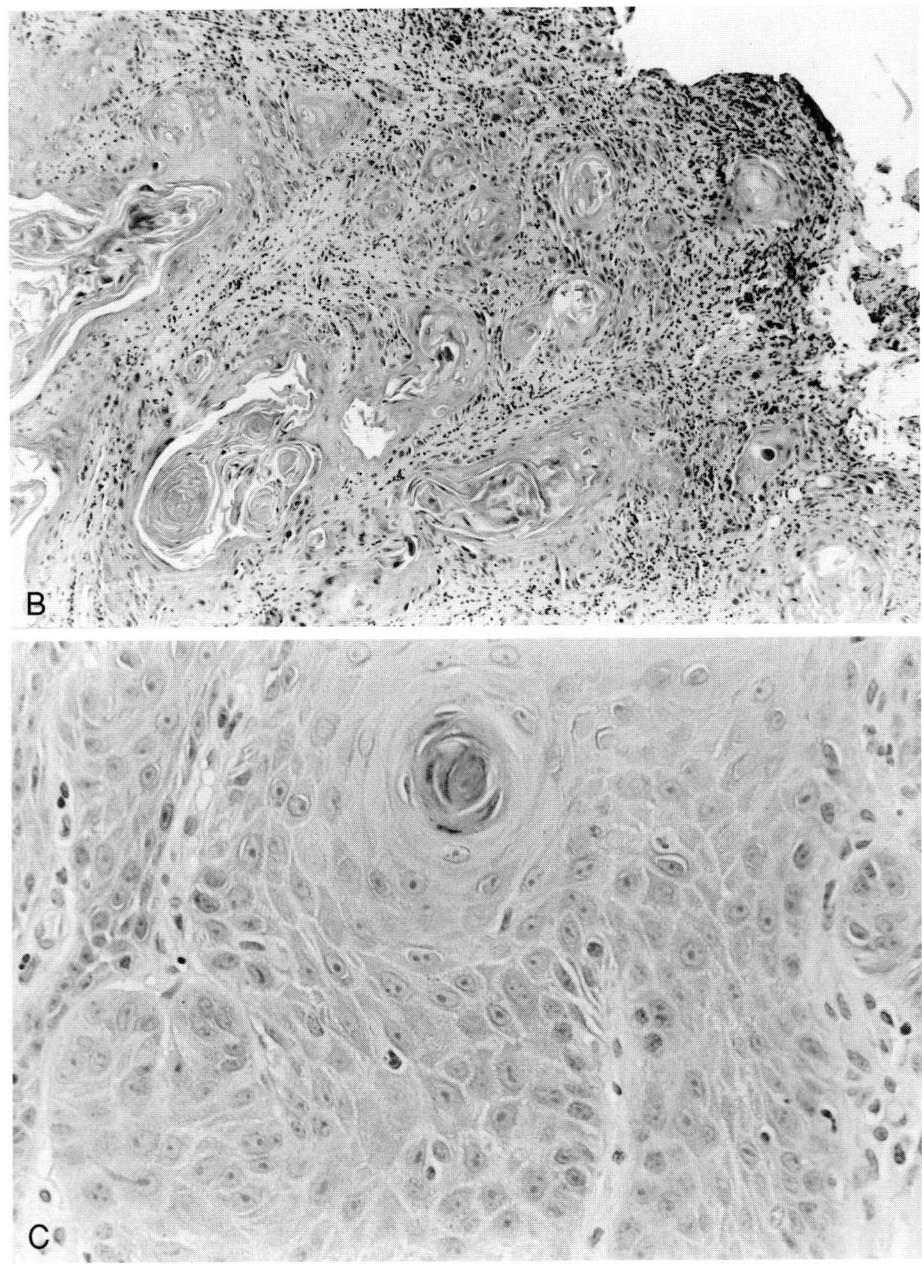

FIGURE 9.14. *(continued)* **B.** Most well-differentiated squamous cell carcinomas are of the large cell, keratinizing type. **C.** A keratin pearl and intracellular bridges are seen.

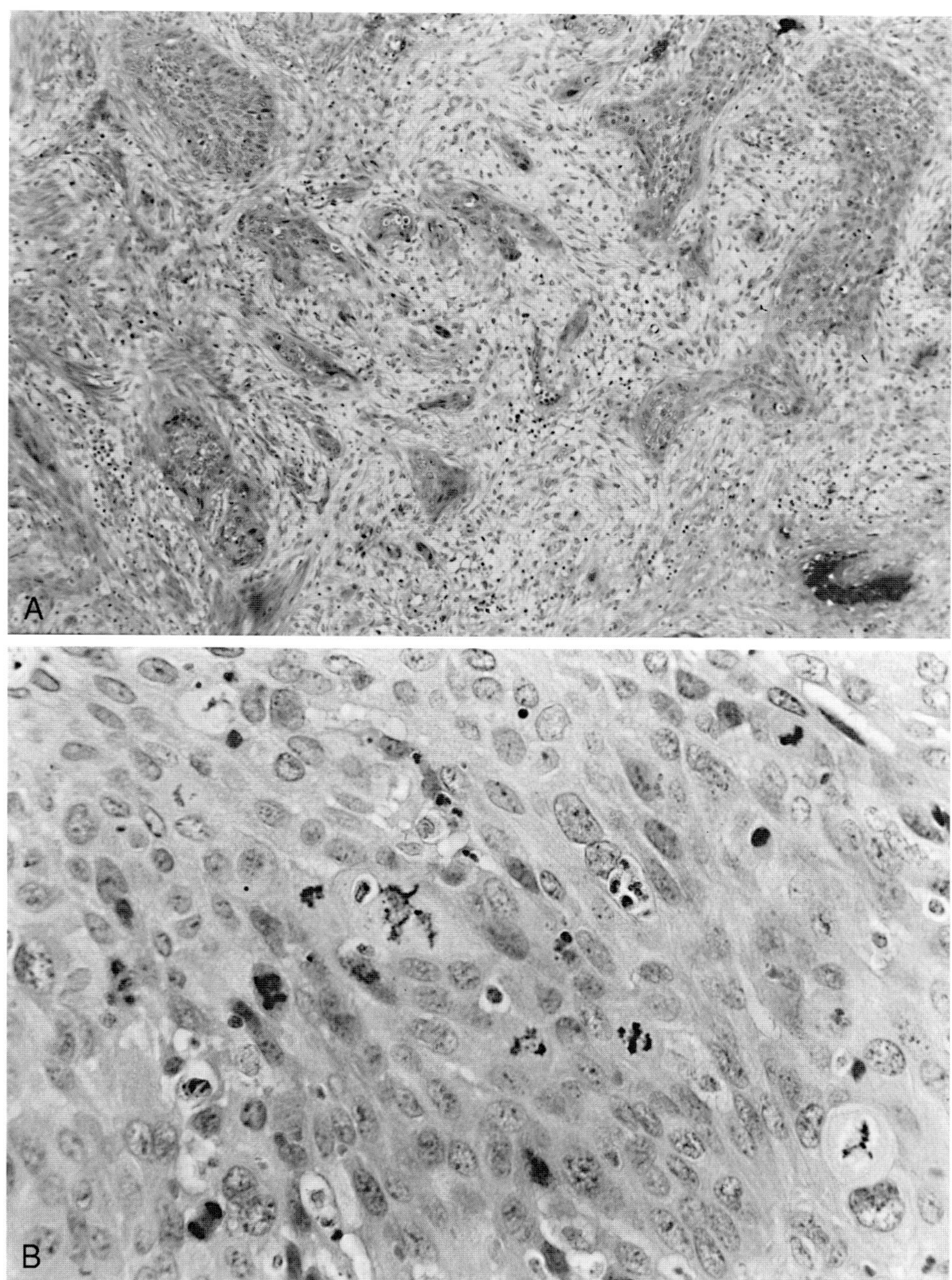

FIGURE 9.15. Moderately differentiated squamous cell carcinoma. **A.** A prominent desmoplastic response is present. **B.** Atypical mitoses are seen.

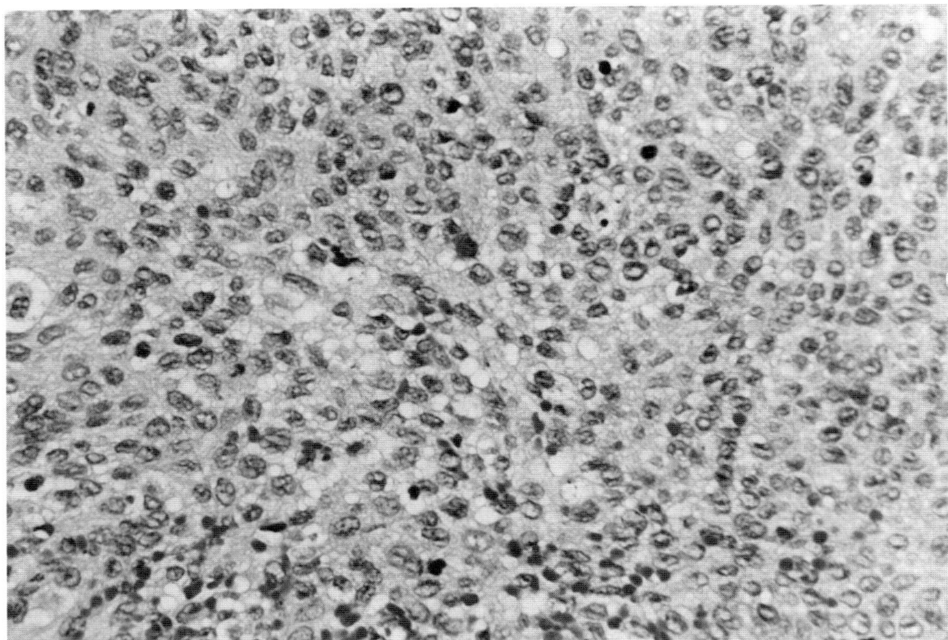

FIGURE 9.16. Poorly differentiated squamous cell carcinoma. This lesion must be distinguished from small cell undifferentiated (neuroendocrine) carcinoma.

ment correlates with tumor size, lymphvascular involvement, and increasing stage. Paraaortic lymph node involvement is often associated with subsequent widespread metastases (15). The gynecological oncologist may request a frozen section on a paraaortic lymph node at the time of a planned radical hysterectomy, and the procedure may be discontinued and radiation planned instead if this node is positive.

There has been some controversy in the literature as to the role of significant eosinophilic tissue reaction in invasive cervical carcinomas. While some investigators found that the presence of a prominent eosinophilic infiltrate did not significantly affect 5-year survival (22), others (23) suggest improved survival in these patients.

THERAPY FOR INVASIVE CERVICAL CARCINOMA

Radical hysterectomy with pelvic lymphadenectomy, radiation therapy, or a combination of both is usually used for treating the disease in its earlier stages. Radiation and sometimes adjuvant chemotherapy are used in cases deemed nonsurgical. Pelvic exenteration is usually reserved for advanced disease with hope of cure, but this procedure has been used palliatively in some cases (Fig. 9.17).

PAPILLARY SQUAMOUS (TRANSITIONAL) CELL CARCINOMA

An infrequent variant of squamous cell carcinoma has a papillary configuration resembling transitional cell carcinoma of the bladder. This tumor is characterized by late metastases and recurrences (24). Thin fibrovascular cores are lined by dysplastic squamous epithelium resembling a high-grade SIL (Fig. 9.18). The tumor occurs in in-situ

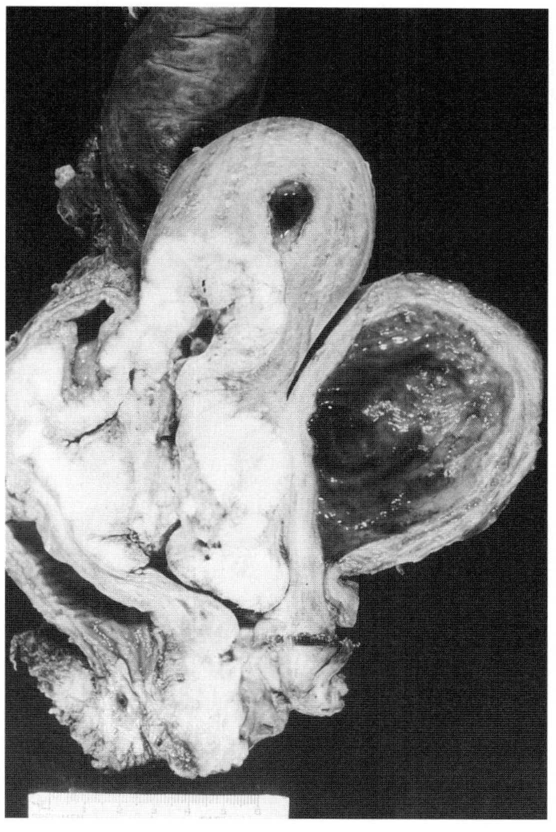

FIGURE 9.17. Pelvic exenteration. The cervical lesion has grossly spread to the uterine corpus, vagina, rectum, and perivesicle tissue.

and microinvasive patterns, and as invasion occurs at the base, deep biopsies may be required to demonstrate invasion. The tumor needs to be distinguished from verrucous carcinoma, which exhibits minimal atypia and a pushing border, and from warty carcinoma, which resembles condyloma but invades like usual squamous cell carcinoma.

VERRUCOUS CARCINOMA OF THE CERVIX

Verrucous carcinoma of the cervix is an extremely well differentiated variant of squamous cell carcinoma that is considerably less common than the vulvar counterpart. Histologically, as in the vulvar tumors, the lesions architecturally resemble large condylomas, but show pushing invasive borders. Verrucous carcinomas also have less koilocytosis and less obvious fibrovascular cores than condylomas (25).

LYMPHOEPITHELIOMA-LIKE CARCINOMA

A rare variant of squamous cell carcinoma, resembling tumors of the head and neck, the lymphoepithelioma-like carcinoma is comprised of cells with eosinophilic cytoplasm and round nuclei with nucleoli in a stroma infiltrated by lymphocytes, eosinophils, and plasma cells (Fig. 9.19). These tumors stain for keratin but are negative for epithelial membrane antigen and leukocyte common antigen (15). Lack of glassy

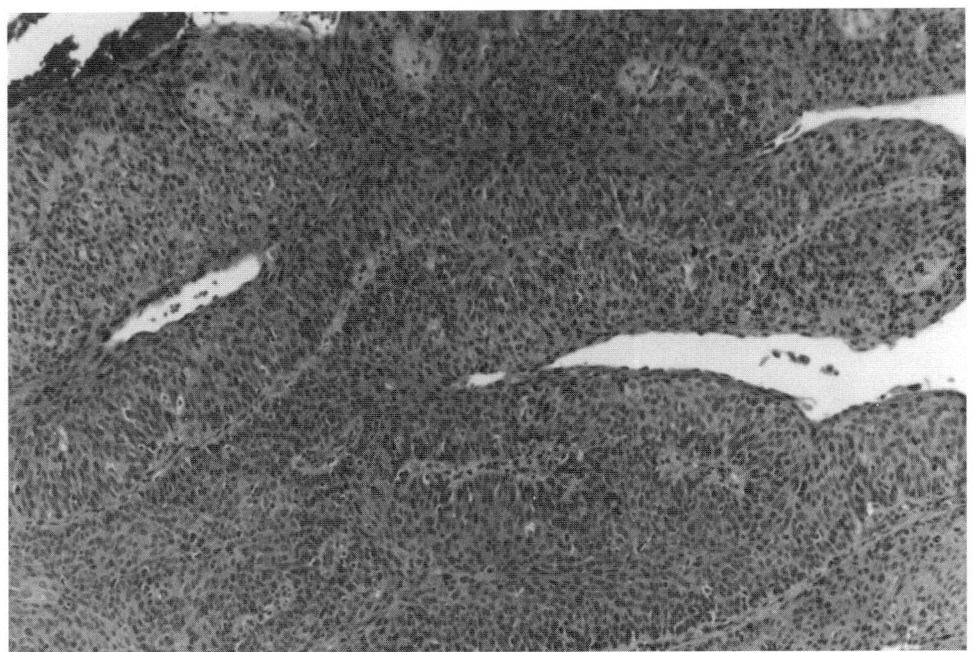

FIGURE 9.18. Papillary squamous (transitional cell) carcinoma. The tumor architecturally resembles transitional cell carcinoma of the bladder. Reprinted with permission of Robboy Associates, Chapel Hill, NC.

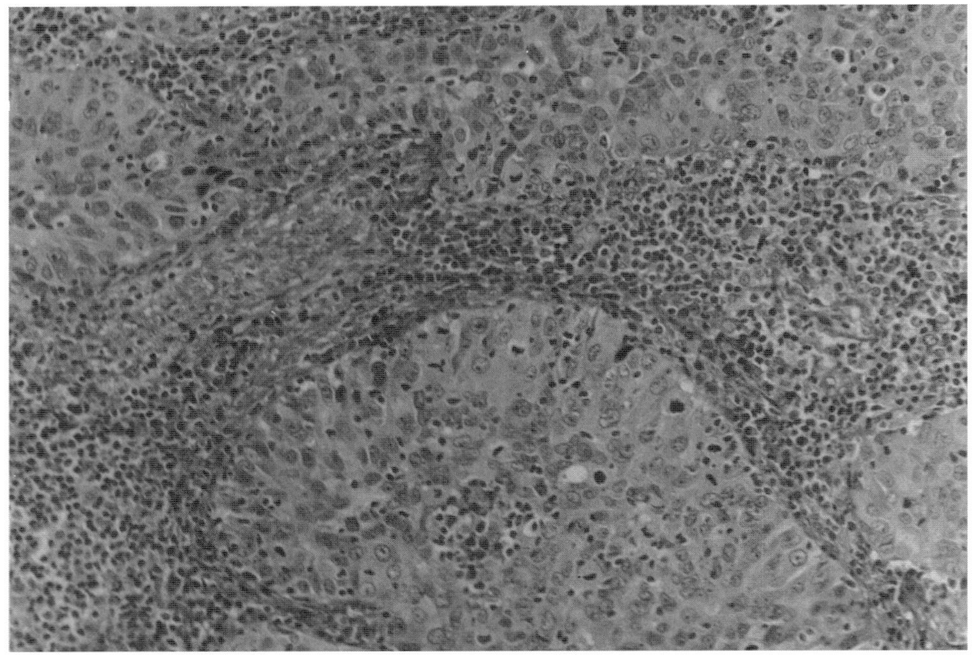

FIGURE 9.19. Lymphoepithelioma-like carcinoma. A prominent lymphoid infiltrate separates nests of tumor cells. Reprinted with permission of Robboy Associates, Chapel Hill, NC.

cytoplasm and less prominent nucleoli help distinguish these lesions from glassy cell carcinoma.

ADENOCARCINOMA OF THE UTERINE CERVIX

Adenocarcinoma of the cervix is increasing in frequency, and this coupled with a decreasing incidence of squamous carcinomas has led to an overall increase in the proportion of invasive cervical malignancies that are adenocarcinomas. As in squamous lesions, HPV plays an important role in the development of these lesions, particularly HPV 18. The most common presenting symptom is abnormal bleeding. Cytology is less sensitive for glandular than squamous cervical lesions (26).

ENDOCERVICAL-TYPE (MUCINOUS) ADENOCARCINOMA

Most invasive cervical adenocarcinomas are of the endocervical type, containing at least focally mucinous cells resembling those seen in endocervical glands (Fig. 9.20). Cellular stratification, nuclear atypia, and mitotic activity are present. Architecturally, glands may be irregular with cribriforming and can invade deeply. A prominent stromal reaction is often present. These lesions have a high association with SIL (26).

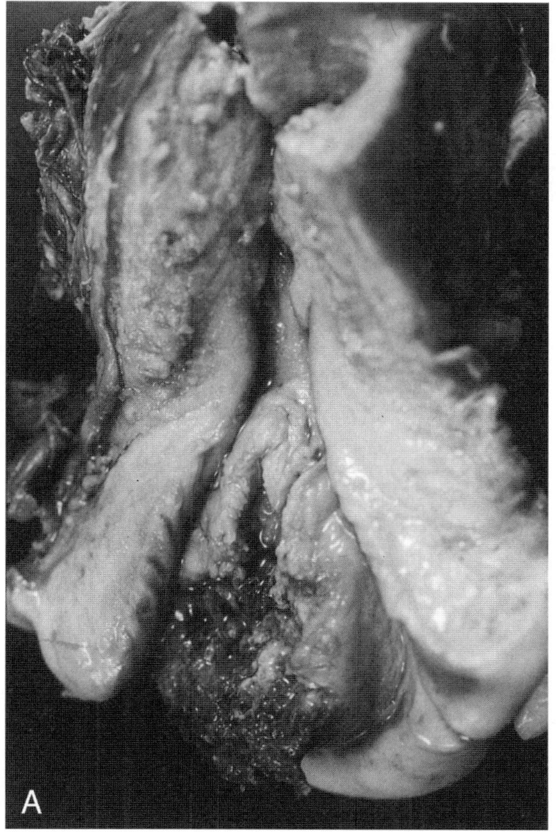

FIGURE 9.20. Endocervical-type (mucinous) endocervical adenocarcinoma. **A.** Tumor arising in the endocervix. The tumor exhibits a complex architecture. *(figure continues)*

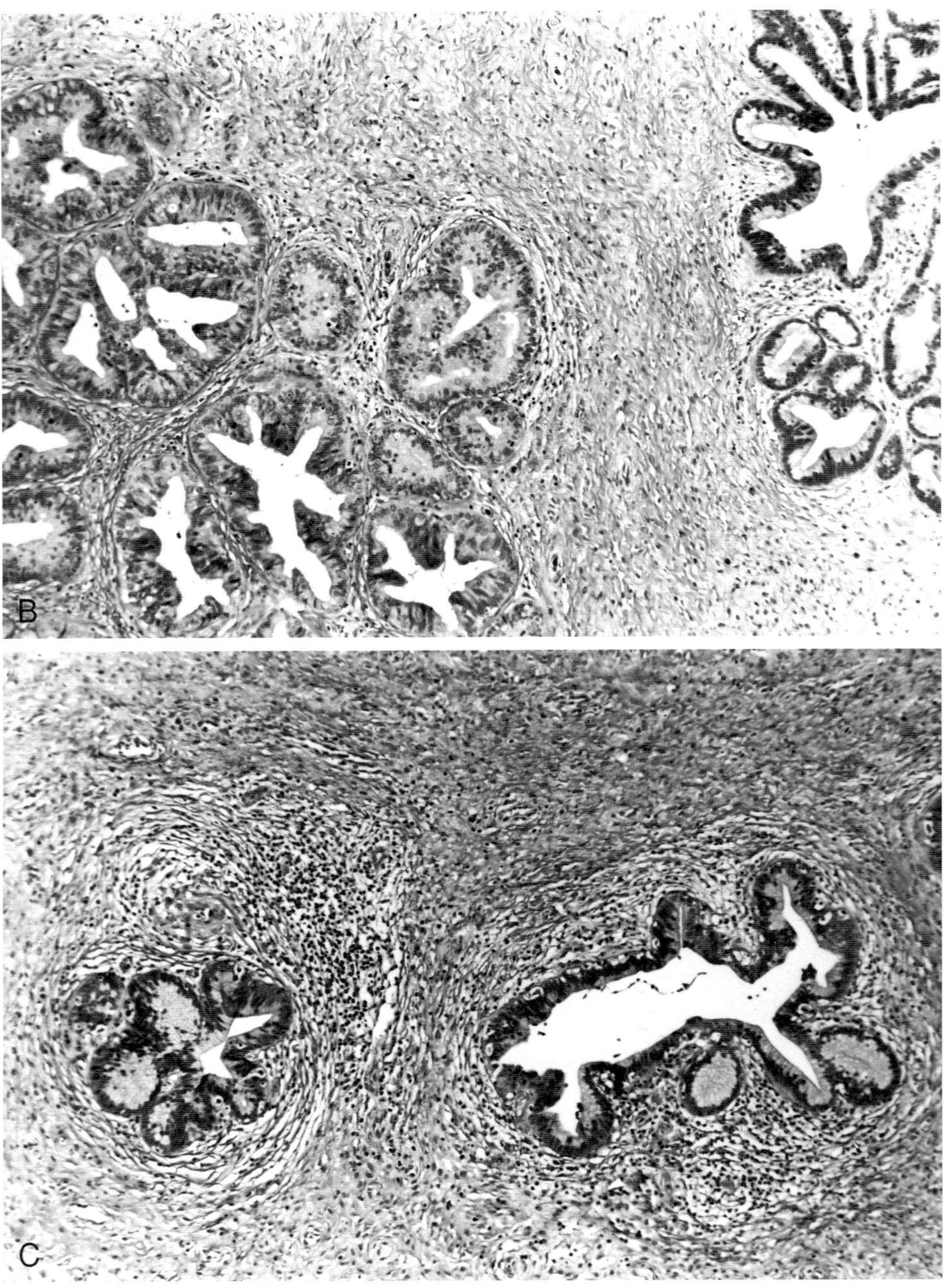

FIGURE 9.20. *(continued)* **(B)** and a prominent stromal reaction **(C)**.

Deeply invasive glands, desmoplasia, and greater architectural and cytological atypia are features to consider in distinguishing invasive endocervical adenocarcinoma from AIS. This distinction can be difficult, and because the patients tend to be somewhat younger that patients with squamous carcinomas, this can pose a clinical dilemma. Invasive adenocarcinoma cannot be ruled out on a cervical punch biopsy. At the very least, an adequate LEEP or cold knife conization specimen is required to make the distinction.

MINIMAL DEVIATION ADENOCARCINOMA (MDA, ADENOMA MALIGNUM)

MDA is a subtype of endocervical type adenocarcinoma that appears deceptively benign. In rare cases, an association with Peutz-Jeghers syndrome exists (26). In MDA, glands are lined by mucinous epithelium with basally located nuclei with minimal atypia. The key to the diagnosis of malignancy is the presence of architecturally complex glands, deep invasion, and at least focal atypia. In addition, there is frequently a stromal response, at least focally (Fig. 9.21)(8).

In an attempt to distinguish MDA from other lesions, Steeper and colleagues (27) noted CEA staining in both MDA and conventional adenocarcinomas of the endocervix, but not in microglandular hyperplasia. CEA may be positive in MDA, and is cytoplasmic as well as luminal when present, in distinction to the luminal only location in normal endocervical glands (26), however CEA is not positive in all cases of endocervical carcinoma regardless of type, limiting clinical utility.

The differential diagnosis of minimal deviation adenocarcinoma also includes mesonephric hyperplasia, tunnel clusters, and deep nabothian cysts. Mesonephric remnants do not contain mucin. Tunnel clusters are rounded rather than irregular and usually contain a flattened epithelium. Deep nabothian cysts are lined by mucinous or flat epithelium but lack atypia, mitoses, and desmoplasia.

The reported prognosis for MDA varies in the literature. While some authors feel this is a particularly aggressive neoplasm (26, 28), others have stated that with optimum therapy the lesion is no more aggressive than other well-differentiated endocervical adenocarcinomas (29).

VILLOGLANDULAR ADENOCARCINOMA

Another subtype of endocervical adenocarcinoma is villoglandular adenocarcinoma. This lesion exhibits a different biologic behavior than other adenocarcinomas of the endocervix, as it occurs in somewhat younger patients and has a better prognosis. A possible relationship to oral contraceptive pills has been suggested, but an etiology has not been established (30). Villoglandular adenocarcinomas are exophytic, exhibiting papillae lined by mildly atypical epithelium of endocervical, endometrioid, or enteric type with occasional mitoses (Fig. 9.22). Infiltration occurs at the base. These tumors tend to be well circumscribed (26). The tumor must be distinguished from the more aggressive serous carcinoma of the cervix, which exhibits significantly more atypia and mitotic activity. Other.lesions in the differential include papillary endocervicitis, papillary adenofibroma, mullerian papilloma, and endocervical polyps, none of which exhibit stratification, invasiveness, atypia, or any significant mitotic activity.

ENDOMETRIOID-TYPE ADENOCARCINOMA

The second most common pattern of endocervical adenocarcinoma is the endometrioid pattern, which histologically resembles the uterine tumor (Fig. 9.23). This can at times present problems identifying a primary site.

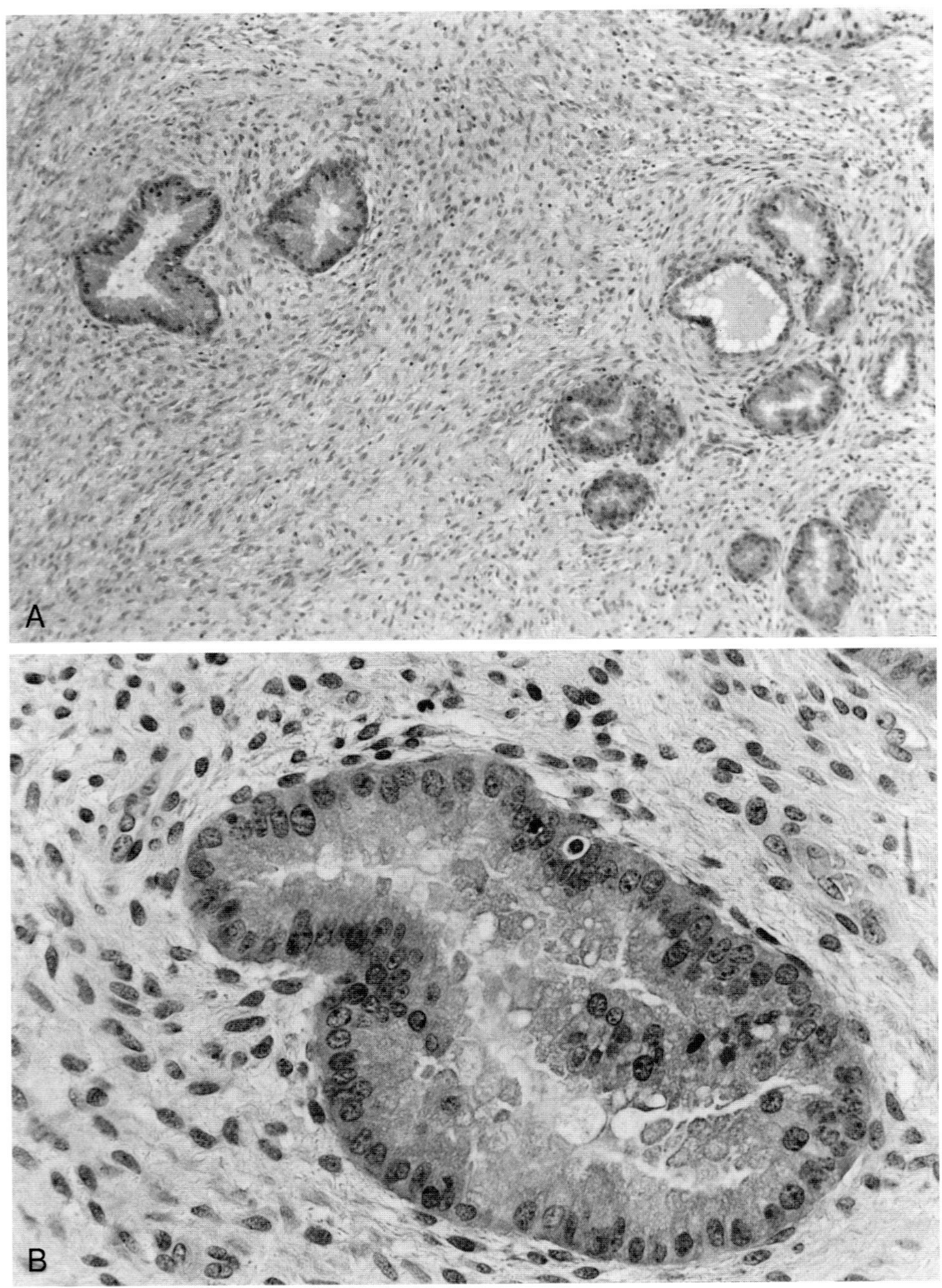

FIGURE 9.21. Minimal deviation adenocarcinoma (adenoma malignum). **A,B.** The tumor appears deceptively benign.

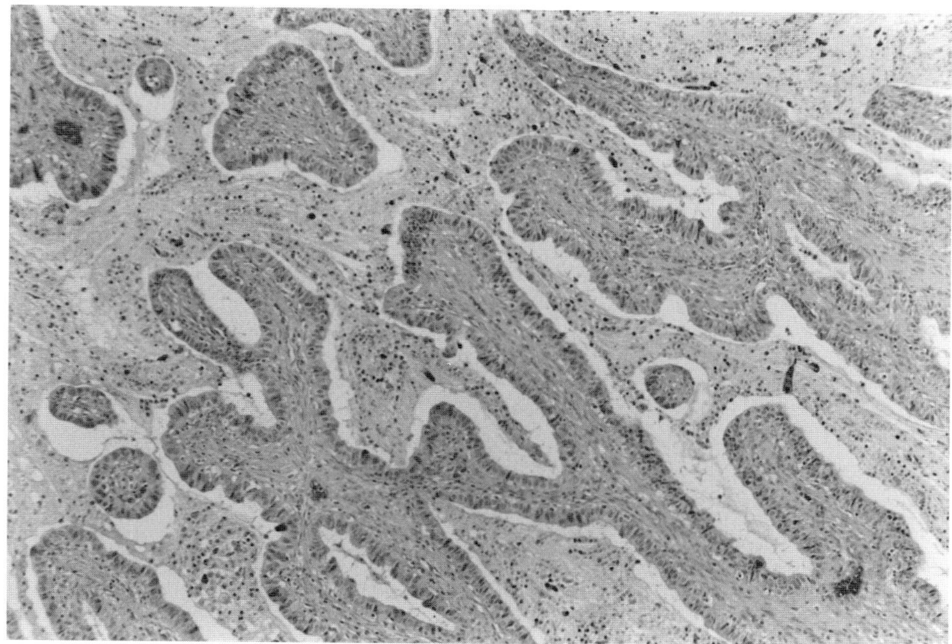

FIGURE 9.22. Villoglandular pattern of adenocarcinoma. Minimally atypical cells line papillae.

An unusual variant of minimal deviation adenocarcinoma with endometrioid features has been described (31), which can be distinguished from a benign lesion by the number, shape, and depth of the glands; moderate nuclear atypia; occasional mitoses; and at least focal stromal reaction. Most of the lesions in this study were incidental findings, and the patients did well.

DISTINGUISHING ENDOCERVICAL FROM ENDOMETRIAL ADENOCARCINOMA

One of the problems that can arise is distinguishing an endocervical-type adenocarcinoma (particularly those with limited mucinous features) from an endometrial adenocarcinoma with spread to the cervix, conditions which may be treated differently. Mucin stains are not helpful in making this distinction although Maes and colleagues (32) suggested that staining with antibody to intestinal mucin supports an endocervical origin, while staining for gastric mucin and absent intestinal mucin favor an endometrial primary. Some authors have found vimentin-staining positivity in some endometrial carcinomas but not cervical ones (33). Others have noted CEA positivity more often in cervical lesions (34). Endocervical lesions are more likely to show cytoplasmic CEA staining whereas endometrial primaries show nonspecific apical staining. Neither vimentin nor CEA will be useful in all cases. Histological examination of all regions of the specimen may reveal more characteristic endometrioid areas as well as areas of hyperplasia in the case of a uterine primary. Squamous metaplasia also points to a uterine lesion (26). In addition, the stroma of the neoplasm may be more characteristic

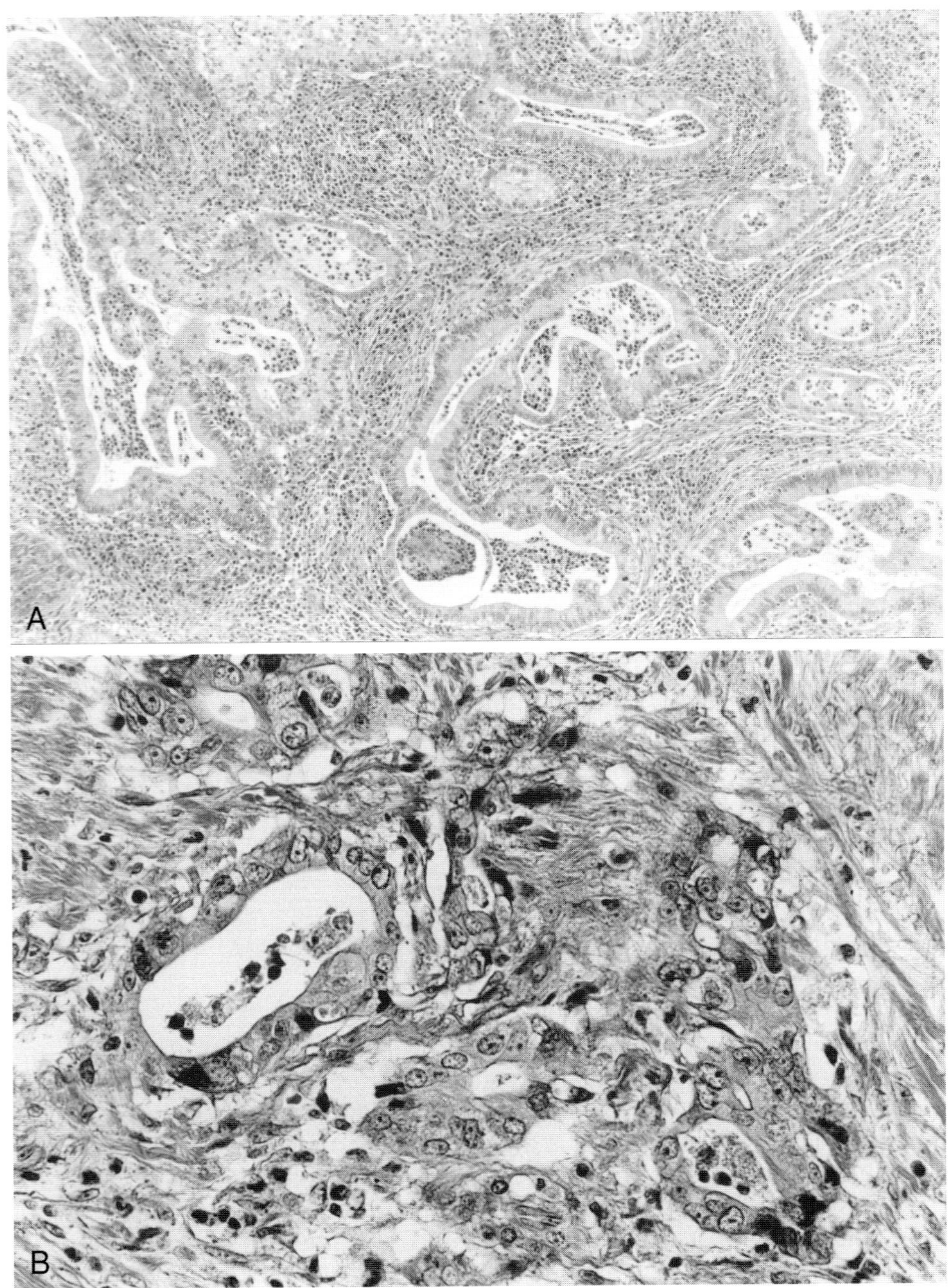

FIGURE 9.23. Endometrioid type endocervical adenocarcinoma. **A,B.** The neoplastic glands resemble endometrial adenocarcinoma of the uterus.

of its region of origin. Examination of nonmalignant endometrial or cervical tissue may contain preinvasive changes, thus pointing to a primary site.

In endometrioid tumors, histology alone may not elucidate the primary site. A recent study (35) detected vimentin in 81.4% of endometrial adenocarcinomas and 13% of endometrioid cervical adenocarcinomas, and CEA in 65.2–95.6% of cervical tumors depending on antibody used, but not in examined endometrial cases. Clinical localization of the main tumor mass by imaging studies or hysteroscopy may be helpful in some cases.

ENTERIC-TYPE ADENOCARCINOMA

Enteric differentiation may be seen in both AIS and invasive endocervical adenocarcinoma, but does not appear to be of prognostic significance (Fig. 9.24) (36).

CLEAR CELL ADENOCARCINOMA

The association between clear cell adenocarcinoma of the cervix and intrauterine diethylstilbestrol exposure has been discussed separately. Clear cell carcinomas of the cervix also arise in the absence of DES exposure. These lesions are histologically identical to other clear cell carcinomas of the female genital tract. The tumor may exhibit single architectural patterns or a combination of tubulocystic, solid, and papillary patterns. Tubulocystic and papillary areas may be lined by hobnail, clear, flat, or cuboidal cells. Solid areas of clear cells are often seen (Fig. 9.25) (37). Stromal hyalinization may be prominent.

Atypical microglandular hyperplasia and the Arias-Stella reaction (ASR) in the cervix

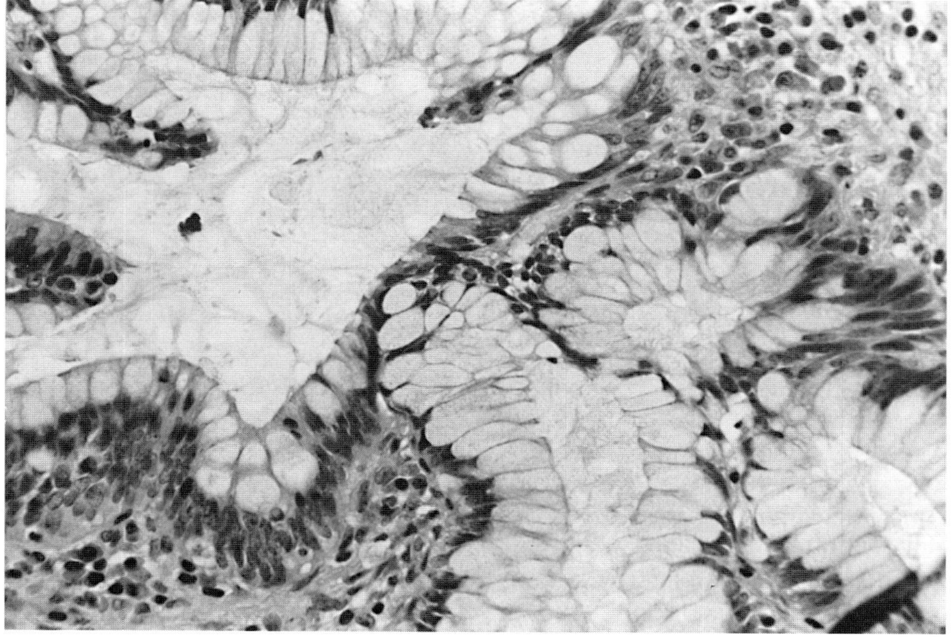

FIGURE 9.24.   Enteric differentiation in AIS. Abundant goblet cells are present.

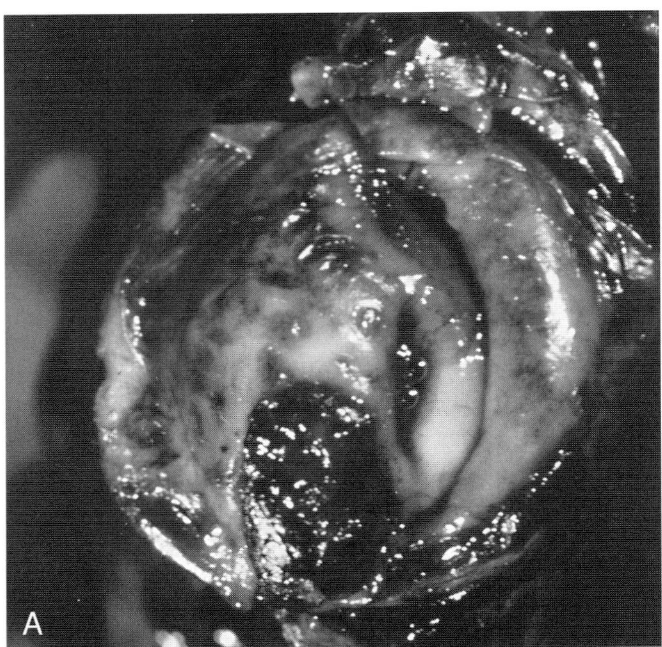

FIGURE 9.25. Clear cell adenocarcinoma. **A.** Clear cell carcinoma of the cervix. Reprinted with permission of Robboy Associates, Chapel Hill, NC. **B–G.** The tumor can show a varied histology including solid with clear cells **(B,C)**, papillary with clear cells **(D,E)**, papillary with hobnail cells **(F)**, and tubulocystic with hobnail cells **(G)**.

should not be mistaken for a clear cell adenocarcinoma. Atypical microglandular hyperplasia may exhibit unusual patterns such as solid, signet-ring like, or reticular, and it may have a prominent myxoid stroma. Clear or hobnail cells may line cystic spaces. The nuclear atypia and mitotic activity of a clear cell adenocarcinoma is absent in microglandular hyperplasia, and areas of more typical microglandular hyperplasia may also be present (8). The Arias-Stella reaction, more common in the endometrium, may be seen in the cervix as well. In addition to history of a pregnancy, there is usually less atypia and little or no mitotic activity in ASR.

MESONEPHRIC DUCT CARCINOMA

Mesonephric carcinomas are rare adenocarcinomas that have a poor prognosis (26). In a study of 29 cases of mesonephric rests and lesions, four cases of carcinoma were described (38). In this study, three out of the four patients died of their disease, and there was insufficient follow-up time on the fourth. Histologically, mesonephric carcinomas arise deep in the cervix, consisting of back-to-back tubules lined by a single layer of atypical cells (Fig. 9.26). The distinction from mesonephric hyperplasia depends upon the nuclear atypia, back-to-back crowding of the tubules, solid areas, and irregular disorderly invasion of the carcinoma. Cytology, architecture, and the presence of normal endocervical glands as well as a background of mesonephric hyperplasia help distinguish mesonephric carcinoma from other endocervical adenocarcinomas.

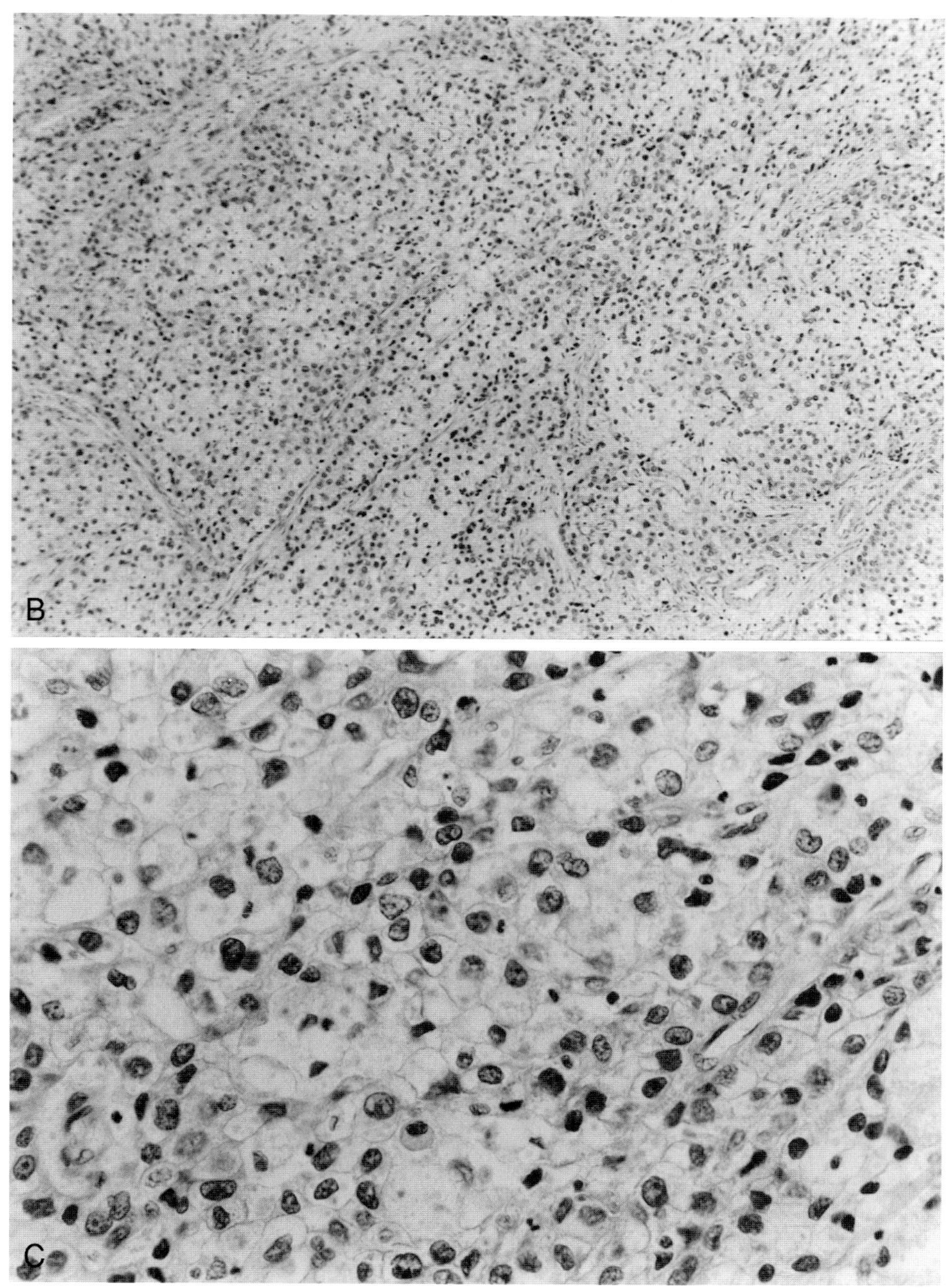

FIGURE 9.25.   *(continued)*

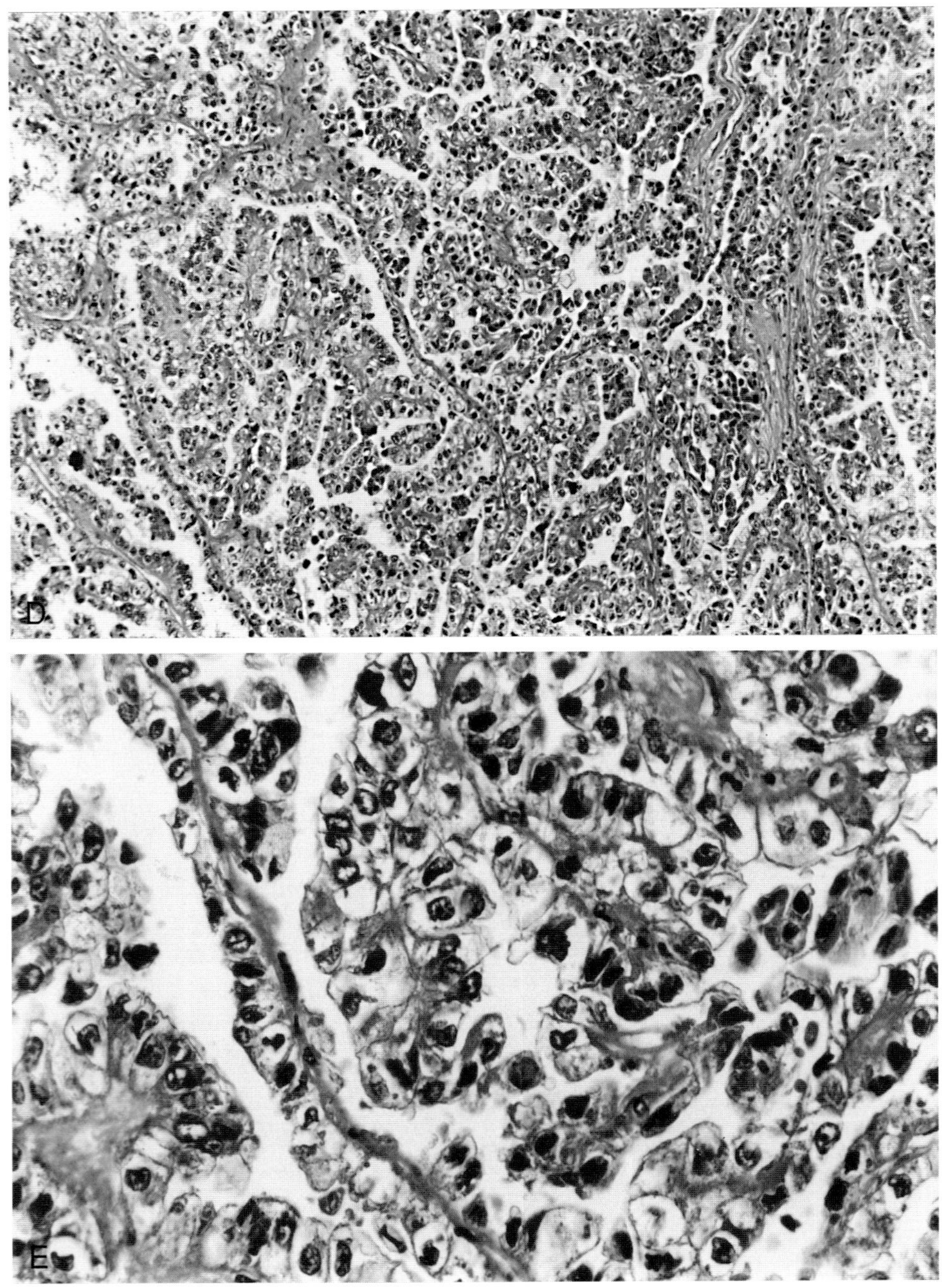

FIGURE 9.25.   *(continued)*

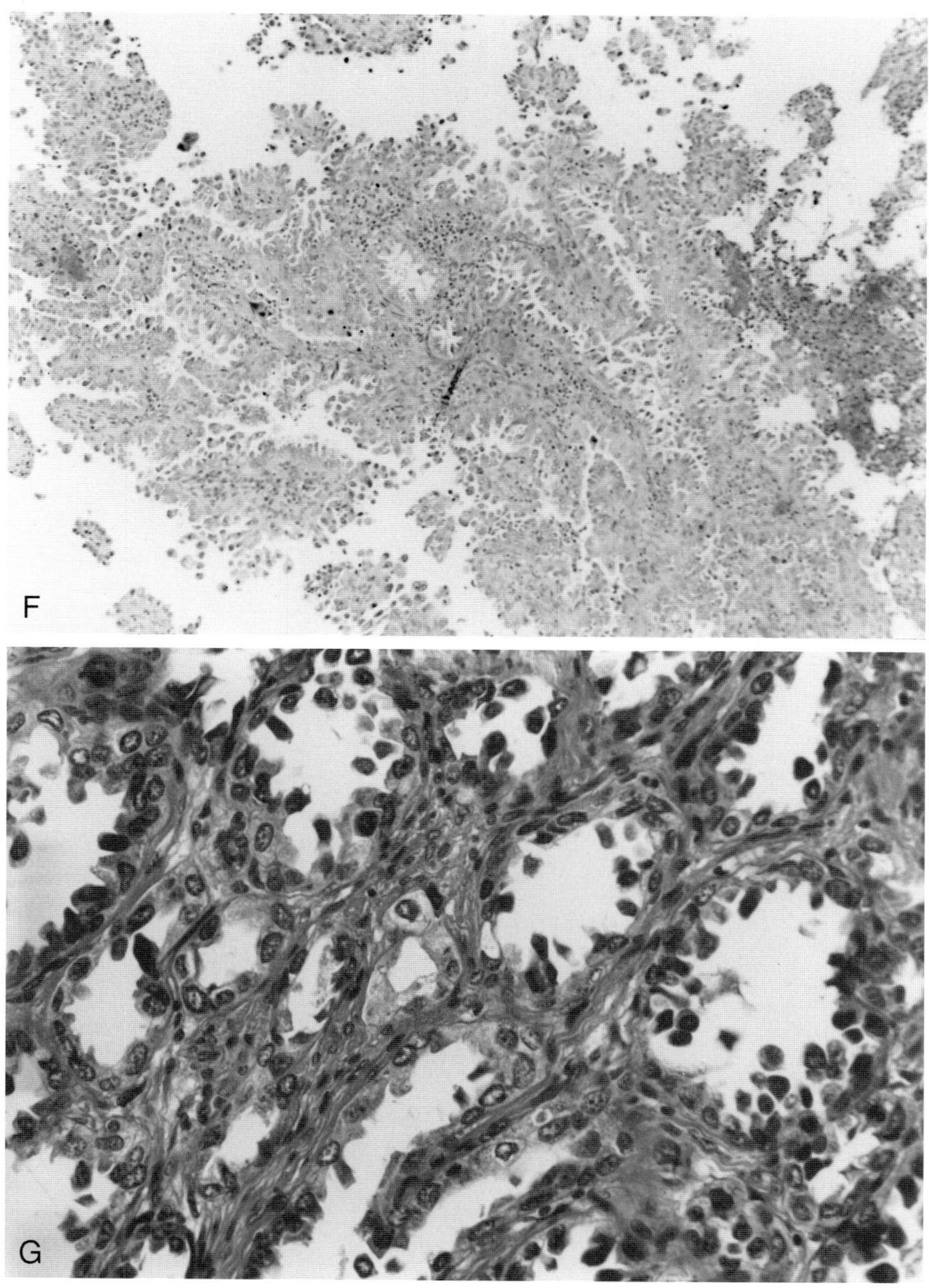

FIGURE 9.25.   *(continued)*

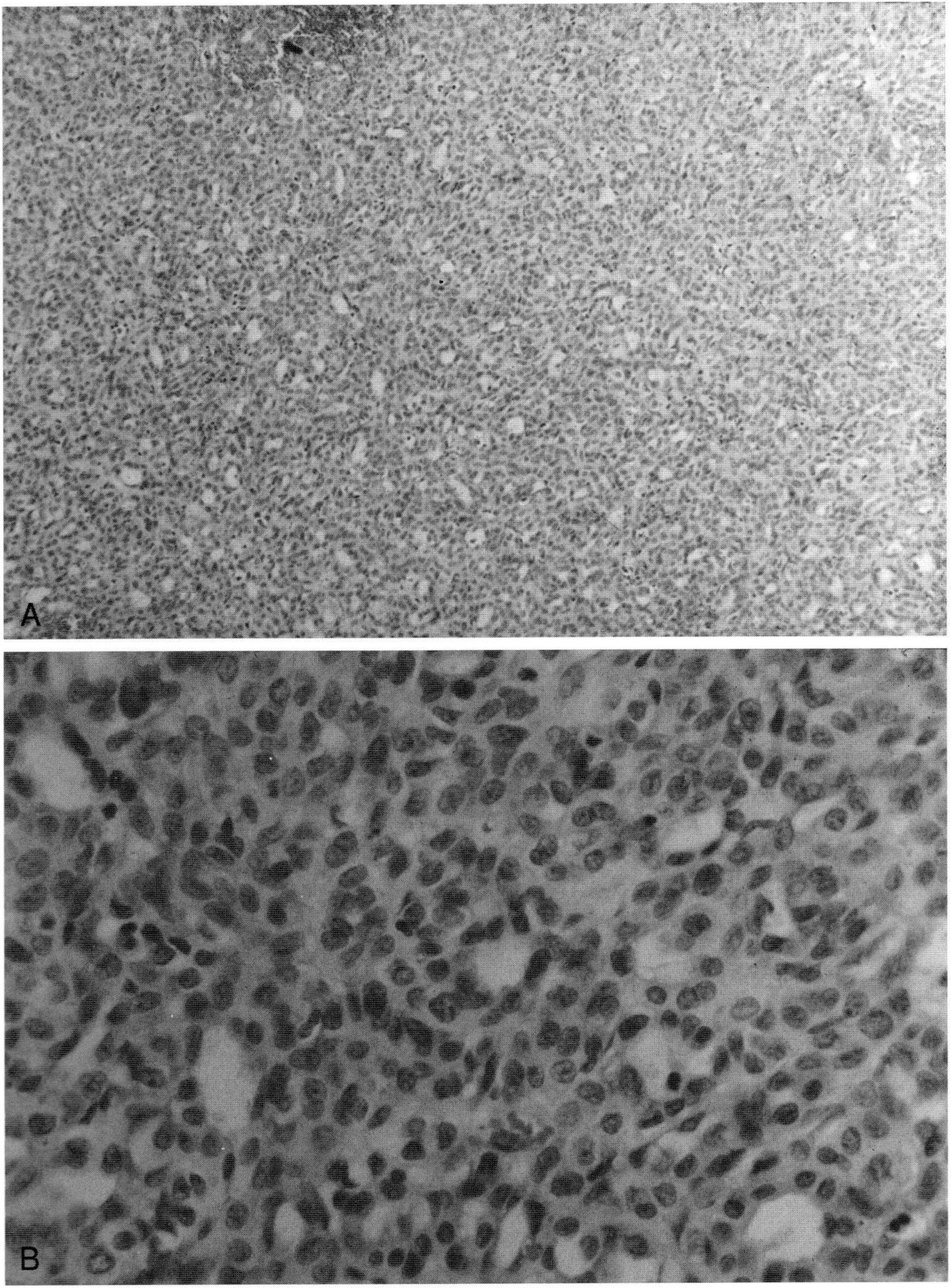

FIGURE 9.26. **A,B.** Mesonephric duct carcinoma, composed of back to back tubules. Reprinted with permission of Robboy Associates, Chapel Hill, NC.

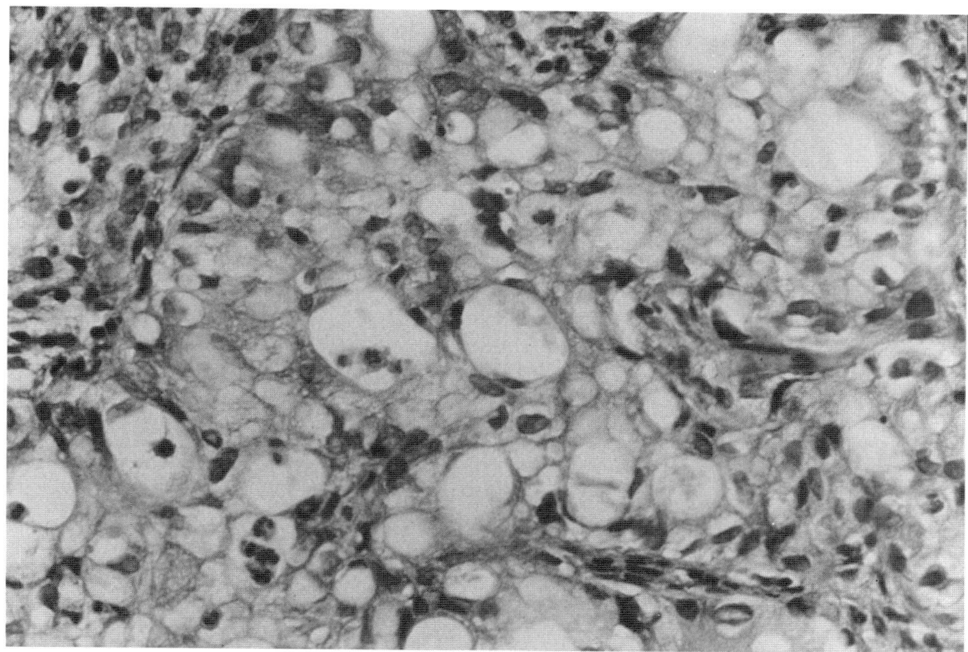

FIGURE 9.27.   Signet ring carcinoma. Numerous signet ring cells are present. Reprinted with permission of Robboy Associates, Chapel Hill, NC.

SIGNET RING CELL ADENOCARCINOMA

Signet ring cells may be seen within cervical adenocarcinomas and adenosquamous carcinomas (26) but rarely present as a pure pattern (Fig. 9.27). In these cases, a metastatic gastrointestinal or breast primary should be considered.

SEROUS CARCINOMA

The rarity of this tumor as a cervical primary dictates ruling out spread from other genital tract sites. Histologically, these tumors resemble papillary serous carcinomas of the ovary and endometrium (Fig. 9.28).

ADENOSQUAMOUS CARCINOMA

Adenosquamous carcinomas have recognizable squamous cell carcinoma and adenocarcinomatous areas (Fig. 9.29). Whether or not there is any prognostic difference between squamous cell carcinoma, adenocarcinoma, and adenosquamous carcinoma is controversial. Shingleton and colleagues (39) found no significant 5-year survival differences between the three types of neoplasm, except in stage 2 patients, where their squamous cell carcinoma patients did significantly better.

SQUAMOUS CELL CARCINOMA WITH MUCIN POSITIVITY

A subset of poorly differentiated squamous cell carcinomas demonstrate mucin positivity, but do not show obvious gland formation. Some pathologists call these lesions

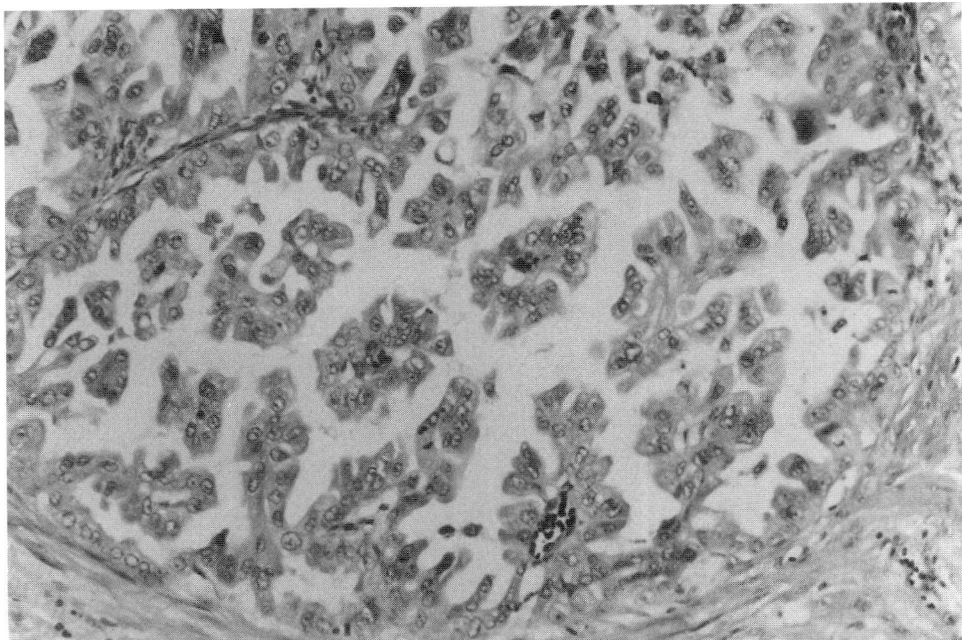

FIGURE 9.28. Serous carcinoma. The tumor resembles the ovarian neoplasm. Reprinted with permission of Robboy Associates, Chapel Hill, NC.

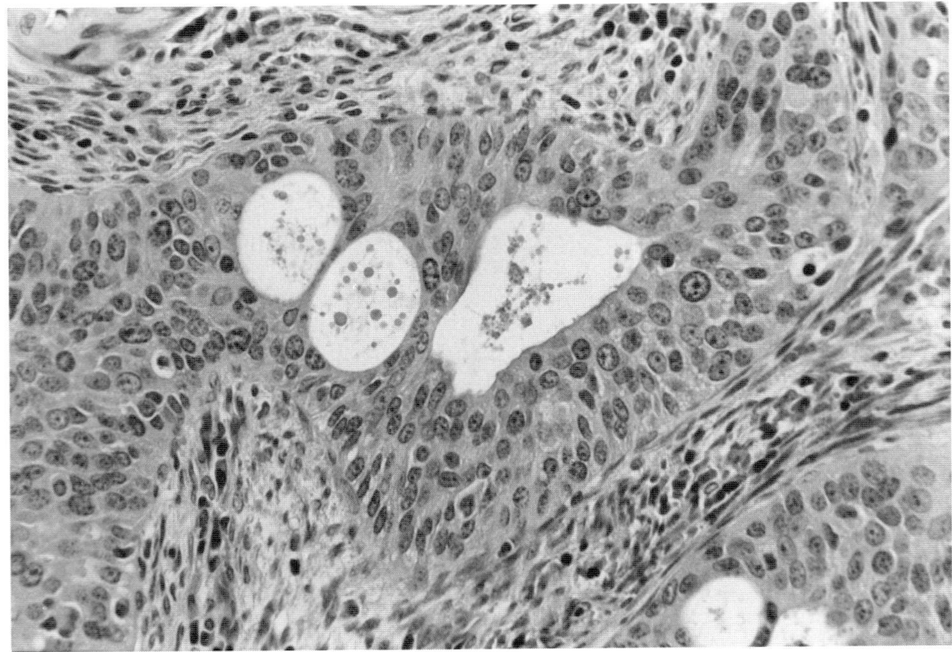

FIGURE 9.29. Adenosquamous carcinoma. The tumor contains mixed squamous and glandular features.

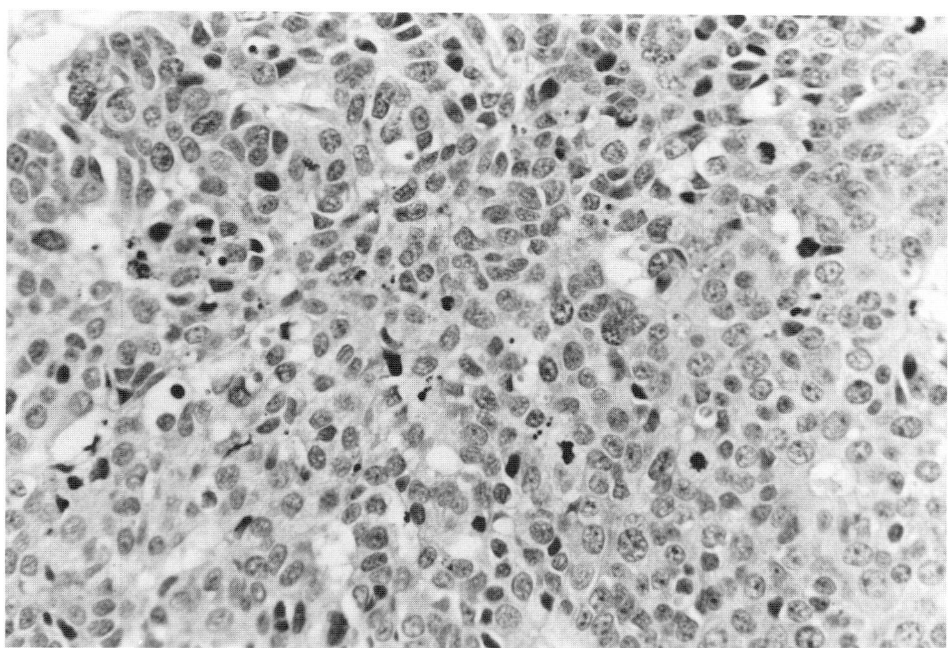

FIGURE 9.30.   SCC with mucin positivity. A few areas suggestive of attempted gland formation are seen.

squamous cell carcinomas with mucin positivity, or mucoepidermoid carcinomas (Fig. 9.30). This tumor has been described as a lesion in younger women, and some authors report a more aggressive behavior (40). In a study of 161 carcinomas of the cervix of at least stage IB, routine mucin staining resulted in reclassification of 38 patients (24%), including identification of 31 mucin producing squamous cell carcinomas. These authors (40) reported a decreased survival in their patients with adenosquamous carcinoma including mucin positive squamous cell tumors as compared to mucin negative squamous cell carcinomas. Others have stated that no significant epidemiological trends are obscured by not separately classifying these tumors (41).

GLASSY CELL CARCINOMA

This aggressive neoplasm is considered by some to be a poorly differentiated variant of adenosquamous carcinoma rather than an independent histologic subtype (42). The tumor contains large cells with abundant eosinophilic or amphophilic "glassy" cytoplasm. Nuclei are large and have prominent nucleoli. Mitotic activity is prominent. The stroma often shows an eosinophilic and plasma cell infiltrate (26) (Fig. 9.31). Mucin is usually absent in these tumors. The outcome of glassy cell carcinomas varies in the literature, which may reflect the variation in criteria for the diagnosis.

OTHER PRIMARY MALIGNANCIES OF THE UTERINE CERVIX

UNDIFFERENTIATED CARCINOMA

Epithelial lesions completely lacking in differentiation are termed "undifferentiated carcinomas" (Fig. 9.32).

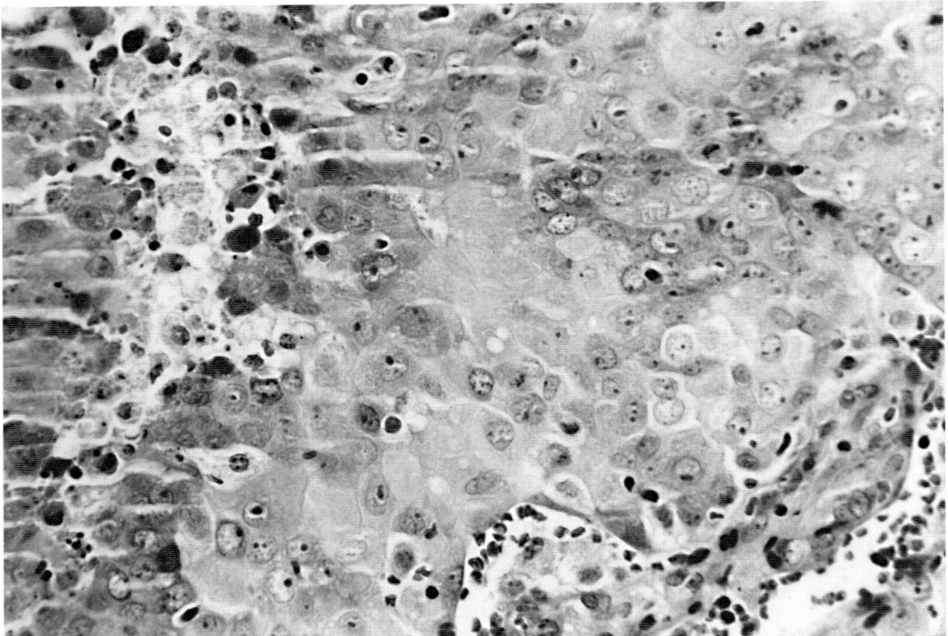

FIGURE 9.31. Glassy cell carcinoma. Poorly differentiated neoplasm with abundant eosinophilic glassy cytoplasm.

SMALL CELL UNDIFFERENTIATED CARCINOMA AND CARCINOID

Some of the tumors that were previously lumped together in the same category as the small cell variant of squamous cell carcinoma were found to have neuroendocrine differentiation and are now separately classified as small cell undifferentiated carcinomas. (Squamous cell carcinomas comprised of small cells are classified as poorly differentiated squamous cell carcinomas.) Small cell undifferentiated neuroendocrine tumors are composed of small undifferentiated cells with minimal cytoplasm and abundant mitotic activity (Fig. 9.33). A crush artifact may be present. These tumors may stain for keratin, EMA, and CEA, and for neuroendocrine markers such as chromogranin, synaptophysin, and NSE. Pure carcinoids of the cervix are rare, and this diagnosis should be reserved for those well-differentiated lesions with the characteristic architecture, uniform nuclei, and infrequent mitotic activity of carcinoids elsewhere in the body (Fig. 9.34) (26). Small cell undifferentiated carcinomas may be distinguished from small cell squamous cell carcinoma by round-to-spindle rather than round-to-oval nuclei, greater hyperchromatism with coarser chromatin, less cytoplasm, the presence of crush artifact, and lack of nucleoli (18). Electron microscopy or immunohistochemistry can demonstrate the neuroendocrine differentiation.

A strong association between small cell undifferentiated carcinomas and HPV type 18 has been reported (43). As well as in small cell undifferentiated carcinomas, neuroendocrine differentiation has also been documented in cases of undifferentiated carcinomas and poorly differentiated adenosquamous carcinomas (44).

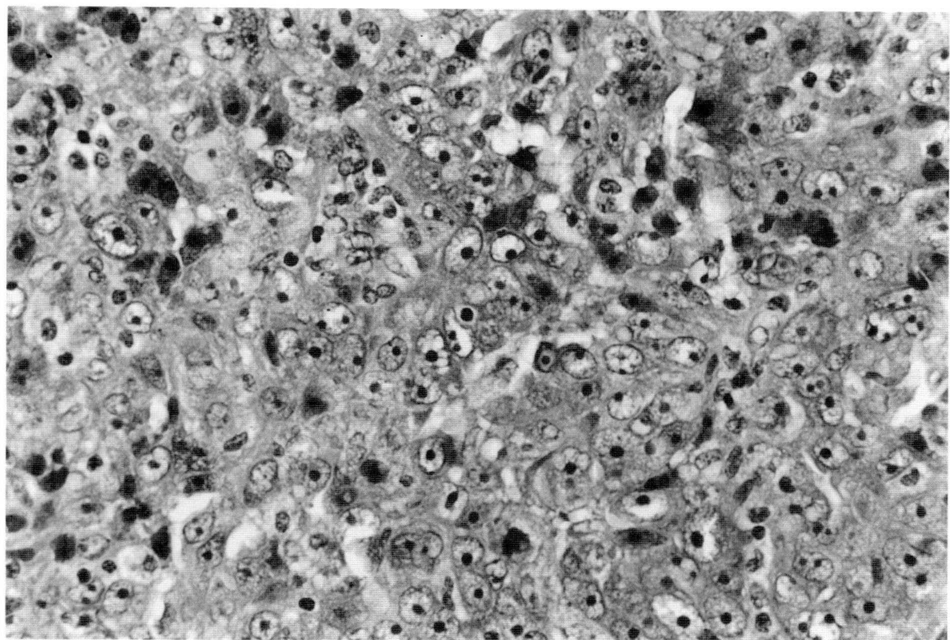

FIGURE 9.32.   Undifferentiated carcinoma. Markedly anaplastic tumor devoid of squamous or glandular differentiation.

ADENOID CYSTIC CARCINOMA

Adenoid cystic carcinoma of the cervix histologically resembles the salivary gland tumor, being composed of small basaloid cells around cystic spaces that may be empty or may contain basophilic or eosinophilic material (Fig. 9.35). Solid areas and cords of tumor cells may also be seen. The tumors exhibit prominent mitotic activity and nuclear pleomorphism. A stromal reaction is usually prominent (8, 45). These lesions are uncommon, and most of the patients are postmenopausal (46). Unlike the better prognosis of adenoid basal carcinoma from which it must be distinguished, adenoid cystic carcinomas behave in an aggressive fashion. The tumors stain for keratin, but do not stain for S100 protein as they lack the myoepithelial differentiation of the salivary gland tumor (26).

ADENOID BASAL CARCINOMA

Adenoid basal carcinomas are low-grade cervical neoplasms. They are characterized by infiltrating nests of small tumor cells, some with central cystic spaces, with palisading of the nuclei peripherally. The cells have scant cytoplasm, uniform hyperchromatic nuclei, and minimal mitotic activity. A stromal reaction is usually absent (Fig. 9.36). Surface ulceration of cervical epithelium often exists. The prognosis of these lesions is considerably better than that of adenoid cystic carcinoma, from which it must be distinguished (45). The tumors stain for keratin and are negative for S100 protein (26).

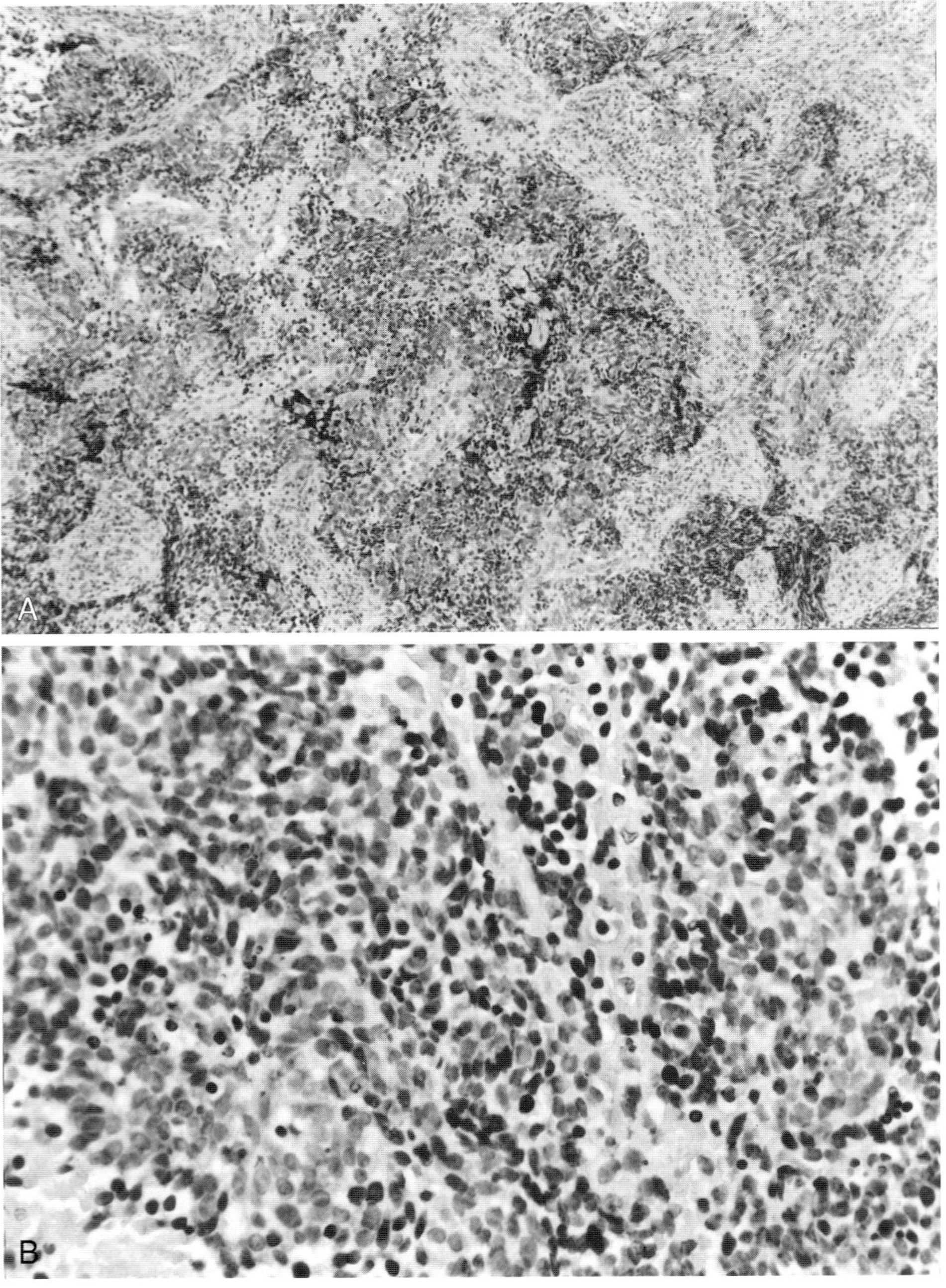

FIGURE 9.33. Small cell undifferentiated carcinoma. **A.** An infiltrating tumor with "crush" artifact. **B.** Small undifferentiated cells with hyperchromatic nuclei and inconspicuous cytoplasm.

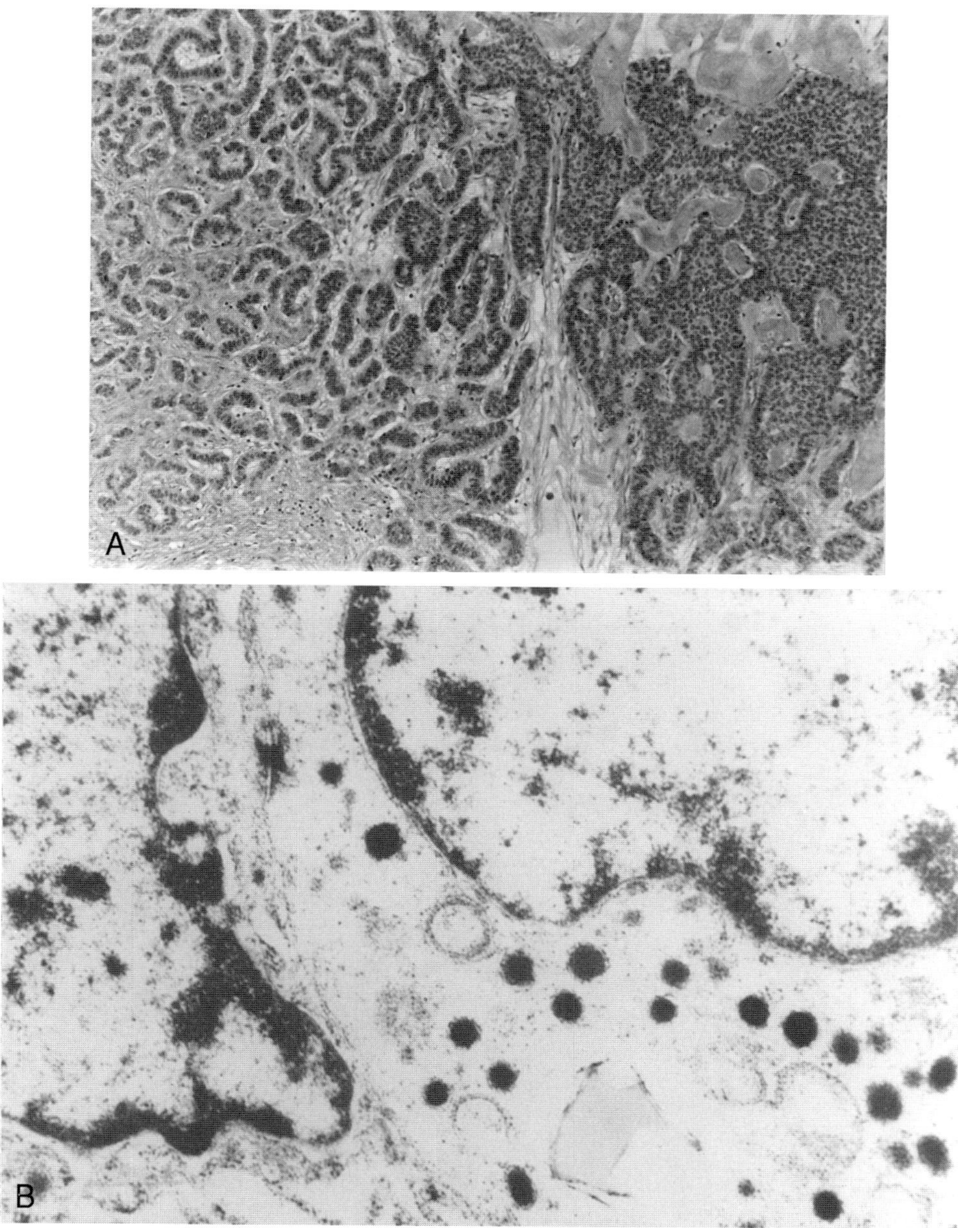

FIGURE 9.34.   Carcinoid. **A.** Typical histology of a carcinoid tumor. **B.** Neurosecretory granules are seen on electron microscopy. Reprinted with permission of Robboy Associates, Chapel Hill, NC.

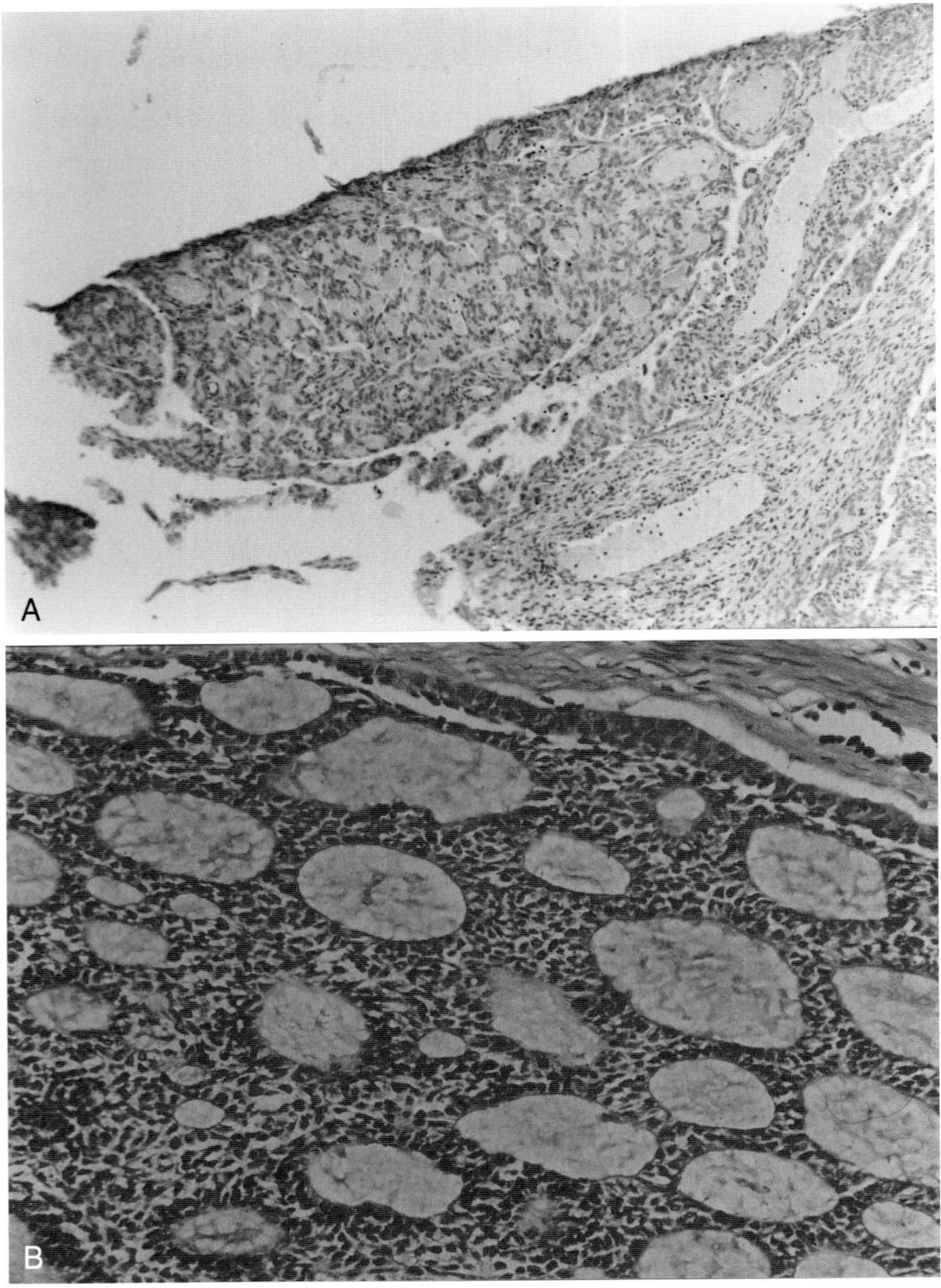

FIGURE 9.35. Adenoid cystic carcinoma. **A,B.** The tumor is similar in appearance to the salivary gland tumor, with cystic spaces containing eosinophilic material surrounded by basaloid tumor cells. B reprinted with permission of Robboy Associates, Chapel Hill, NC.

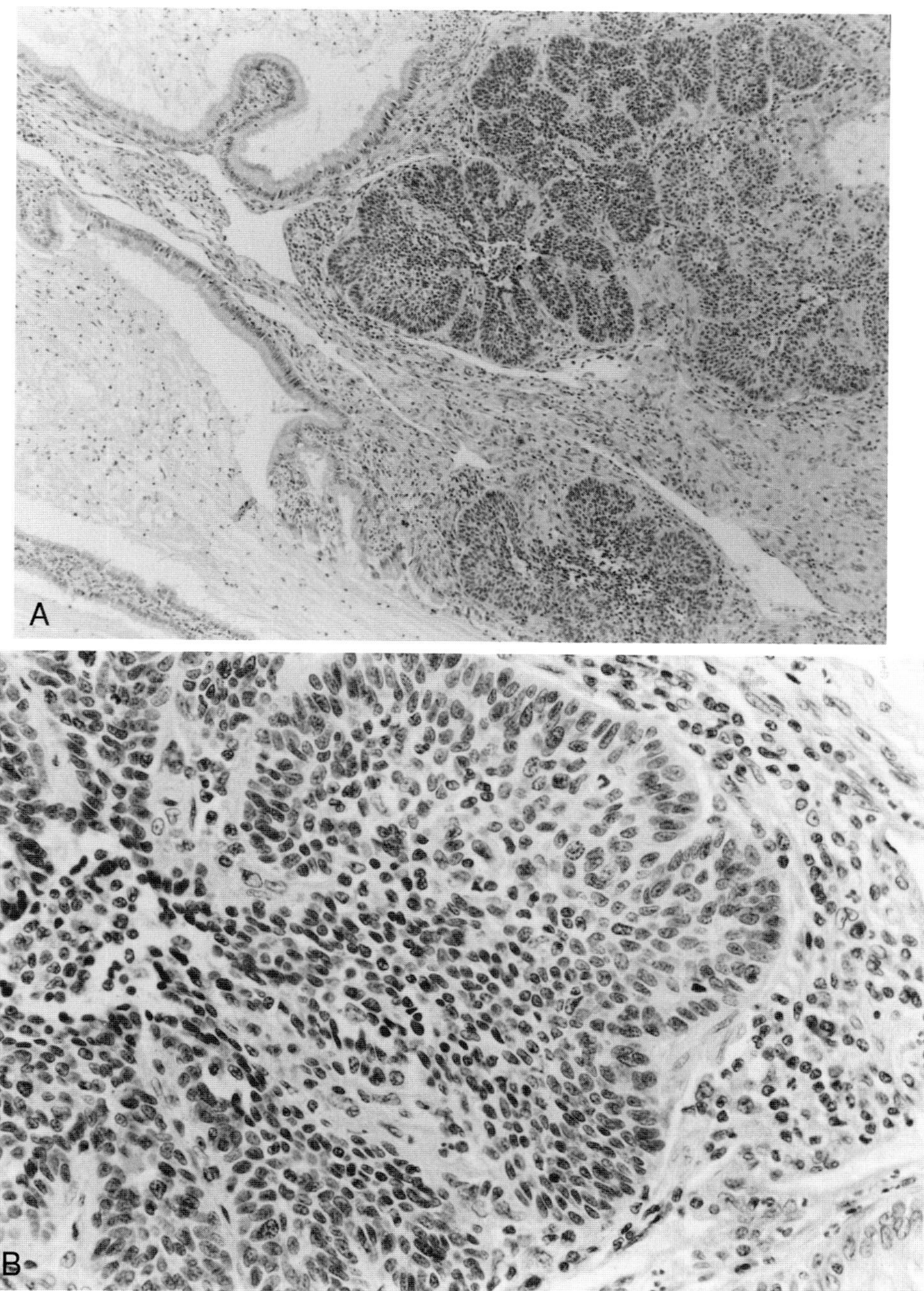

FIGURE 9.36.   Adenoid basal carcinoma. **A.** Infiltrating nests of basaloid cells with no stromal reaction. **B.** There is peripheral palisading of nuclei.

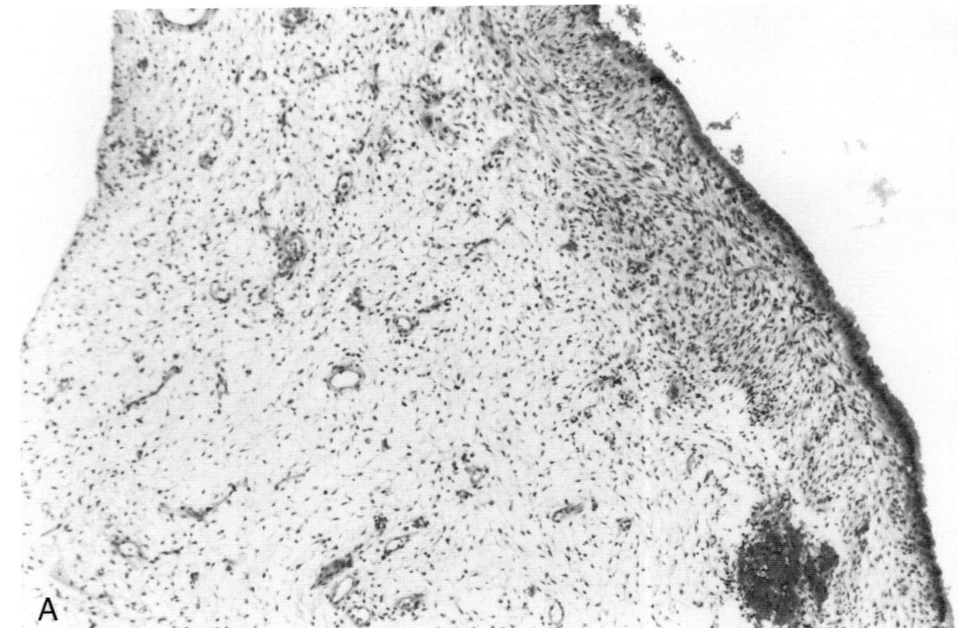

FIGURE 9.37.   Embryonal rhabdomyosarcoma. **A.** Most of this lesion was polypoid and grossly resembled an endocervical polyp. The cambium layer is seen under the epithelium, and the rest of the stroma appears deceptively benign.

CERVICAL MELANOMA

Although melanocytes have occasionally been demonstrated in the cervix, primary cervical melanoma is exceedingly rare. Melanoma should not be confused with the more common blue nevus of the cervix (47).

CERVICAL LYMPHOMAS

Lymphoma in the cervix may be mistaken for chronic inflammation. Other areas of confusion include granulocytic sarcoma and small cell carcinomas. Markers such as leukocyte common antigen help establish the hematopoietic nature of the infiltrate. A mixed lymphoid infiltrate favors an inflammatory process over a lymphoma. A monoclonal proliferation is characteristic of a lymphoma. Granulocytic sarcoma, a tumor having a poor prognosis, will stain with the chloroacetate esterase stain or with an immunohistochemical stain for lysozyme. Small cell squamous cell carcinoma will stain for epithelial markers, and the neuroendocrine small cell undifferentiated carcinoma will stain for neuroendocrine markers. In cervical lymphoma, a barrel-shaped cervix or submucosal mass may present and give rise to suspicion of a neoplasm (47). The prognosis for a primary cervical lymphoma is usually good (47).

EMBRYONAL RHABDOMYOSARCOMA (SARCOMA BOTRYOIDES)

Sarcoma botryoides arising in the uterine cervix occurs in young women with a mean age of 18 years (48), as opposed to the vaginal tumor that occurs in infants. The cervical

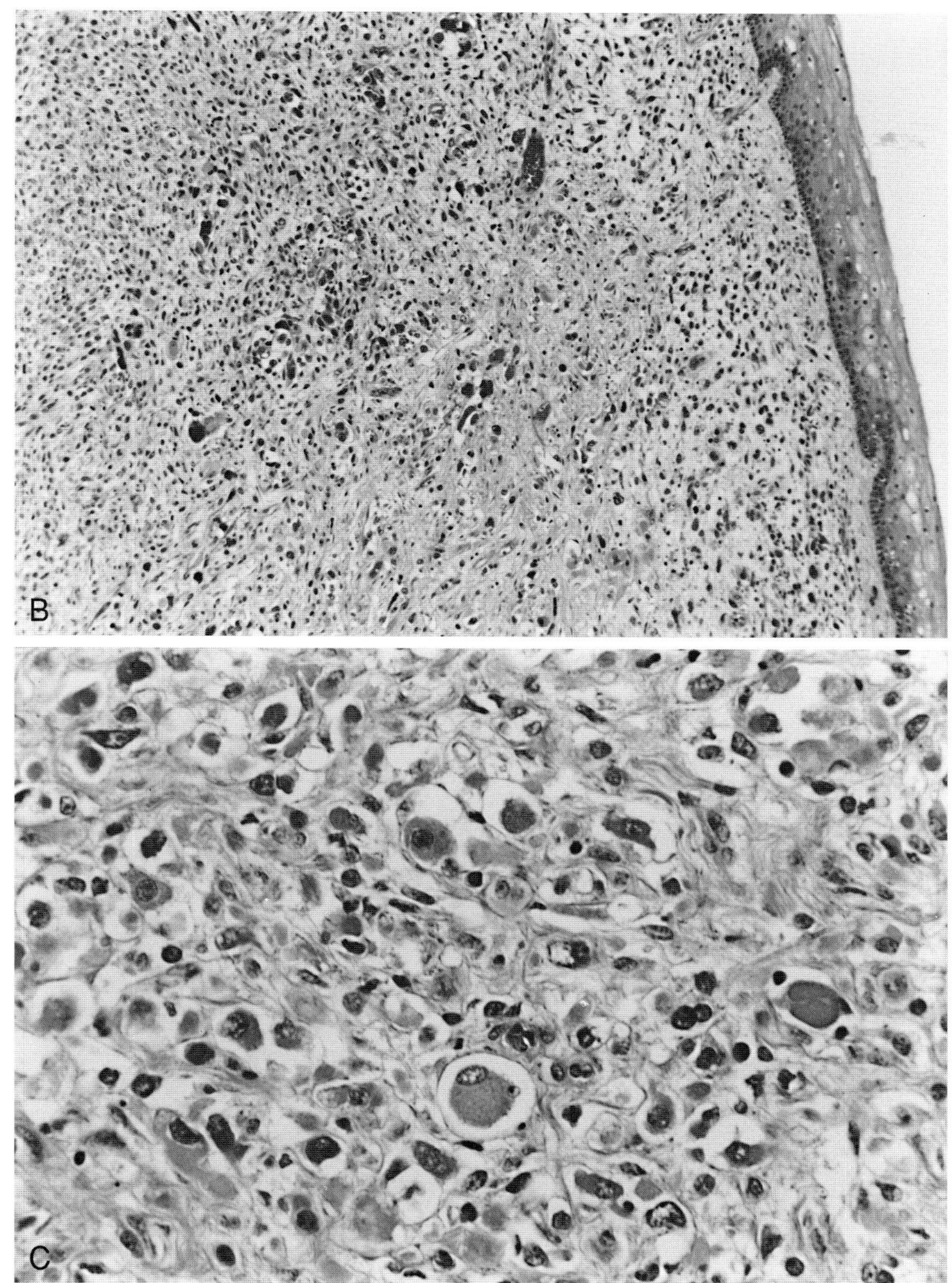

FIGURE 9.37.   *(continued)* **B,C.** Focally, the lesion invades cervical stroma, where a more atypical appearance with primitive rhabdomyoblasts is present.

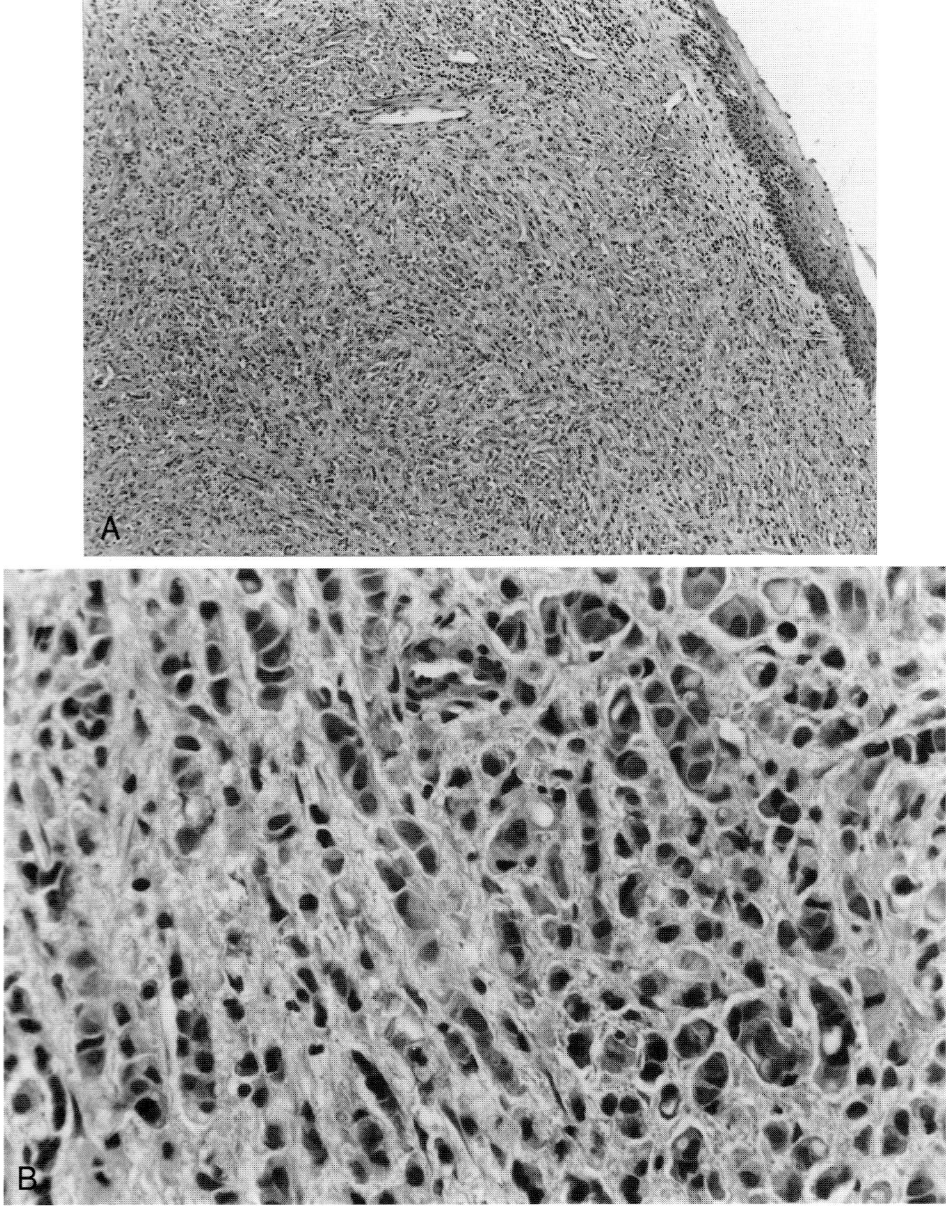

FIGURE 9.38. Metastatic breast carcinoma to cervix. **A.** Tumor infiltrating cervical stroma. **B.** Indian File pattern with occasional signet ring cells, consistent with metastatic invasive lobular carcinoma of the breast.

TABLE 9.2.   Malignant Tumors of the Uterine Cervix

Squamous cell carcinoma
  Squamous cell carcinoma
  Warty (condylomatous) carcinoma
  Verrucous carcinoma
  Papillary squamous (transitional) cell carcinoma
  Lymphoepithelioma-like carcinoma
Adenocarcinoma
  Endocervical-type (mucinous) adenocarcinoma of the endocervix
  Minimal deviation adenocarcinoma
  Villoglandular adenocarcinoma
  Endometrioid-type adenocarcinoma of the endocervix
  Enteric-type adenocarcinoma of the endocervix
  Signet ring carcinoma
  Clear cell adenocarcinoma
  Serous carcinoma
  Mesonephric carcinoma
Adenosquamous carcinoma
  Adenosquamous carcinoma
  Glassy cell carcinoma
Undifferentiated carcinoma
Other Uncommon Epithelial Malignancies
  Neuroendocrine carcinomas
    Carcinoid
    Small cell undifferentiated carcinoma
  Adenoid cystic carcinoma
  Adenoid basal carcinoma
Other Uncommon Primary Malignancies of the Cervix
  Embryonal rhabdomyosarcoma
  Lymphoma
  Melanoma
  Stromal sarcoma
  Leiomyosarcoma
  Adenosarcoma
  Malignant mixed mesodermal tumor
  Malignant fibrous histiocytoma
  Liposarcoma
  Alveolar soft part sarcoma
  Malignant schwannoma
  Endodermal sinus tumor
  Osteosarcoma
  Wilm's tumor
Tumors metastatic to the cervix

tumor usually presents with vaginal bleeding or a protruding mass, and it has a similar histology to the vaginal tumor (Fig. 9.37). The tumors stain for myoglobin and desmin, and foci of cartilage may be present. Cervical embryonal rhabdomyosarcoma usually has a favorable prognosis (47). The most common misdiagnosis is a benign endocervical polyp, which lacks rhabdomyoblasts and a cambium layer.

METASTATIC TUMORS TO THE UTERINE CERVIX

The most common metastatic tumors to the cervix are from other genital primaries. If the cervix is the first presentation of a nongenital tumor, a signet ring or "Indian file" pattern, trapped benign glands, and extensive lymphvascular space involvement should be looked for. The most common extragenital tumors to spread to the cervix are from the breast (Fig. 9.38), stomach, and colon (47). For an overview of the malignant tumors of the cervix, please see Table 9.2.

REFERENCES

1. Richart RM. Cervical intraepithelial neoplasia: a review. In Sommes SC, ed. Pathology Annual 1973. New York: Appleton Century Crofts, 1973:301–328.
2. Nuovo G, Friedman D, Richart RM. In situ hybridization analysis of human papillomavirus DNA segregation patterns in lesions of the female genital tract. Gynecol Oncol 1990;36:256–262.
3. Richart RM. A modified terminology for cervical intraepithelial neoplasia. Obstet Gynecol 1990;75:131–133.
4. Tidbury P, Singer A, Jenkins D. CIN 3: the role of lesion size in invasion. Br J Obstet Gynaecol 1992;99:583–586.
5. Leung KM, Chan WY, Hui PK. Invasive squamous cell carcinoma and cervical intraepithelial neoplasia III of uterine cervix. Morphologic differences other than stromal invasion. Am J Clin Pathol 1994;101:508–513.
6. Al-Nafussi AI, Hughes D. Histological features of CIN 3 and their value in predicting invasive microinvasive squamous carcinoma. J Clin Pathol 1994;47:799–804.
7. Alejo M, Macedo I, Matias-Guiu X, et al. Adenocarcinoma in situ of the uterine cervix: clinicopathological study of nine cases with detection of human papillomavirus DNA by in situ hybridization and polymerase chain reaction. Int J Gynecol Pathol 1993;12: 219–223.
8. Lawrence WD. Advances in the pathology of the uterine cervix [review]. Hum Pathol 1991;22:792–806.
9. Kobal KH, Roman LD, Felix JC, et al. The role of endocervical curettage at cervical conization for high-grade dysplasia. Obstet Gynecol 1995;85:197–201.
10. Jansen FW, Trimbos JB, Hermans J, et al. Persistent cervical intraepithelial neoplasia after incomplete conization: predictive value of clinical and histological parameters. Gynecol Obstet Invest 1994;37:270–274.
11. Wolf JK, Levenback C, Malpica A, et al. Adenocarcinoma in situ of the cervix: the significance of cone biopsy margins. Obstet Gynecol 1996;88:82–86.
12. Creasman W. New gynecologic cancer staging. Gynecol Oncol 1995;58:157–158.
13. Kurman RJ, Norris H. Tumors of the Cervix, Vagina and Vulva: Atlas of Tumor Pathology. 3rd series. Washington, DC:AFIP, 1992:55.
14. van Nagell JR Jr., Greenwell N, Powell DF, et al Microinvasive carcinoma of the cervix. Am J Obstet Gynecol 1983;145:981–991.
15. Robert ME, Fu YS Squamous cell carcinoma of the uterine cervix-a review with emphasis on prognostic factors and unusual variants [review]. Semin Diagn Pathol 1990;7:173–189.

16. McLachlin CM, Devine P, Muto M, et al. Pseudoinvasion of vascular spaces: report of an artifact caused by cervical lidocaine injection prior to loop diathermy. Hum Pathol 1994; 25:208–211.
17. Wentz WB, Reagan JW, Heggie AD, et al. Survival in cervical cancer with respect to cell type. Cancer 1959;12:384–388.
18. Reagan JW. The cellular manifestation of uterine carcinogenesis. In Norris HJ, Hertig AT, Abell MR eds. The Uterus. Baltimore: Williams & Wilkins, 1973:320–324.
19. Crissman JD, Makuch R, Budhraja M. Histopathologic grading of squamous cell carcinoma of the uterine cervix. An evaluation of 70 stage IB patients. Cancer 1985;55:1590–1596.
20. Broders AC. Carcinoma-grading and practical application. Arch Pathol 1926;2:376–381.
21. Young RH, Kurman RJ, Scully RE. Proliferations and tumors of intermediate trophoblast of the placental site [review]. Semin Diagn Pathol 1988;5:223–237.
22. Ayhan A, Altintas A, Tuncer ZS, et al. Predictive value of mitotic activity, eosinophilic and inflammatory reaction in stage I cancer of the uterine cervix. Eur J Surg Oncol 1992;18: 264–266
23. Bethwaite PB, Holloway LJ, Yeong ML, et al. Effect of tumor associated tissue eosinophilia on survival of women with stage 1B carcinoma of the uterine cervix. J Clin Pathol 1993; 46:1016–1020.
24. Randall ME, Anderson WA, Mills SE, et al. Papillary squamous cell carcinoma of the uterine cervix: a clinicopathologic study of nine cases. Int J Gynecol Pathol 1986;5:1–10.
25. Wong WS, Ng CS, Lee CK. Verrucous carcinoma of the cervix. Arch Gynecol Obstet 1990; 247:47–51.
26. Young RH, Scully RE. Invasive adenocarcinoma and related tumors of the uterine cervix [review]. Semin Diagn Pathol 1990;7:205–227.
27. Steeper TA, WicK MR. Minimal deviation adenocarcinoma of the uterine cervix ("adenoma malignum"): an immunohistochemical comparison with microglandular hyperplasia and conventional endocervical adenocarcinoma. Cancer 1986;58:1131–1138.
28. Gilks CB, Young RH, Aguirre P, et al. Adenoma malignum (minimal deviation adenocarcinoma) of the uterine cervix: a clinicopathological and immunohistochemical analysis of 26 cases. Int J Surg Pathol 1989;13:717–729.
29. Silverberg S, Hurt W. Minimal deviation adenocarcinoma ("adenoma malignum") of the cervix. A reappraisal. Am J Obstet Gynecol 1975;121;971–975.
30. Jones MW, Silverberg SG, Kurman RJ. Well-differentiated villoglandular adenocarcinoma of the uterine cervix: a clinicopathological study of 24 cases. Int J Gynecol Pathol 1993; 12:1–7.
31. Young RH, Scully RE. Minimal deviation endometrioid adenocarcinoma of the uterine cervix: a report of five cases of a distinctive neoplasm that may be interpreted as benign. Am J Surg Pathol 1993;17:660–665.
32. Maes G, Fleuren GJ, Bara J, et al. The distribution of mucins, carcinoembryonic antigen and mucus-associated antigens in endocervical and endometrial adenocarcinomas. Int J Gynecol Pathol 1988;7:112–122.
33. Dabbs DJ, Geisinger KR, Norris HT. Intermediate filaments in endometrial and endocervical carcinomas: the diagnostic utility of vimentin patterns. Am J Surg Pathol 1986;10:568–576.
34. Wahlstrom T, Lingren J, Korhonen M, et al. Distinction between endocervical and endometrial adenocarcinoma with immunoperoxidase staining of carcinoembryonic antigen in routine histological tissue specimens. Lancet 1979;2:1159–1160.
35. Dabbs DJ, Sturtz K, Zaino RJ. The immunohistochemical discrimination of endometrioid adenocarcinomas. Hum Pathol 1996;27:172–177.
36. Savargaonkar PR, Hale RJ, Pope R, et al. Enteric differentiation in cervical adenocarcinomas and its prognostic significance. Histopathol 1993;23:275–277.
37. Herbst AL, Anderson D. Clear cell adenocarcinoma of the vagina and cervix secondary to intrauterine exposure to diethylstilbestrol [review]. Semin Surg Oncol 1990;16:343–346.

38. Ferry JA, Scully RE. Mesonephric remnants, hyperplasia and neoplasia of the uterine cervix: a study of 49 Cases. Am J Surg Pathol 1990;14;1100–1111.
39. Shingleton HM, Bell MC, Fremgen A, et al. Is there really a difference in survival of women with squamous cell carcinoma, adenocarcinoma and adenosquamous cell carcinoma of the cervix? Cancer 1995;76:1948–1955.
40. Bethwaite P, Yeong ML, Holloway L, et al. The prognosis of adenosquamous carcinomas of the uterine cervix. Br J Obstet Gynaecol 1992;99:745–750.
41. Colgan TJ, Auger M, McLaughlin JR. Histopathologic classification of cervical carcinomas and recognition of mucin-secreting squamous cell carcinomas. Int J Gynecol Pathol 1993; 12:64–69.
42. Costa MJ, Kenny MB, Hewan-Lowe K, et al. Glassy cell features in adenosquamous carcinoma of the uterine cervix. Histologic, ultrastructural, immunohistochemical, and clinical findings. Am J Clin Pathol 1991;96:520–528.
43. Stoler MH, Mills SE, Gersell DJ, et al. Small-cell neuroendocrine carcinoma of the cervix. A human papillomavirus type 18–associated cancer. Am J Surg Pathol 1991;15:28–32.
44. Barrett RJ 2nd, Davos I, Leuchter RS, et al. Neuroendocrine features in poorly differentiated and undifferentiated carcinomas of the cervix. Cancer 1987;60:2325–2330.
45. Kudo R. Cervical adenocarcinoma [review]. Curr Topics Pathol 1992;85:81–111.
46. Dixit S, Singhal S, Vyas R, et al. Adenoid cystic carcinoma of the cervix [review]. J Postgrad Med 1993;39:211–215.
47. Clement PB. Miscellaneous primary tumors and metastatic tumors of the uterine cervix [review]. Semin Diagn Pathol 1990;7:228–248.
48. Daya DA, Scully RE. Sarcoma botryoides of the uterine cervix in young women: a clinicopathological study of 13 cases [review]. Gynecol Oncol 1988;29:290–304.

DIETHYLSTILBESTROL (DES) AND THE LOWER GENITAL TRACT

Stanley J. Robboy, MD, Rex C. Bentley, MD,
Hannah R. Krigman, MD,
and Malcolm C. Anderson, FRCPath, FRCOG

■

Clear Cell Adenocarcinoma
Pathogenesis
Nonneoplastic Changes
Preneoplastic Changes
Lesions of Statistical Chance
New Investigative Techniques

Diethylstilbestrol (DES), a nonsteroidal estrogen first synthesized in 1937, was widely prescribed by the mid-1940s and 1950s to gravid women who were thought to be at high risk for early pregnancy loss. Up to two (1) to three (2, 3) million women had been born with a history of prenatal exposure when, in 1971, DES became linked to the extremely rare development of clear cell adenocarcinoma of the vagina and cervix in some of the young female offspring who had been exposed in utero (1).

The DES story, as it has since evolved, has provided a fertile opportunity to examine many aspects of developmental biology, human disease processes, experimental animal models and their relevance to humans, and even forays into governmental regulatory processes and tort law (3–14). The DES story has led to reevaluations of concepts about carcinogenesis and teratogenesis and provided new insights into mechanisms of disease involving both women who were DES-exposed as well as the general population who were never exposed to DES or related synthetic drugs with a stilbene core. It has also led to new assessments of the effects on females of other agents possessing estrogenic activity but having diverse chemical structures. Since DES was the first drug discovered to cause teratogenic effects transplacentally and only after a long latent period, retrospective historical analyses have been made (14, 15); some have lead to revisionist interpretations of original data and even somewhat contentious beliefs based on animal experimentation that some sequelae later found should have been foreseeable. For an insight into the research studies using DES during the 1940s and 1950s, see the 30-year historical perspective by Dr. Edith Potter (16), an international authority on obstetrical and pediatric pathology at the University of Chicago who was intimately involved in many of these research efforts.

This chapter summarizes current knowledge of the role of DES in the development of clear cell adenocarcinoma, adenosis (benign glands found in the vagina) and its healing process, reports of chance occurrences of a diversity of lesions in exposed women, and some new experimental models in which human tissue has been used to recreate the DES syndrome in laboratory animals. For an extensive atlas depicting the various lesions described in this chapter, see reference 17. Functional reproductive changes and long-term effects in the female offspring (5, 18), breast cancer in exposed mothers (19), health status of male offspring (18, 20), and possible multigenerational effects are covered in other publications (8–10), including proceedings of symposia and workshops (21, 22).

CLEAR CELL ADENOCARCINOMA

Shortly after a history of drug exposure was associated with the development of vaginal clear cell adenocarcinoma, the International Registry for Research on Hormonal Transplacental Carcinogenesis was formed to accumulate information rapidly on this extremely rare tumor. Currently, about 600 patients with clear cell carcinoma of the lower genital tract have been registered, with estimates that about 25–50 new cases are developing each year (23). Most are from the United States, but some women with documented histories of exposure have been born in Canada, Mexico, Europe, Australia, and Africa. Smaller registries have also been established in other countries with findings similar to that of the International Registry (24).

Because the number of patients with clear cell adenocarcinoma is so small, the Registry has sought to obtain information from all diseased women, regardless of their drug history. About three-fifths of the patients in the Registry have some evidence suggesting exposure in utero to DES, hexestrol or dienestrol. Another one-tenth were exposed to unknown medications, usually for a high-risk pregnancy. A few women had been exposed to steroidal estrogens or progesterone alone. While the relative risk of a vaginal cancer being associated with stilbestrol usage is high (25), the proportion of women lacking a history of drug exposure is still substantial (12–22% [26, 27]), confirming that this tumor occurs spontaneously. For cervical tumors alone, the majority of women have no drug history. In the Registry data, 54% were negative for drug history (27), and other sources have suggested that this percentage may be higher. This finding is in accord with clear cell adenocarcinoma of the cervix in young women being a well-recognized entity long prior to the DES era. Clear cell adenocarcinoma of the vagina in women under the age of 20 was known before the synthesis and use of DES in pregnancy, but its occurrence was much less frequent at that time.

The median and mode ages at the time of diagnosis are both 19 years (Fig. 10.1), which remains remarkably uniform regardless of the patient's year of birth. Although a rare patient has been as young as 7 years of age, only after the age of 14 does the age-incidence curve rise sharply, which strongly suggests a pathogenesis related in part to puberty. The curve plateaus between ages 17 and 22 years and then declines rapidly, with few women developing this form of cancer in their thirties or forties. Despite the

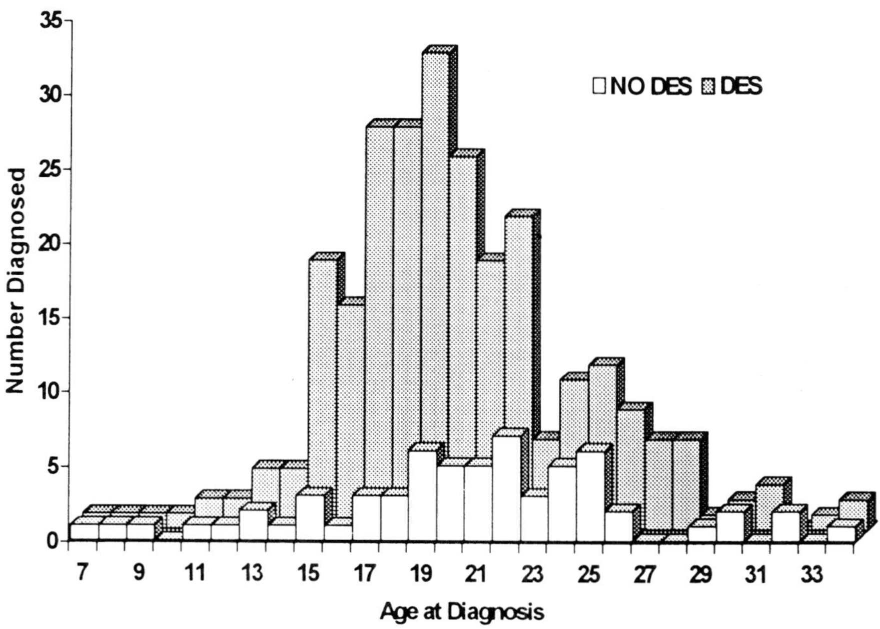

FIGURE 10.1. Age-incidence curve. Age at diagnosis of clear cell adenocarcinoma of the vagina only for both DES-exposed and DES-unexposed women. Reprinted with permission from Waggoner SE, Mittendorf R, Biney N, et al. Gynecol Oncol 1994;55:238–244.

strong association between drug and tumor, clear cell adenocarcinoma develops in only about 0.01% to 0.1% of exposed women through the age of 34 years (28). Based upon currently accessioned cases with prenatal drug exposure and the total population believed exposed in utero, the cumulative incidence to date is at least 0.02% (1 per 5000). Multiple studies of large groups of women specifically examined because of their known history of prenatal DES exposure have confirmed the rarity of the neoplasm (i.e., no tumors encountered) (2, 22, 29–31). The greatest number of DES-exposed patients with these tumors were born in 1951–1953, the years when the drug appears to have been prescribed most frequently for pregnancy support. The final incidence will very likely prove to be slightly greater than Registry estimates (but still less than 0.1%) because cases are known to have been misclassified and thus unreported (32) and because some new tumors are still being discovered in DES-exposed women (33, 34). Epidemiological studies indicate that the risk of tumor development is higher when the drug was started early in pregnancy or a history of prior miscarriage exists (2). The risk is also increased in women who were taller or more obese than their contemporaries at ages 14–15 years (35), findings of interest since height and body mass are risk factors for endometrial cancer, the most common glandular cancer of the female reproductive tract. Rare reports of tumor formation in only one of two monozygotic twins underscore that many factors, including perhaps unidentified environmental ones, operate in carcinogenesis.

PATHOLOGY

The tumor may involve any portion of the vagina (Fig. 10.2) and/or cervix (Fig. 10.3). Most vaginal tumors arise on the anterior wall, usually in the upper third, corresponding

FIGURE 10.2. Vaginal cancer. Polypoid clear cell adenocarcinoma bordered by dark zone of adenosis lies on the anterior vaginal wall. Another patch of adenosis occupies the posterior wall. The vaginal adenosis and the extensive ectropion appeared red in the fresh state. Reprinted with permission from CANCER, Vol. 25, 1970, 745–757. Copyright 1970 American Cancer Society. Reprinted by permission of Wiley-Liss, Inc., a susidiary of John Wiley & Sons, Inc.

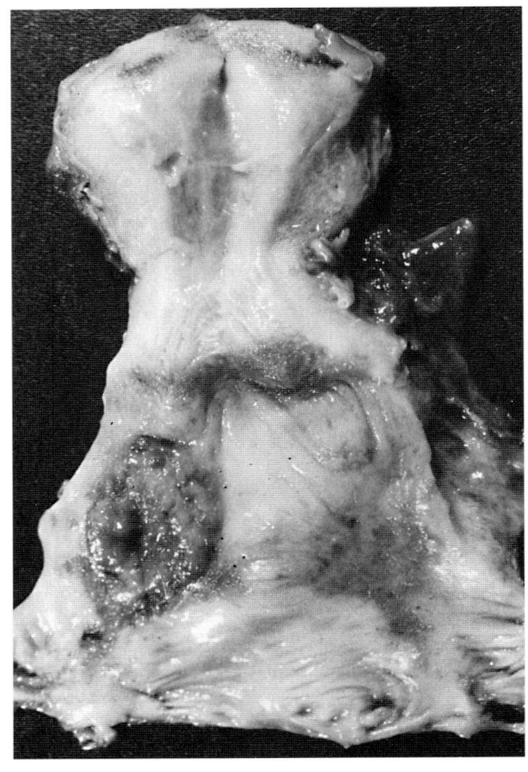

FIGURE 10.3. Clear cell adenocarcinoma confined to exocervix. Reprinted with permission from Robboy SJ, An atlas of findings in the human female after intrauterine exposure to diethylstilbestrol. DHEW publication 84-2344, 1984.

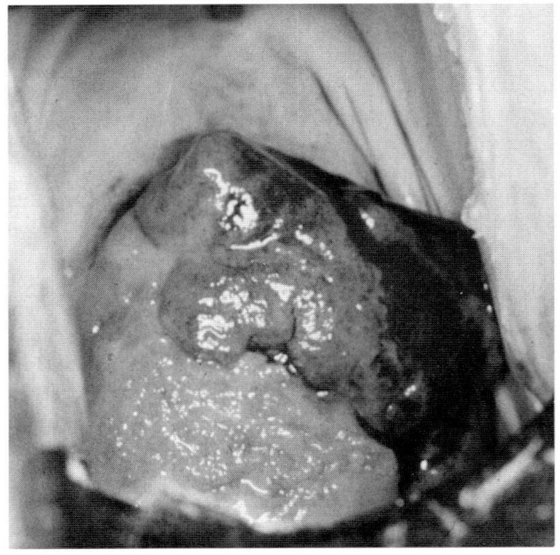

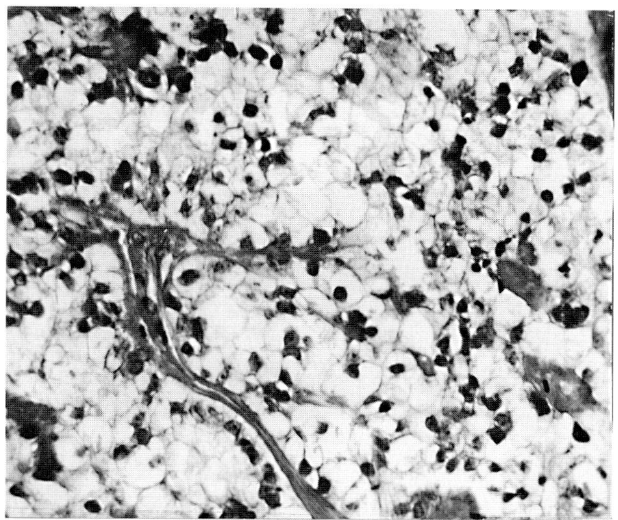

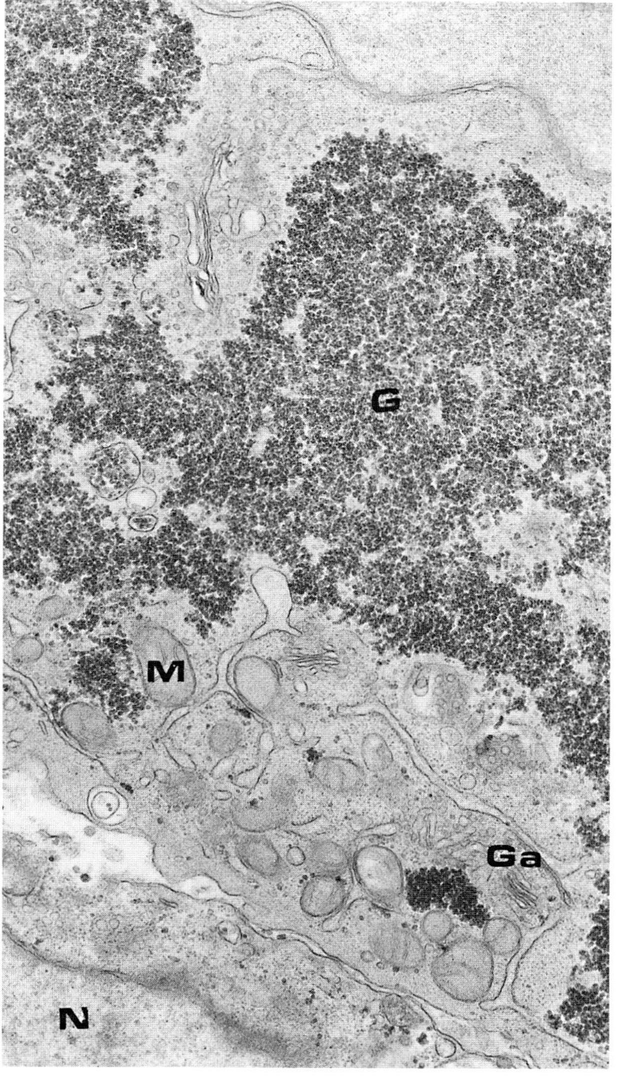

FIGURE 10.4. Clear pattern of clear cell adenocarcinoma, which resembles by light microscopy the clear cell carcinoma of the ovary and endometrium. Special processing of the specimen for electron microscopy demonstrates the glycogen particles (G) in large collections in the cytoplasm. Nuclei (N) and cytoplasmic organelles, such as mitochondria (M) and Golgi apparatus (Ga), are less electron-dense by this technique. Top-hematoxylin-eosin, x300; bottom-osmium tetroxide, x12,000. Reprinted with permission from (top) Scully RE, Robboy SJ, Herbst AL. Ann Clin Lab Sci 1974;4: 222–233 and (bottom) CANCER, Vol. 45, 1980, 1615–1624. Copyright 1980 American Cancer Society. Reprinted by permission of Wiley-Liss, Inc., a subsidiary of John Wiley & Sons, Inc.

to the most frequent site of adenosis. The lateral and posterior walls and, occasionally, the middle and lower third of the vagina may also be involved. On occasion, multicentric tumors have been demonstrated on microscopic examination. Whereas a multicentric origin has been suspected grossly in some larger tumors since the tumor is seen in differing surface areas, continuity of the tumor in the submucosa has often been found on microscopic examination in these cases. Tumors have also been found on the wall opposite the main tumor, presumably a result of implantation ("kissing lesion").

The tumors have varied in size from microscopic to large. During the early period when tumors were being reported to the Registry, many were of substantial size, which reflected the infrequency of pelvic exams in asymptomatic and sometimes even symptomatic young women. Most of the larger cancers were polypoid and nodular. Some were flat or ulcerated, having a granular or indurated surface. With increasing awareness that periodic examinations in exposed women should begin early in the teenage period, the tumors subsequently were discovered more often when they were small. While usually palpable, they may still be invisible on colposcopic examination if confined to the lamina propria and if covered by intact normal or metaplastic squamous epithelium. Although most cancers are superficial and invade only a few millimeters into the vaginal or cervical wall, some penetrate far more deeply or extend more centrifugally than might be anticipated on gross examination.

By light and electron microscopy, the clear cell adenocarcinomas of the vagina and cervix are identical to the clear cell adenocarcinomas of the ovary and endometrium, both of which occur sporadically in older women. Several histologic patterns may be observed, either existing alone or in combination. A characteristic pattern, for which the tumor is named, consists of solid sheets of clear cells (Fig. 10.4); the clear appearance of the cytoplasm is caused by the dissolution of glycogen when the specimen is processed for microscopic examination. A second pattern, the tubulocystic pattern, exhibits tubules and cysts lined by hobnail cells (Fig. 10.5), by flat cells (Fig. 10.6), or by cells

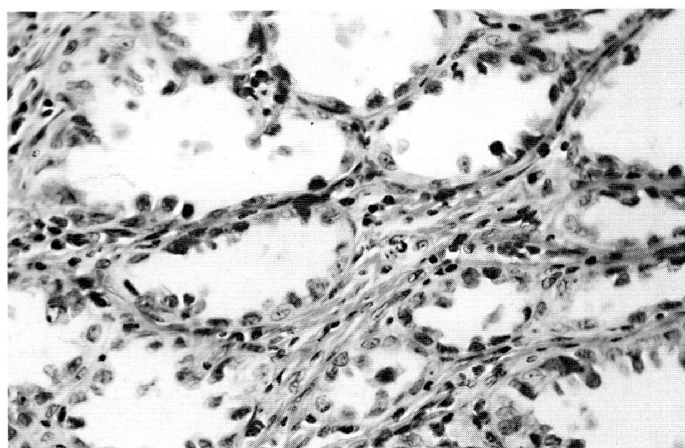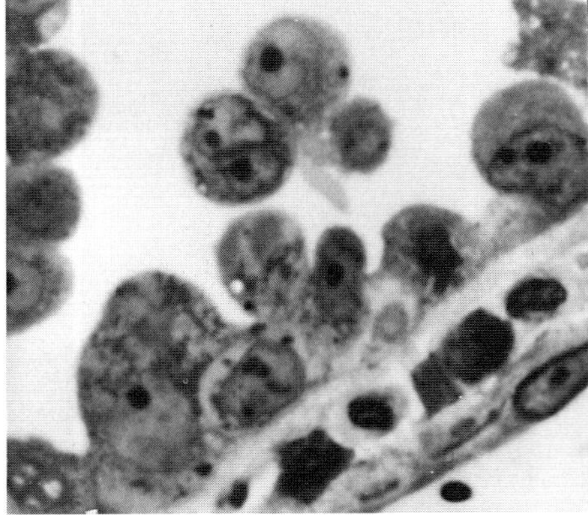

FIGURE 10.5. Hobnail cells. Tubulocystic pattern of clear cell adenocarcinoma in which small tubules are lined by neoplastic hobnail, columnar or cuboidal cells. Right—Detail of hobnail cell showing luminal protrusion of nucleus and scant apical cytoplasm. Left—hematoxylin-eosin, x300; right-Giemsa, x690. Reprinted with permission from (left) Zaino R, Robboy SJ, Bentley R, et al. In: Kurman RT, ed. Blaustein's Pathology of the Female Genital Tract. 4th ed. New York: Springer-Verlag, 1994:131–185 and (right) Dickersin GR, Welch WR, Erlandson R, et al. Cancer 1980;45:1615–1624.

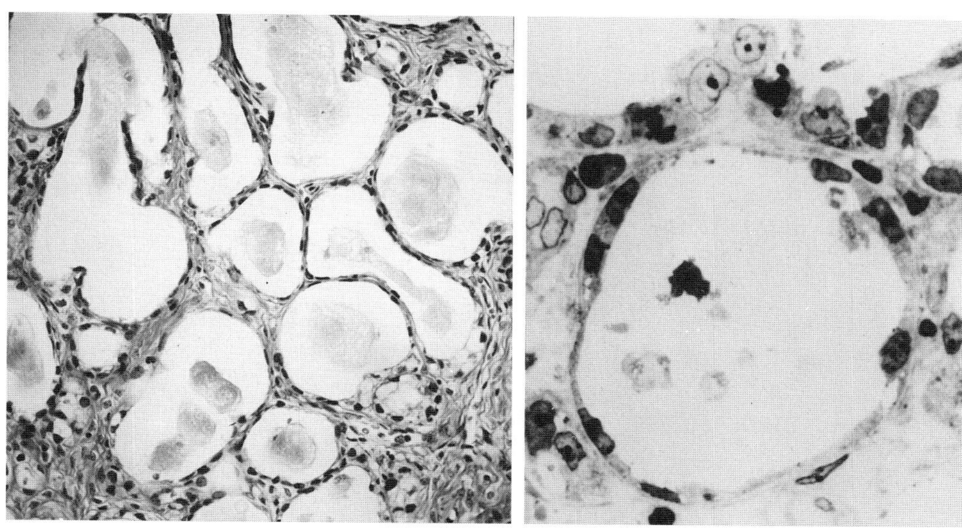

FIGURE 10.6.   Dilated cysts lined by flat cells in clear cell carcinoma. Right—Detail of neoplastic flat cells one of which has an atypical mitosis. Small clear spaces in the cytoplasm are vestiges of glycogen. Left—hematoxylin-eosin, x100; right—Giemsa, x540). Reprinted with permission from (left) Zaino R, Robboy SJ, Bentley R, et al. In: Kurman RT, ed. Blaustein's Pathology of the Female Genital Tract. 4th ed. New York: Springer-Verlag, 1994:131–185 and (right) CANCER, Vol. 45, 1980, 1615–1624. Copyright 1980 American Cancer Society. Reprinted by permission of Wiley-Liss, Inc., a subsidiary of John Wiley & Sons, Inc.

that resemble mullerian-type epithelium to varying degrees. The hobnail cell displays a bulbous nucleus that protrudes into the lumen beyond the apparent cytoplasmic limits of the cell. Flat cells often appear innocuous. When only this latter epithelium is present in a small biopsy, it may be difficult to differentiate tumor from adenosis. Less common appearances include a papillary pattern (Fig. 10.7), a tubular pattern resembling endometrial carcinoma (Fig. 10.8), and a pattern composed of cords of cells with eosinophilic cytoplasm (Fig. 10.9). Mitoses usually are rare. In any of these patterns, the lumina may contain mucin, but the cytoplasm is mucin-free.

Using electron microscopy, it can be seen that the neoplastic cells from each of the tumor patterns are of the same basic type, with glycogen and microvilli being prominent features. Intracellular glycogen is abundant in clear cells in the solid areas (Fig. 10.4) and is present in varying but lesser amounts in the other cell types, including areas in which it is not apparent at the light microscopic level.

Clear cell adenocarcinoma is often detected cytologically, especially in the cervix (80% detection rate in the cervix versus a 33% rate in the vagina [24]). Occasionally, a suspicious or positive smear may be the first indication that an asymptomatic woman has the tumor. The cancerous cells often resemble large endocervical cells or nonspecific adenocarcinoma cells (Fig. 10.10), but these cells vary greatly and may appear even as undifferentiated carcinoma (Fig. 10.11).

NATURAL HISTORY

The tumor spreads locally and also metastasizes via lymphatic channels and blood vessels. Approximately one-sixth of tumors confined clinically to the lower genital tract

FIGURE 10.7. Papillary pattern of clear cell adenocarcinoma. Hematoxylin-eosin, x140. Reprinted with permission from Zaino R, Robboy SJ, Bentley R, et al. In: Kurman RT, ed. Blaustein's Pathology of the Female Genital Tract. 4th ed. New York: Springer-Verlag, 1994:131–185.

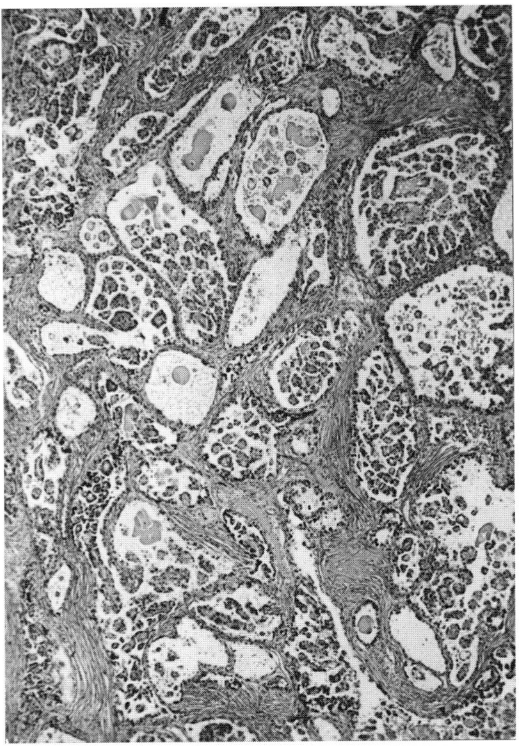

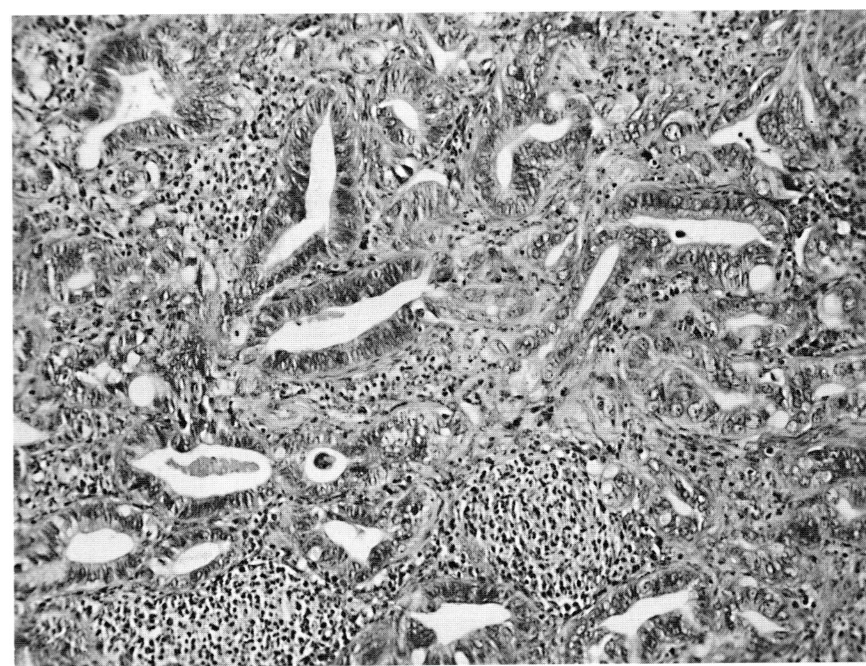

FIGURE 10.8. Endometrioid pattern of clear cell adenocarcinoma. Hematoxylin-eosin, x140. Reprinted with permission from Zaino R, Robboy SJ, Bentley R, et al. In: Kurman RT, ed. Blaustein's Pathology of the Female Genital Tract. 4th ed. New York: Springer-Verlag, 1994:131–185.

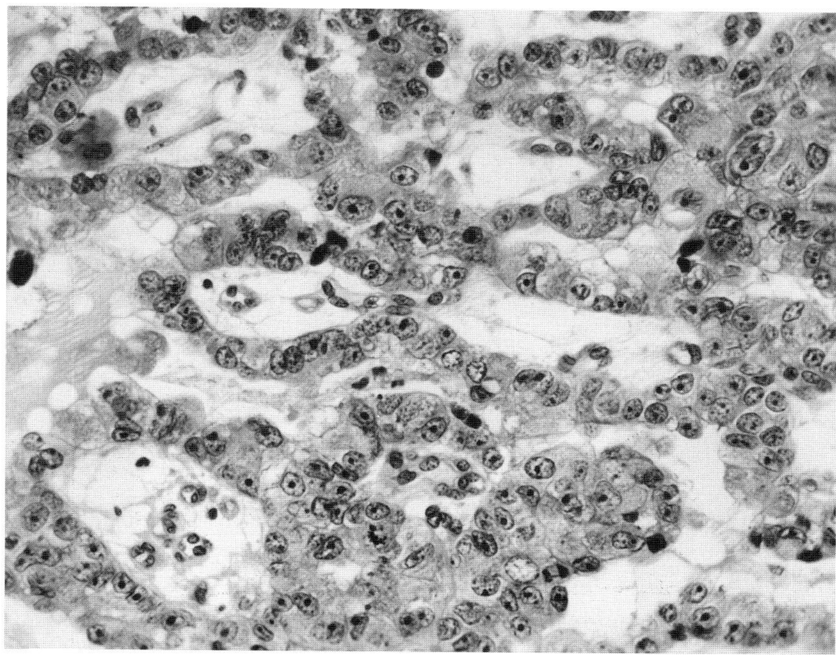

FIGURE 10.9. Cords and solid tumor with unusually deeply eosinophilic cytoplasm and nuclei with prominent nucleolus and delicate chromatin. Hematoxylin-eosin, x290. Reprinted with permission from Zaino R, Robboy SJ, Bentley R, et al. In: Kurman RT, ed. Blaustein's Pathology of the Female Genital Tract. 4th ed. New York: Springer-Verlag, 1994: 131–185.

(stage I) will have metastasized to the pelvic lymph nodes on exploration. The frequency of nodal involvement reaches 50% when clinical stage II tumors are considered. Clear cell adenocarcinoma extends outside the abdominal cavity more frequently than does squamous cell carcinoma of the vagina or cervix. Thirty-six percent of the initial recurrences of clear cell carcinomas are in the lung or supraclavicular lymph nodes, in contrast to less than 10% for squamous cell carcinomas.

The actuarial survival rate for all patients with clear cell adenocarcinoma is high, at about 93% at 5 years and 87% at 10 years when the tumor is stage 1. In patients with asymptomatic tumors or those discovered by an examination performed solely for a history of DES exposure, survival with appropriate therapy approaches 100%. Other factors associated with a better prognosis are an older age (19 years or older) at the time of diagnosis and a tubulocystic microscopic pattern (36). Large size and/or deep invasion into the wall are associated with a poorer prognosis, but small or superficial tumors also may recur or metastasize. While nuclear aneuploidy has no effect on prognosis, nuclear atypia may be associated with a worse prognosis (24). Pregnancy at the time of diagnosis does not affect outcome adversely (37). Recurrences develop most often within 3 years after primary therapy; however, recurrences as late as 19 years after treatment have been observed (38). After treatment of the recurrence, approximately one-fifth of the patients survive an additional 3 years or more.

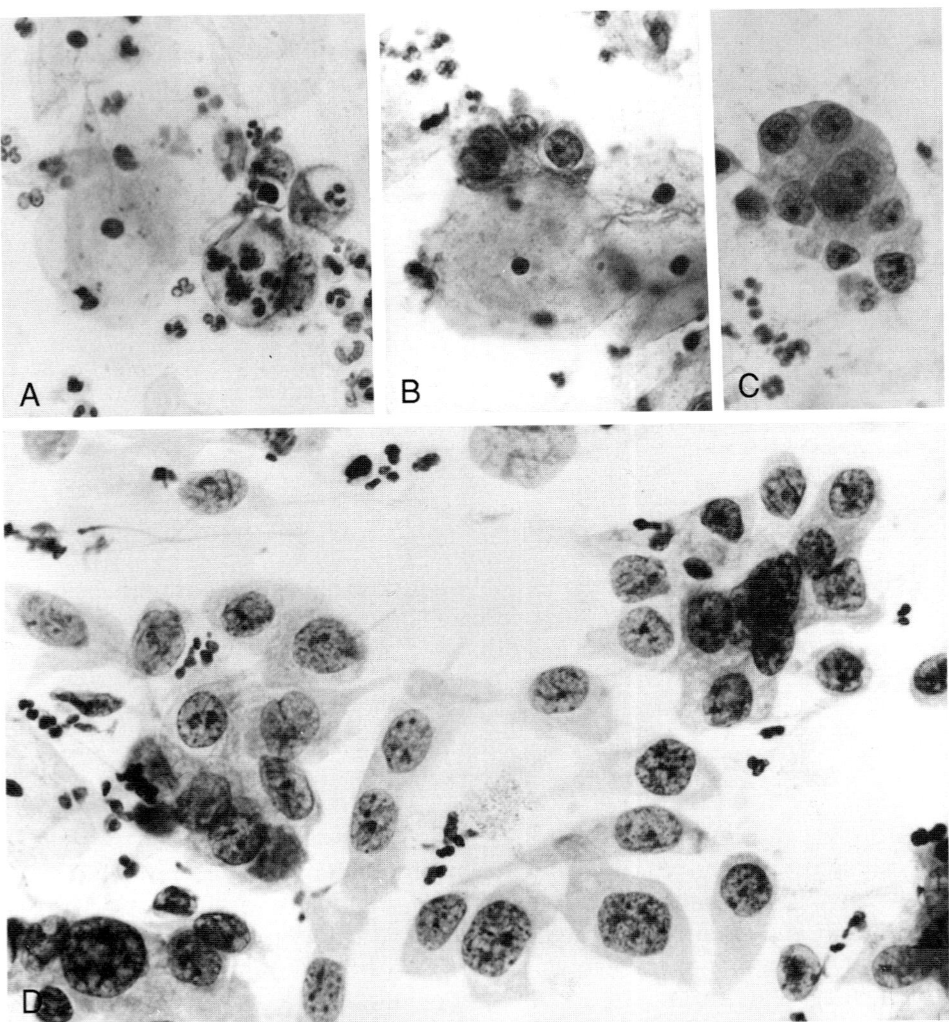

FIGURE 10.10. Vaginal and cervical smears of clear cell adenocarcinoma. **A.** A clump of adenocarcinoma cells varies markedly in size; large cytoplasmic vacuoles are filled with polymorphonuclear leukocytes. **B.** A cluster of four tumor cells with prominent nucleoli. **C.** A clump of tumor cells with strikingly large nucleoli. The nuclei vary in size more than in shape. Their borders are delicate and the chromatin is granular. The cytoplasm is finely vacuolated with indefinite borders. **D.** Well-preserved adenocarcinoma cells with large nuclei, course chromatin, and multiple nucleoli. The cytoplasm is variable; several nuclei are naked. Papanicolaou stain, x540. Reprinted with permission from Taft PD, Robboy SJ, Herbst AL, et al. Acta Cytol 1974;19:279–290.

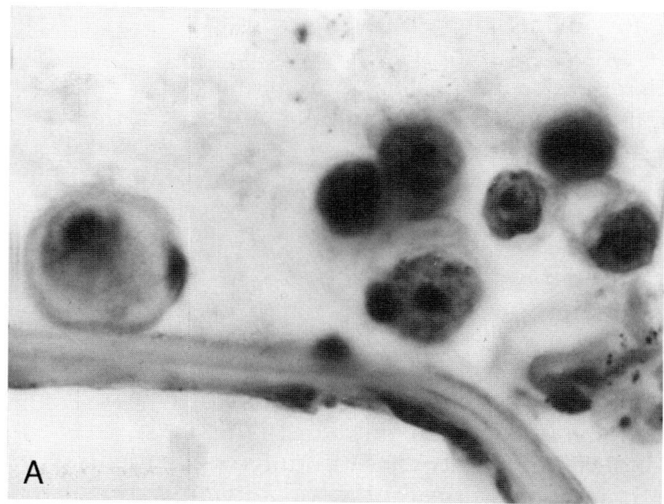

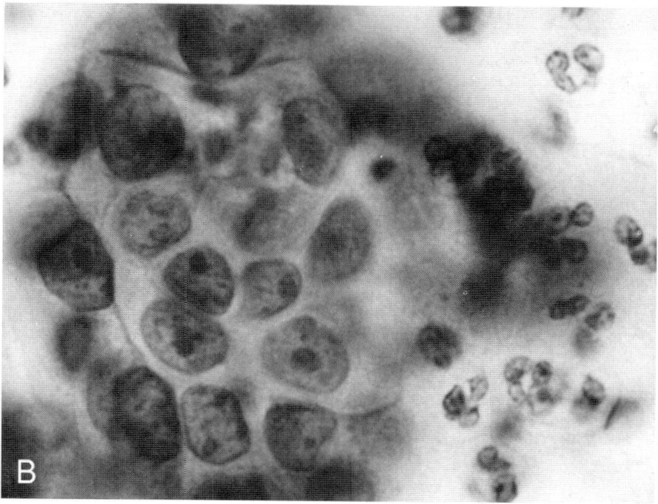

FIGURE 10.11. Clear cell adenocarcinoma cells with macronucleoli and clear cytoplasm (top) and a clump of cells with strikingly prominent nucleoli. Papanicolaou stain, x1,000 & x1,100. Reprinted with permission from Taft PD, Robboy SJ, Herbst AL, et al. Acta Cytol 1974;19:279–290.

PATHOGENESIS

To date, numerous animal models have been studied to help to unravel the mechanisms and interrelations that permit the tumor to develop. Few studies use or have used human tissues. Unlike squamous cell carcinoma of the genital tract in which the etiology is generally considered established and caused by human *Papillomavirus* (HPV) (39), no such correlations have been found associated with clear cell adenocarcinoma (40). HPV type 31, an oncogenic HPV type, occurs in one-fourth of the clear cell cancers, but in none of its metastases. A further genetic alteration commonly associated with human cancers is loss of normal p53 function. The normal function of the p53 oncogene (called wild-type in the normal person) is to inhibit cellular proliferation or initiate programmed cell death in response to DNA damage. Loss can occur by mutation, gene deletion, or degradation by viral oncoproteins. While over two-thirds of clear cell cancers display altered expression of the tumor suppressor protein p53, no case of clear cell cancer has been documented in which mutated p53 and the HPV virus have existed in combination (40). Other oncogenes found not to have mutated include the K-ras and H-ras protooncogenes, the Wilms' tumor (WT1) tumor suppressor gene, and the estrogen receptor gene (41). A recent report describes genetic instability as manifesting as somatic mutation of microsatellite repeats in all DES-associated tumors examined, and in half of those clear cell cancers occurring in women who were never exposed prenatally to DES (41). Researchers have raised the possibility that induced genomic instability may be an important mechanism in the genesis of clear cell cancer, regardless of the prenatal history to drug exposure.

Differences Between Tumors Associated with DES Exposure and Those Without

Prior to the DES era, clear cell adenocarcinoma was a tumor well recognized to develop sporadically in the lower genital tract of young women—usually in the cervix, but even rarely in the vagina. Registry data indicate differences exist in tumors in patients with and without DES history (26), even though the histopathology of both is indistinguishable. For example, while the mean ages are similar, the mode ages for the unexposed were greater at the time of discovery (DES-negative at 22 years versus DES-positive at 19 years). Most features were similar (i.e., stage, grade, and histologic patterns of growth), but several differences were strikingly apparent. Positive paraaortic lymph nodes were found in 8.6% (3/35) of DES-negative cases but only in 1.2% (2/161) of DES-positive cases. DES-negative cases developed distant tumor in lungs (24% vs 9%) and metastases to supraclavicular lymph nodes (8% versus 1.6%) more often. Survival rates also differed substantially. Probability of survival at 5 years was much better for DES-positive cases (84% versus 69%). Although the mechanisms involved are not yet understood and one interpretation might suggest that patients lacking a history of DES exposure have more aggressive tumors than patients with known exposure, some of the observations might possibly reflect more aggressive surveillance of the DES-exposed population.

DIFFERENTIAL DIAGNOSIS

Based upon consultation cases received, several conditions that are easily confused with clear cell adenocarcinoma have been found.

Microglandular hyperplasia is a benign condition that can resemble clear cell adenocarcinoma on gross and microscopic examination. Usually associated with the use of oral contraceptives or occasionally with pregnancy, it is rarely observed in their absence. Although microglandular hyperplasia almost always develops in the cervix of unexposed women (42), cases also have been described arising in foci of the mucinous form of vaginal adenosis (Fig. 10.12), usually in young women who have histories of prenatal exposure to DES. Initially, the lesions were misinterpreted as a clear cell adenocarcinoma. Grossly, the lesions are soft, granular, tan-yellow, and usually flat. Occasionally, they may be cauliflower-like and multicentric (Fig. 10.13). Microscopic examination demonstrates the presence of many small, closely packed glands devoid of intervening stroma. The presence of extensive nests of metaplastic squamous cells with pale eosinophilic cytoplasm may make such a lesion difficult to distinguish from the solid pattern of clear cell carcinoma. A clue to the diagnosis is the presence of clefts lined by mucinous epithelium that course through the metaplastic squamous epithelium. That the glands have been observed in continuity with the clefts suggests that the glands result from

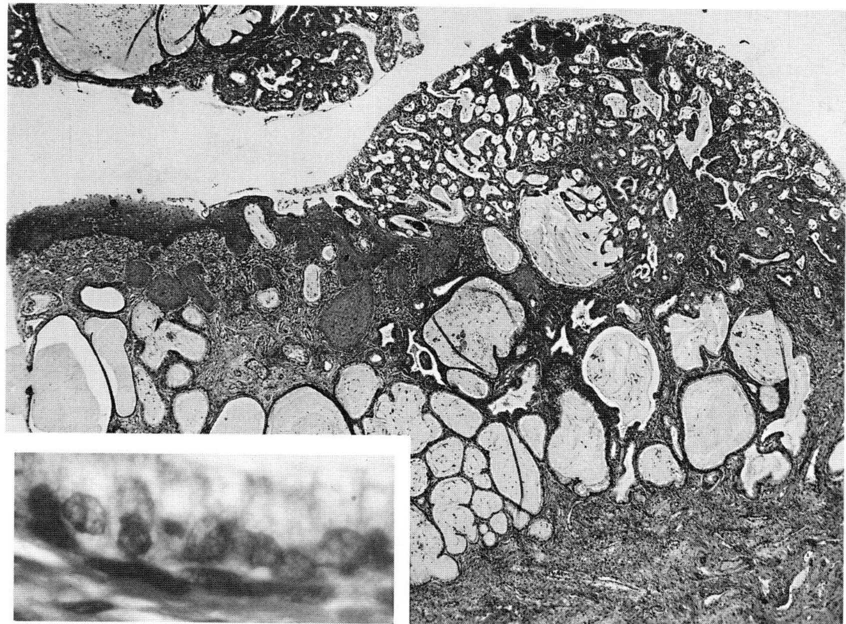

FIGURE 10.12.   Microglandular hyperplasia arising from mucinous adenosis. The adenosis, characterized by cysts lined by mucinous columnar cells, lies deeps to the small glands of microglandular hyperplasia. (Inset) Detail of mucinous glandular epithelium forming the mucinous adenosis. Hematoxylin-eosin, x28, x490. Reprinted with permission from The American College of Obstetricians and Gynecologists (Obstetrics and Gynecology 1977; 49:430–434).

budding and arborization of the mucinous epithelium that constitutes one type of vaginal adenosis as well as the lining of the normal endocervix. Microglandular hyperplasia has not been shown to arise from the tuboendometrial type of adenosis. The lesion generally regresses when oral contraceptives are discontinued.

The Arias-Stella reaction, which sometimes occurs in pregnant women, must be distinguished from clear cell adenocarcinoma. Although usually encountered in the endometrium (Fig. 10.14), the Arias-Stella reaction has been observed in the endocervix and occasionally in vaginal adenosis of the tuboendometrial type. Characteristically, hypersecretory glands are lined by cells with markedly enlarged nuclei resembling hobnail cells. However, in clear cell adenocarcinoma, the presence of sheets of clear cells or prominent papillae should enable the two lesions to be distinguished. In addition, the hobnail-like nuclei in the Arias-Stella reaction commonly are smudged, lack mitotic activity, and appear to be degenerative.

NONNEOPLASTIC CHANGES

A variety of nonneoplastic changes are associated with intrauterine DES exposure. Deformities found in the upper reproductive tract (T-shaped uterine cavity, constrictions of the uterine cavity, hypoplasia of the uterine cavity and uterine corpus [43]) are not discussed in this chapter. Approximately one-fifth of exposed women demonstrate gross structural changes in the cervix or vagina (44, 45). Descriptive designations include

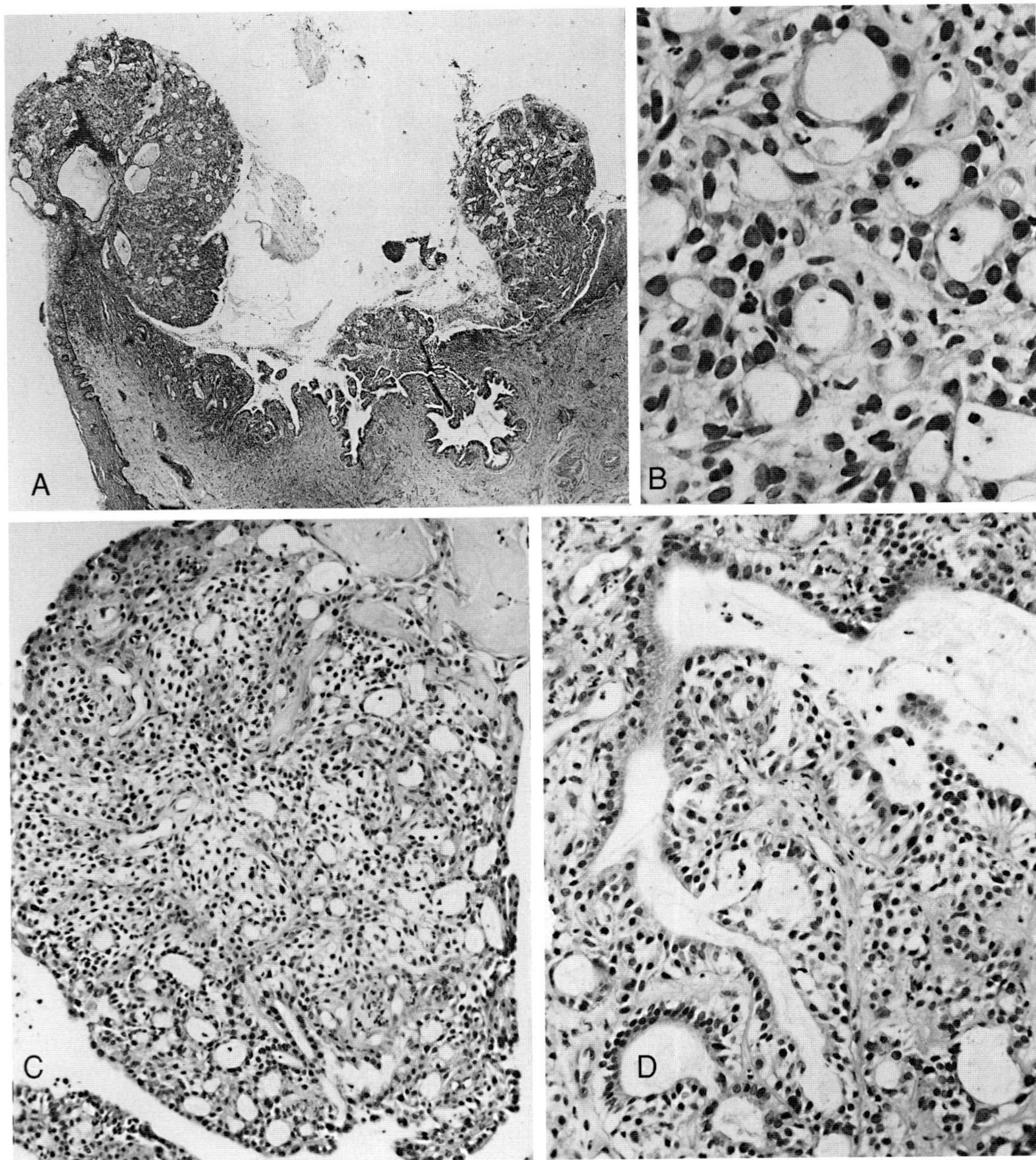

FIGURE 10.13. Microglandular hyperplasia. **A.** Polypoid mass in which irregular clefts lined by mucinous columnar cells are continuous with the mucinous glandular epithelium of the adenosis in the lamina propria of the vagina. **B.** Detail of glands that are closely packed and are separated by little or no stroma. The nuclei are uniform and have relatively fine, evenly dispersed chromatin. **C.** Nests composed largely of metaplastic squamous cells. **D.** Cleft lined by mucinous cells is continuous with the microglands. Hematoxylin-eosin, x29, x490, x150, x288. Reprinted with permission from The American College of Obstetricians and Gynecologists (Obstetrics and Gynecology, 1977;49:430–434).

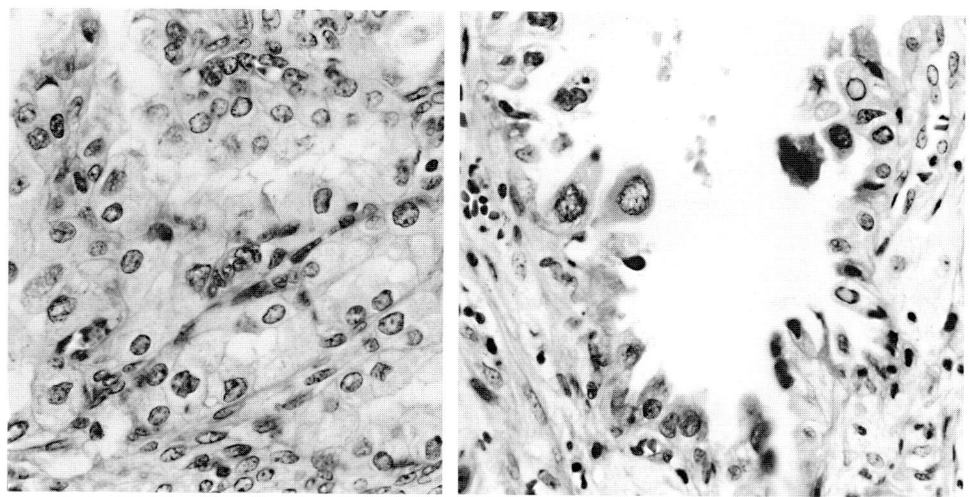

FIGURE 10.14.   Arias-Stella phenomenon in the normal gestational endometrium from women not exposed prenatally to DES. The stimulus by hCG can result in glands which resemble the clear cells (left) and hobnail (right) of clear cell adenocarcinoma (see figures 10.4 and 10.5, respectively). Hematoxylin-eosin, x325, x400.

coxcomb (hood) (Fig. 10.15), collar (rim), pseudopolyp (Fig. 10.16), hypoplastic cervix/altered fornix, and ridge (Fig. 10.17). All of these conditions also occur in approximately 2–4% of women with no prenatal drug history. A few forms of structural changes, such as cervical vascular malformations that give rise to polyps, have been reported in DES-exposed women (46), but these are so rare that their occurrence must be relegated to happenstance. Over time, many structural changes disappear as the cervix remodels with age (Fig. 10.18) (47). As many as two-thirds of all such structural changes disappear after pregnancy (44).

Most women exposed prenatally to DES have some form of microscopic change in the inner half of their exocervix; in studies relatively free of selection bias, a substantial number of women also have shown changes in the vagina. The presence of glandular tissue in the vagina is called "adenosis." In addition, many involved areas often disclose squamous metaplasia, which from a mechanistic viewpoint, represents the normal healing process by which adenosis transforms, ultimately to be replaced by a normal squamous epithelium. Collectively, these glandular and squamous cell changes in the vagina are designated "vaginal epithelial changes" (VEC). Clinically, adenosis in its adult microscopic form should be suspected when the vaginal mucosa contains red granular spots or patches (Fig. 10.2) and fails to stain with an iodine solution (Fig. 10.19). On colposcopy, adenosis appears as glandular or metaplastic epithelium replacing the native squamous epithelium of the vaginal mucosa.

Adenosis, with or without squamous metaplasia, involves the upper third of the vagina in 34% of DES-exposed women. The anterior wall is involved more frequently than the posterior wall. These changes extend into the middle third of the vagina in 9% and the lower third in 2% of exposed women. In unexposed women, adenosis of the adult type is rare (48), but when present, it is identical to that which occurs in exposed women (49, 50). As is discussed in the following, an embryonic form of adenosis

FIGURE 10.15. Cervical cockscomb and ectropion. Top—Colpophotograph of anterior cervical cockscomb covered with metaplastic squamous epithelium in the pattern of mosaicism (M). The grape-like structures on the inner half of the cervix are composed of fibrovascular cores covered by mucinous columnar epithelium (ectropion) (E). Bottom—Photomicrograph of the mucinous columnar cells lining the fibrovascular papillae. The same microscopical pattern in the vagina is called adenosis. Hematoxylin-eosin, X378. Reprinted with permission from Zaino R, et al. In: Kurman RT, ed. Blaustein's Pathology of the Female Genital Tract. 4th ed. New York: Springer-Verlag, 1994:131–185.

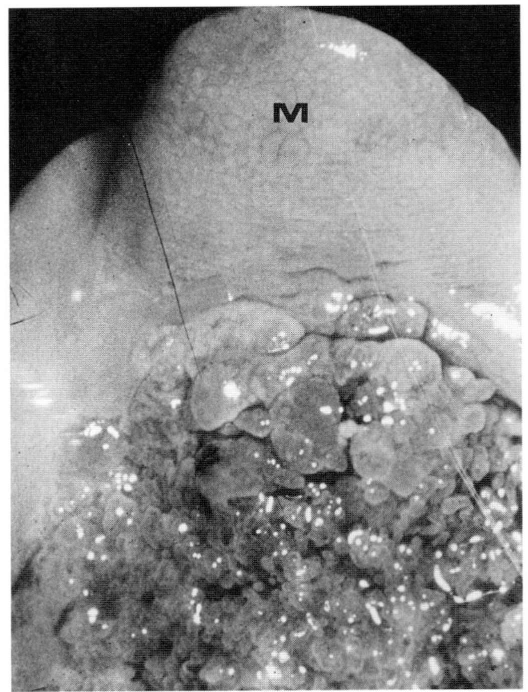

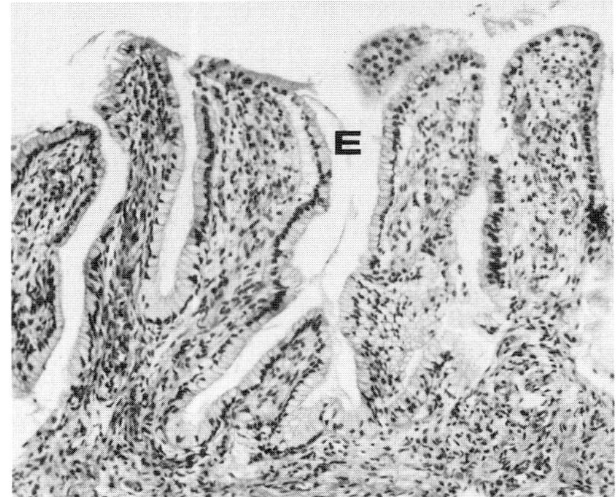

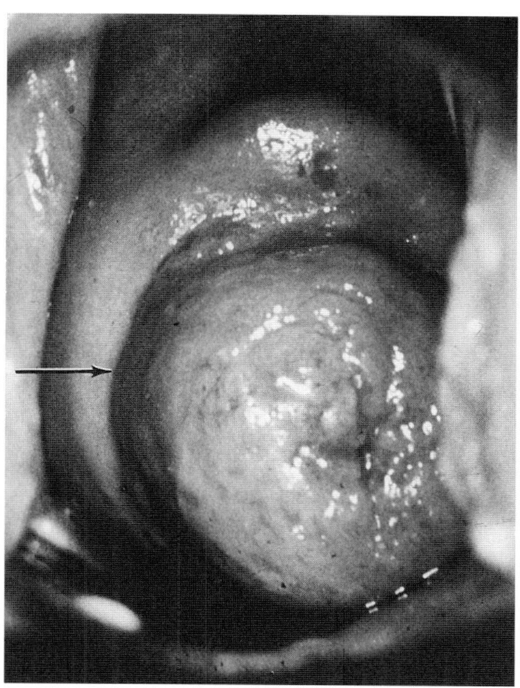

FIGURE 10.16. Concentric ridge (arrow) in the cervix creating the appearance of a "pseudopolyp" in the center of which is the external os. A circular fold gives the appearance of a hood covering the cervix. Reprinted with permission from Robboy SJ, Scully RE, Herbst AL. J Reprod Med 1975; 15:13–18.

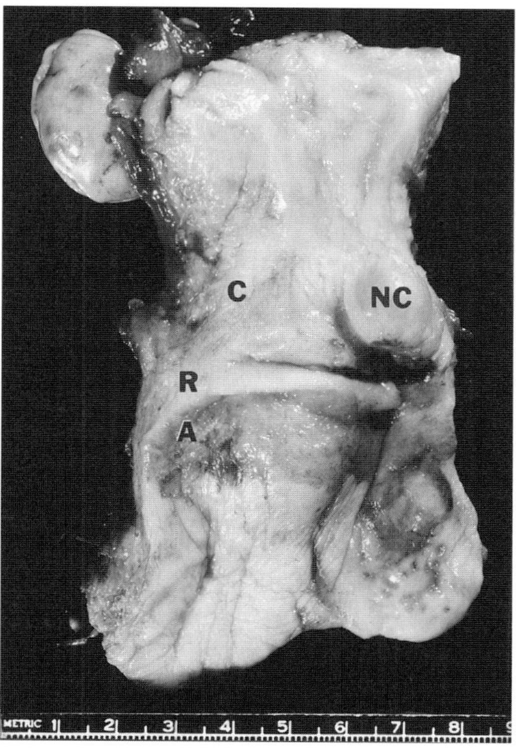

FIGURE 10.17. Opened uterus and vagina with transverse vaginal ridge (R), cervix (C), and zone of adenosis (A) which macroscopically appears as a patch of red granularity. A Nabothian cyst (NC) of the cervix is also visible along the right margin of the specimen. Reprinted by permission of *The New England Journal of Medicine.* Herbst AL, Kurman RJ, Scully RE, et al. Clear cell adenocarcinoma of the genital tract in young females. Registry report. New Eng J Med 1972; 287:1259–1264. Copyright 1972, Massachusetts Medical Society.

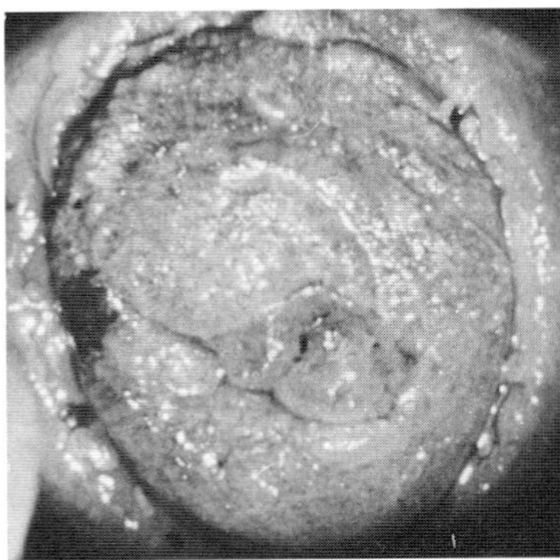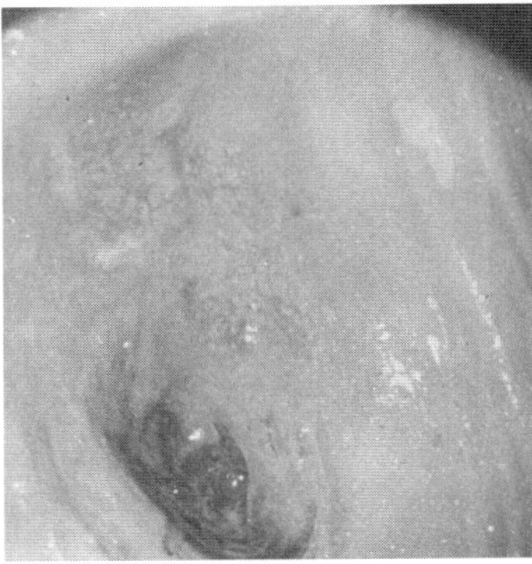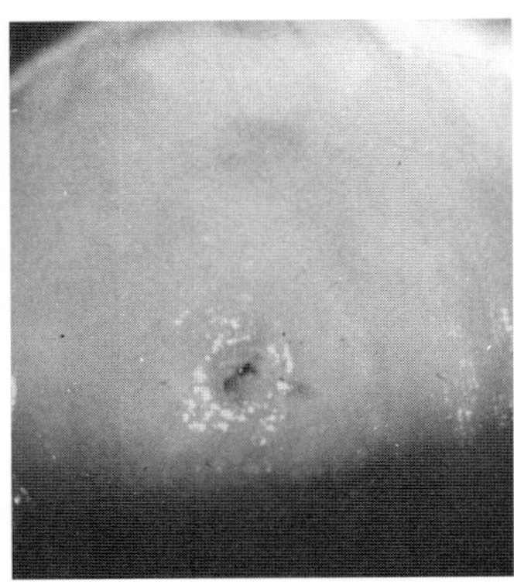

FIGURE 10.18.   Serial colpophotographs of cervix showing disappearance of structural changes over time. Left—The portio of the cervix displays extensive ectropion. The cervical rim is circumferential and covered with columnar epithelium. The groove demarcating it from the portio vaginalis is prominent. Middle—After 24 months much of the rim has disappeared and 70% of the ectropion has been replaced by metaplastic epithelium. The groove is obliterated between 9 and 4 o'clock. Right—Forty-two months after initial observation, the entire portio vaginalis is covered by metaplastic epithelium and the rim has been completely obliterated. All colpophotographs x8. Reprinted with permission from Antonioli DA, Burke L, Friedman EA. Amer J Obstet Gynecol 1980;137:847–853.

FIGURE 10.19. Abnormal iodine (Schiller) stain in which aglycogenated (nonstaining) areas in both the vagina and the cervix appear white in the photograph and represent the so-called transformation zone. The glycogenated vaginal epithelium stains black. Arrows demarcate the staining from the nonstaining areas. Reprinted with permission from Robboy SJ, Scully RE, Herbst AL. J Reprod Med 1975;15:13–18.

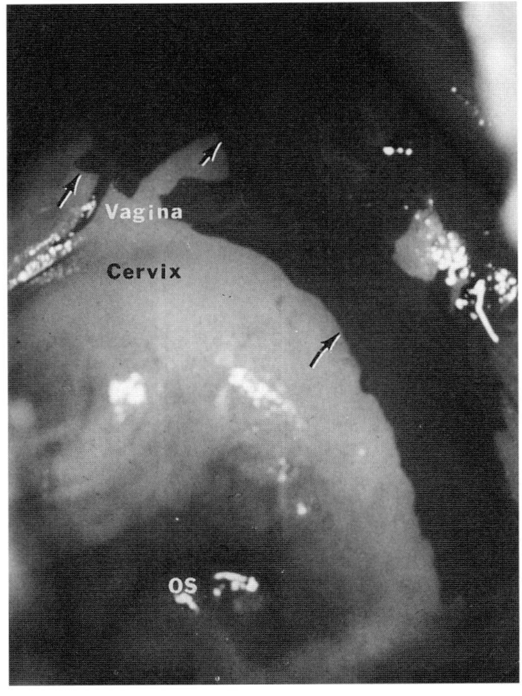

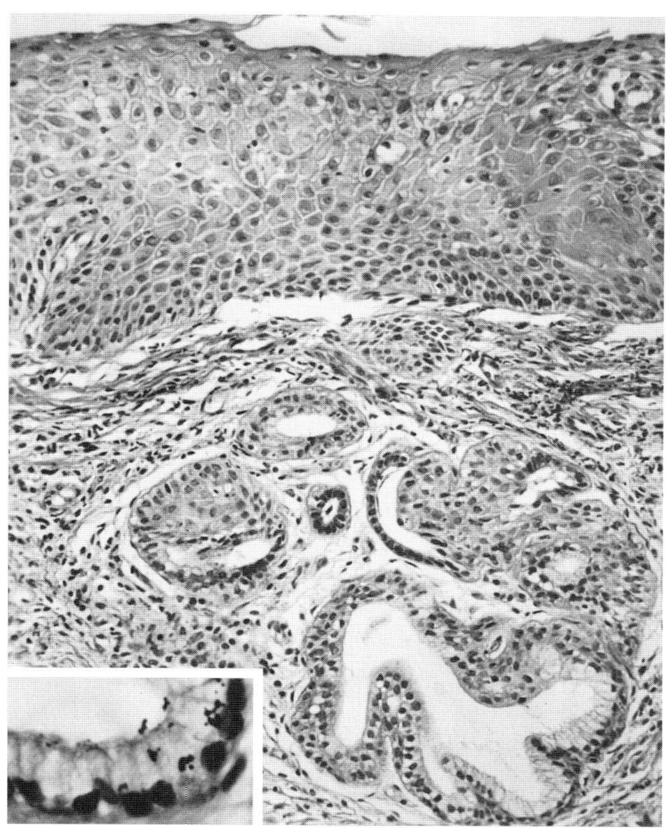

FIGURE 10.20. Mucinous form of vaginal adenosis. Mucinous gland with focal squamous metaplasia in lamina propria. Inset-Detail of individual mucinous columnar cells. Hematoxylin-eosin, x160, Inset-x640. Reprinted with permission from Zaino R, Robboy SJ, Bentley R, et al. In: Kurman RT, ed. Blaustein's Pathology of the Female Genital Tract. 4th ed. New York: Springer-Verlag, 1994:131–185.

is also encountered on occasion (51); it occurs naturally in tiny foci and has been found during late fetal life and childhood (52) and even in adults.

The adult (or differentiated) forms of adenosis have two cytologic types: mucinous (Fig. 10.20) and tuboendometrial (Fig. 10.21). Mucinous columnar cells, which by light and electron microscopy resemble those of the normal endocervical mucosa, comprise the glandular epithelium most frequently encountered in adenosis (62% of biopsy specimens with vaginal adenosis). As this epithelium frequently lines the surface of the vagina, it is the type of glandular epithelium most commonly seen by colposcopy and seemingly the type also found lining the exocervix and upper vagina in stillbirths exposed in utero to DES (53). Commonly, the mucinous columnar cells also line glands within the lamina propria itself.

Tuboendometrial cells, often ciliated and resembling the cells lining the fallopian tube and endometrium, are found in 21% of specimens with adenosis (Fig. 10.21). These cells are usually found in glands in the lamina propria and not on the surface of the vagina. Although adenosis in the middle vagina is uncommon and even more rare in the lower vagina, the percentage of biopsy specimens with adenosis that exhibit tuboendometrial cells in comparison to mucinous cells increases proportionally. Mucinous and tuboendometrial cells are found together only occasionally in biopsy material.

The third type of cell found in adenosis is embryonic, i.e., a fetal form of adenosis (Fig. 10.22). The putative precursor from which the adult form of adenosis develops

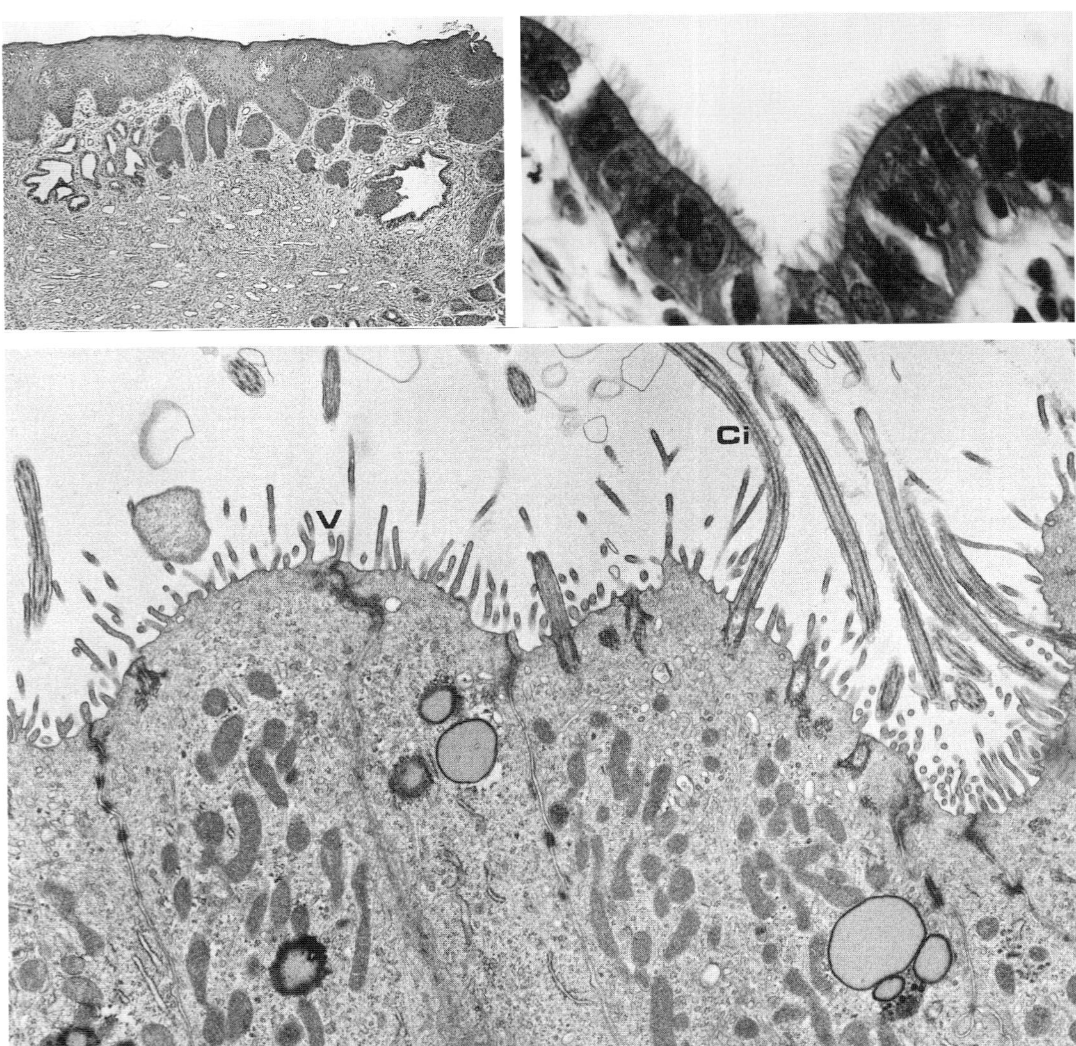

FIGURE 10.21.   Tuboendometrial form of vaginal adenosis. Upper left—Glands lined by ciliated dark cells similar to tubal or endometrial epithelium are present in the inflamed lamina propria and merge with squamous pegs. The surface epithelium is composed of glycogen-free squamous cells that account for the abnormal iodine staining. Upper right—Detail of ciliated dark (tuboendometrial) cells. Bottom—The tuboendometrial cells are tall columnar and have an orderly arrangement and distribution of organelles, some of which, such as mitochondria, are in a supranuclear location. The many cilia (Ci) are in the apex. Microvilli (V) are numerous and regularly distributed along the luminal surface. Hematoxylin-eosin, x41, x1,122; ultrastructure x12,800). Reprinted with permission from (top right and left) Zaino R, Robboy SJ, Bentley R, et al. In: Kurman RT, ed. Blaustein's Pathology of the Female Genital Tract, 4th ed. New York: Springer-Verlag, 1994:131–185 and (bottom) CANCER, Vol. 45, 1980, 1615–1624. Copyright 1980 American Cancer Society. Reprinted by permission of Wiley-Liss, Inc., a subsidiary of John Wiley & Sons, Inc.

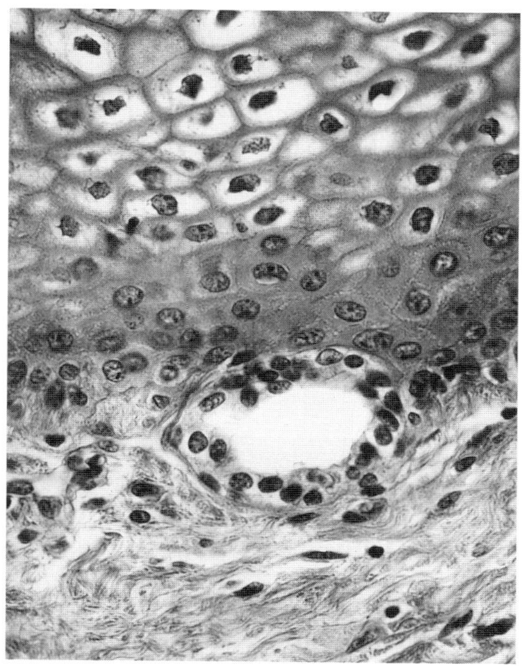

FIGURE 10.22. Embryonic form of vaginal adenosis. The glands, which typically are single and small, lie at the interface between the mucosa and submucosa, and are composed of indifferent cytoplasm which has not yet differentiated towards a mucinous or tuboendometrial form. Hematoxylin-eosin, x640.

postpubertally, this form of adenosis is found in up to 15% of fetuses and stillbirths (52), occasionally in adult women regardless of DES history (51), and finally experimentally in human embryonic vagina grown in an athymic mouse host in a DES milieu (54).

In most biopsy specimens, metaplastic squamous cells replace adenosis to some degree (Fig. 10.23), indicating the manner by which adenosis regresses. Squamous metaplasia, a normal reactive and physiological process that occurs at one time or another in all women regardless of whether or not they have a history of prenatal exposure, is believed to be the process by which the body heals itself of the presence of glandular tissue anywhere on the ectocervix or in the vagina (adenosis). Whether or not the metaplastic epithelium in a DES exposed child is more (or less) susceptible to other disease processes than a truly uninvolved vaginal epithelium remains unclear.

Remnants of columnar cells, which appear as intercellular pools of mucin surrounded by metaplastic squamous cells or as intracellular droplets of mucin in metaplastic squamous cells (Figs. 10.24 and 10.25), constitute the evidence for adenosis in 48% of biopsy specimens with adenosis. Squamous metaplasia begins as reserve cell proliferation and then progresses through immature (Fig. 10.26) and mature stages. The glandular epithelium gradually disappears, and intercellular pools of mucin (Fig. 10.27) and intracellular droplets (Figs. 10.28 and 10.29) remain as the final vestiges of adenosis. When completely replaced by squamous epithelium, obliterated glands appear in the lamina propria as squamous pegs, which are continuous with the metaplastic squamous epithelium covering the surface. Cytologically, the reparative process manifests as increased relative proportions of metaplastic squamous cells to mucinous columnar cells.

The paucity or total lack of glycogen in the early stages of squamous metaplasia often accounts for the failure of the epithelium to stain with iodine, whereas the increased vascularity, the slightly tortuous arrangement of the vessels surrounding the pegs in

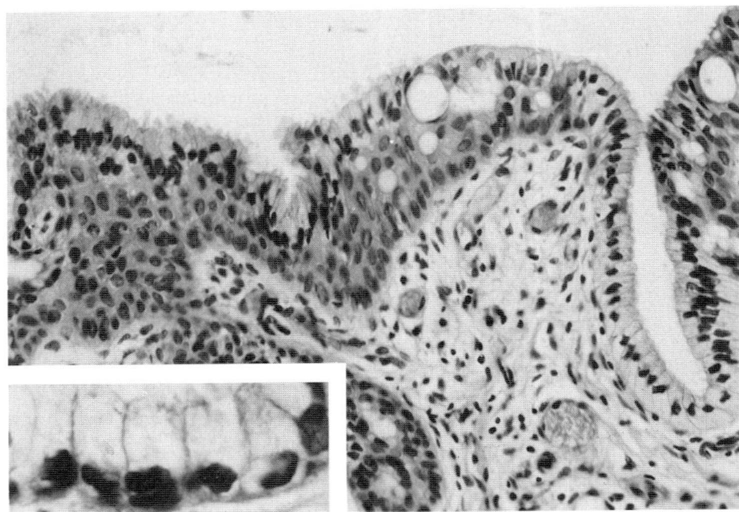

FIGURE 10.23. Metaplastic squamous cells replacing mucinous form of adenosis. Inset—Detail of individual mucinous columnar cells. Hematoxylin-eosin, x160, Inset—x640. Reprinted with permission from Zaino R, Robboy SJ, Bentley R, et al. In: Kurman RT, ed. Blaustein's Pathology of the Female Genital Tract. 4th ed. New York: Springer-Verlag, 1994: 131–185.

FIGURE 10.24. Vaginal adenosis in squamous pegs. The lamina propria exhibits numerous nests of metaplastic squamous cells in which there are numerous pools of mucin and intracellular droplets of mucin. These nest reflect the healing process of adenosis, and should not be mistaken for invasive squamous cell carcinoma. Hematoxylin-eosin, x35. Reprinted with permission from Herbst AL, Robboy SJ, MacDonald GJ et al. Amer J Obstet Gynec 1974;118:607–615.

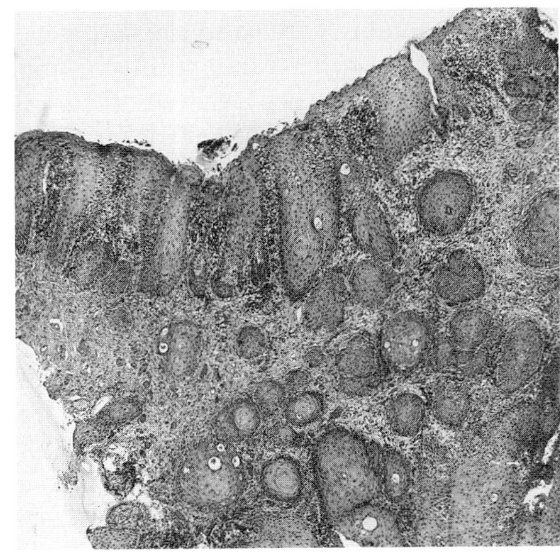

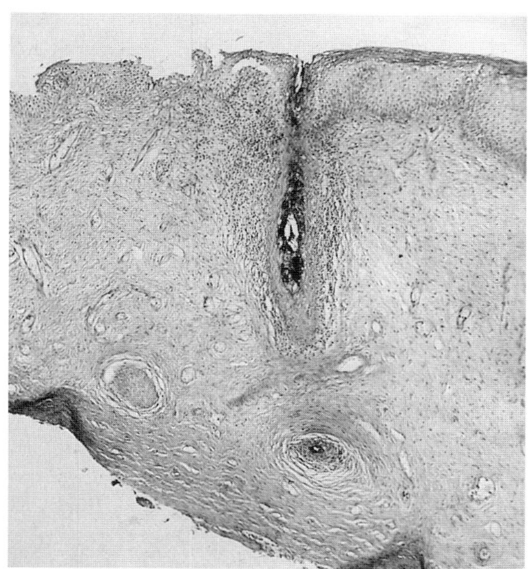

FIGURE 10.25. Sagittal section through a squamous peg in which the central core, lined by mucinous epithelium, is the neck of a gland. Periodic acid-Schiff x55. Reprinted with permission from Robboy SJ, Noller KL, Kaufman RH. An atlas of findings in the human female after intrauterine exposure to diethylstilbestrol. DHEW publication 84-2344, 1984.

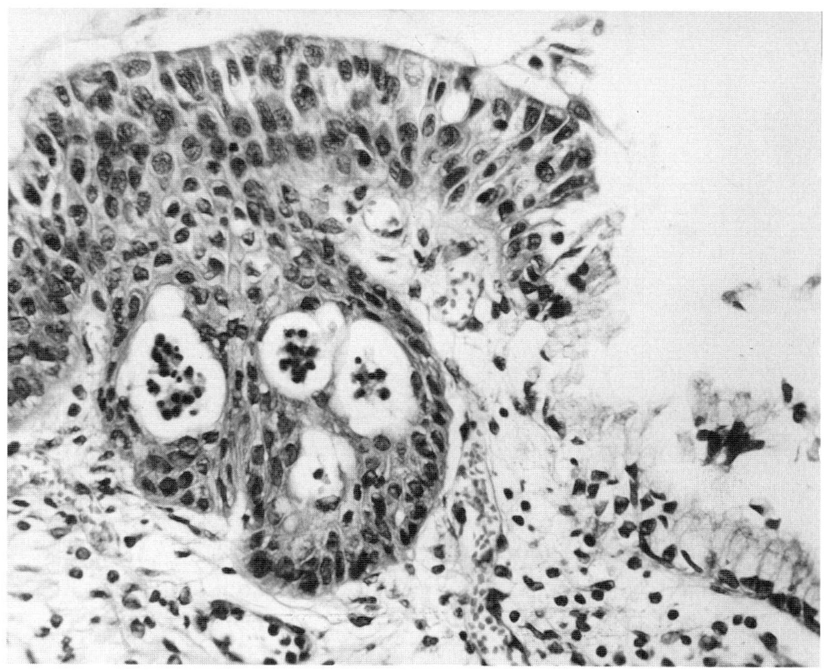

FIGURE 10.26.   Immature squamous metaplasia in mucinous form of vaginal adenosis. Although the immature squamous cells have large nuclei, they are uniform in size and shape and have finely dispersed chromatin and should not be misdiagnosed as dysplastic. Hematoxylin-eosin, x310. Reproduced with permission. Herbst AL, Robboy SJ, Scully RE, et al. Malignant and non-malignant changes in the female genital tract associated with maternal DES ingestion. HOSPITAL PRACTICE 1975;10:51–57. Copyright 1975 The McGraw-Hill Companies, Inc.

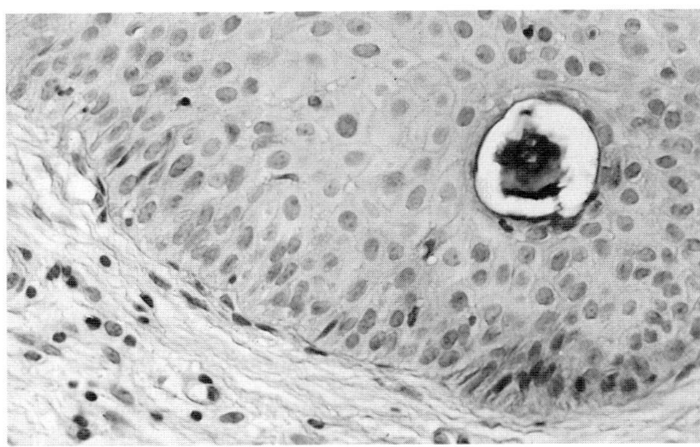

FIGURE 10.27. Vaginal adenosis with pool of mucin surrounded by flat cells with mucinous cytoplasm obvious only with mucin stains. Mucicarmine stain, x259. Reprinted with permission from Robboy SJ, Scully RE, Herbst AL. J Reprod Med 1975;15: 13–18.

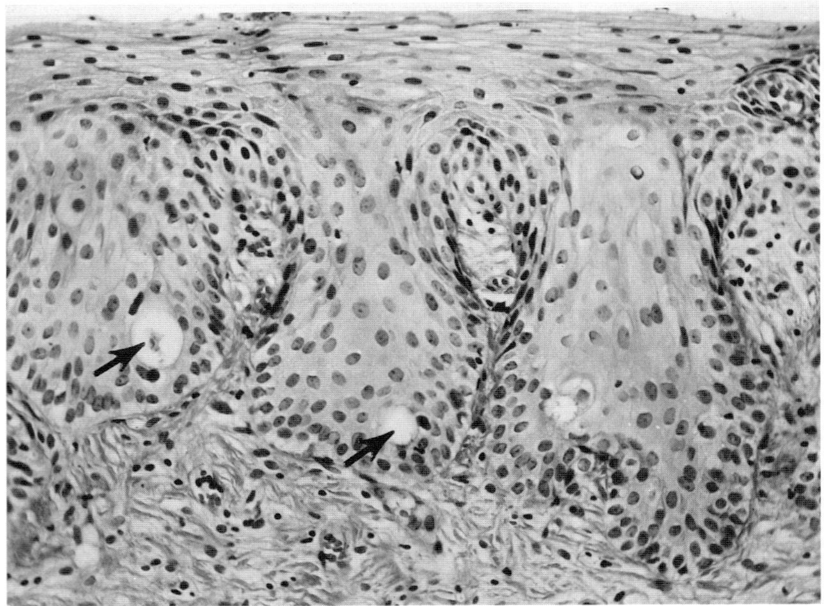

FIGURE 10.28.   Vaginal adenosis in squamous pegs. Nests of metaplastic squamous cells are present in the lamina propria and are continuous with the surface epithelium. Intracellular droplets of mucin (arrows) represent the final vestiges of the healing process of adenosis. Hematoxylin-eosin, x610. Reprinted with permission from The American College of Obstetricians and Gynecologists (Obstetrics and Gynecology, 1979;53:309–317).

the lamina propria, the chronic inflammatory infiltrate, and the tile-like patterns are responsible for atypical colposcopic motifs (55), such as mosaicism and punctation, which are seen so often in patients with adenosis. Hyperkeratosis accounts for the colposcopic finding of leukoplakia. Eventual maturation of the metaplastic squamous epithelium with acquisition of glycogen makes it indistinguishable from the normal (native) squamous epithelium.

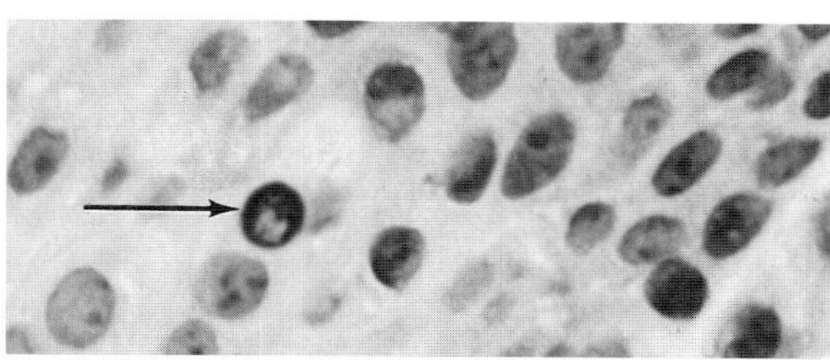

FIGURE 10.29. Vaginal adenosis with a single mucin droplet. The droplet (arrow) is bright red, the nuclei of the cells are brown-black, and the cytoplasm is pale yellow in the tissue slide. Mucicarmine stain, x1,350. Reprinted with permission from Robboy SJ, Scully RE, Herbst AL. J Reprod Med 1975;15:13–18.

PRENEOPLASTIC CHANGES
ATYPICAL ADENOSIS

Atypical adenosis, characterized by glands with cellular stratification, nuclear pleomorphism, hyperchromasia, and prominent nucleoli (Fig. 10.30), has been identified near the periphery of most clear cell carcinomas in which the excised vagina has been serially blocked for microscopic examination (56). Atypical cells with large, irregular nuclei have also been identified in approximately 0.5% of cervical and vaginal smears from DES-exposed women. The frequent finding of tuboendometrial-type glandular cells adjacent to the tumors and the rare presence of mucinous cells (57) suggest that the clear cell adenocarcinoma, if it is linked to atypical adenosis, is most likely from the tuboendometrial-type. However, any such relation must at this time be considered speculative as no cases are yet known in which, over time, microscopically proven atypical adenosis has progressed to carcinoma.

SQUAMOUS CELL LESIONS (DYSPLASIA AND CANCER)

Squamous metaplasia, a mechanism of repair and a common finding in the cervix, may give rise to dysplasia, which is the forerunner of squamous cell carcinoma-in-situ and, later, squamous cell carcinoma. During the mid-1970s, the postulate was first raised that DES-exposed offspring might be at risk for increased rates of dysplasia because metaplastic tissue was present extensively in the cervix and vagina of some patients. Multiple studies subsequently conducted indicated that the prevalence rates of dysplasia in both the exposed and unexposed populations were not significantly different. In the largest controlled study conducted, the unexposed women, in fact, had higher rates (1.9% versus 4.0%) (58). Factors complicating determination of true rates included the following: morphologic criteria or application of the criteria used to diagnose dysplasia (some investigators overestimated the severity of lesions), bias in selection of groups of patients used (women referred because of known exposure have much higher rates than women randomly picked for evaluation), and discord between biopsy and cytology findings. The colposcopic appearance of squamous metaplasia has also been misinterpreted in some studies as being indicative of dysplasia, further complicating the determination of expected frequency (55,59). Small tiles of squamous epithelium that are uniform and surrounded by vessels of small caliber, now called "pseudomosaicism," are benign; however, in the past they were often interpreted as true tiles, which are associated with dysplasia (55).

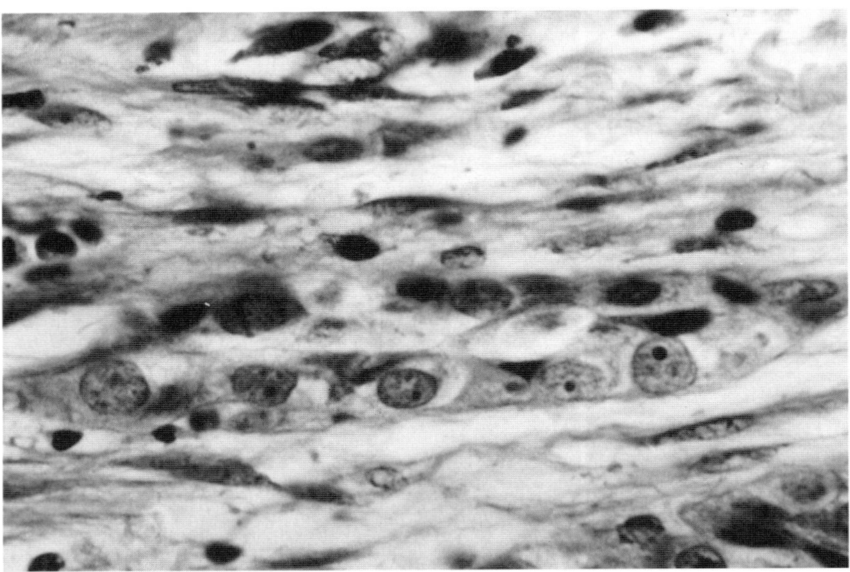

FIGURE 10.30.   Atypical adenosis of the vagina. The nuclei vary both in size and in shape and the cells are stratified. Hematoxylin-eosin, x500. Reprinted with permission from CANCER, Vol. 54, 1984, 869–875. Copyright 1984 American Cancer Society. Reprinted by permission of Wiley-Liss, Inc., a subsidiary of John Wiley & Sons, Inc.

The DESAD Project, after reporting lower prevalence rates in exposed women in a 1981 report (58), found in subsequent years that the incidence rates were slightly higher in exposed than in unexposed women (60). Thus, the new occurrence of squamous cell dysplasia in women under observation developed twice as frequently in DES-exposed women when compared to the women who were never exposed in utero. Interpretation of this finding has been controversial. First, the discord between the prevalence and incidence rates has never been resolved. Since the actual frequency of incident cases was less in comparison to the number of women, both exposed and unexposed, who had dysplasia detected during the prevalence exam, simple arithmetic would indicate that during the first few years of follow-up, high rates in the exposed group might simply bring the overall lifetime rates in both groups to equality. A longer follow-up period, clearly, was to be required if the true rates and the significance for health care were to be determined.

Second, the researchers were uncertain regarding the coexistence of HPV infection and how it may have affected interpretation of the DESAD findings. During the late 1970s and early 1980s, the time of the DESAD reports, relatively little was known about HPV infection and hence understood about its manifestations. Even today, a compounding factor related to HPV regards differing criteria for dysplasia in cytologic smears and biopsy, a subject beyond the scope of this review. A third and related factor concerns what degrees of dysplasia are biologically significant. As most DESAD cases had only low-grade squamous epithelial lesions (SIL) (as they are now reported under the Bethesda system) and since many—if not most—cases of low-grade SIL spontaneously resolve, especially if related to the benign HPV infections with types 6 and 11, many would argue that the only meaningful interpretations about rates should be confined to high-grade lesions, which were uncommon in the DESAD project in both exposed and unexposed women. The clearest insight into the role of HPV in the etiology of dysplasia is the absence of the latter in all women in the DESAD studies who never had intercourse. Even if the mechanism by which prenatal exposure to DES was associated with higher rates related to expanding the transformation zone (enlarging the target zone), this would apply potentially if a woman had few partners, for with multiple partners, the incidence rates of dysplasia in both exposed and unexposed women are similar.

To date, reports of invasive squamous cell cancer are exceeding rare (61–63). Thus, some investigators believe that the DESAD findings are artifactual and that the increased rates of dysplasia, especially of the mild forms, were due to overinterpretation or misinterpretation of the HPV-infected tissue for dysplasia (64), especially since much of the DESAD study was conducted at a time before HPV was fully understood. Both then and now, DES has not been perceived to be the etiologic cause of dysplasia.

LESIONS OF STATISTICAL CHANCE

During the past 25 years, periodic articles have appeared describing various rare abnormalities with the admonition that each might also have developed due to prenatal DES use. Included are cancers of both the lower and upper genital tracts plus multiple other organ systems. Also included are benign neoplasms, cysts, and other lesions. Given estimates that more than 5% of the U.S. population was exposed during the 1940s and 1950s, and approximately 1% in the 1960s up to 1971, it would seem axiomatic that, on a statistical basis alone, virtually every disease currently known in the medical lexicon should have been encountered in substantial numbers.

One rare tumor we have seen occasionally in unexposed women and recently was reported in an exposed woman (65) is the mucin-secreting adenocarcinoma of the vagina. Composed of glands resembling intestinal epithelium, this cancer, unlike the clear cell carcinoma, occurs in older women and more often involves the lower vagina. Cancer of the endometrium has also been reported in DES-exposed women (66).

Sporadic articles report ovarian and paraovarian lesions (67, 68) and peritoneal tumors resembling those arising in the ovary (69). One report suggested that as parovarian cysts are of Wolffian (mesonephric) duct origin, prenatal DES exposure, at critical moments in embryogenesis, might therefore affect the normal development of the male duct system (68).

Given both the many years that have elapsed since the DES story first began and the intensity with which possible associations have been sought, the extreme rarity of each such alleged association effectively negates any such potential relation to DES.

NEW INVESTIGATIVE TECHNIQUES

The DES story has opened new avenues of investigation useful in basic, applied, and clinical research. An extensive literature now exists to show that rodents and several other species, when neonatally or prenatally exposed to DES or other estrogens, develop adenosis plus other genital tract disorders (7, 11, 12). Although cancers have been produced, none resemble the clear cell adenocarcinoma found in humans.

Reassessment of the embryology of genital systems in light of the DES story has led to new concepts or confirmations (70) of how the lower genital tract forms in the human. Based on a personal review of embryo slides known as the Carnegie Collection of Embryology (University of California at Davis), new specimens prepared, and a study of accidents of nature (congenital anomalies), the senior author and colleagues postulated that the embryonic transitional-squamous epithelium of the urogenital sinus grows up the muscular scaffold of the vagina and outer cervix to replace the original columnar epithelium (of mullerian origin) lining these organs (51, 71). Estrogen appears to affect the stroma (72), which then inhibits the upgrowth, leading to the development of adenosis from persistent residual embryonic glandular epithelium.

A byproduct of DES research is a new model for studying organ growth, whereby organs from aborted human fetuses grown in immunologically deficient athymic ("nude") mice can be exposed to drugs under controlled laboratory conditions (54, 73). The developing organs can then be maintained to grow normally (without exposure), or they can be exposed to various drugs, such as DES. Using this system, for example, clomiphene and tamoxifen, both hormonally active triphenylethylene compounds that exhibit estrogenic and antiestrogenic activities, were shown to manifest effects, including adenosis (Fig. 10.31), similar to those caused by DES (74). Progesterone, in contrast, elicits no such changes (75). Such studies have recreated aspects of the DES syndrome, and offer no indication that adenosis is other than a normal tissue that is in an abnormal location. No study has disproved the hypothesis that the development of adenosis is caused by a failure of squamous tissue to replace the mullerian epithelium originally

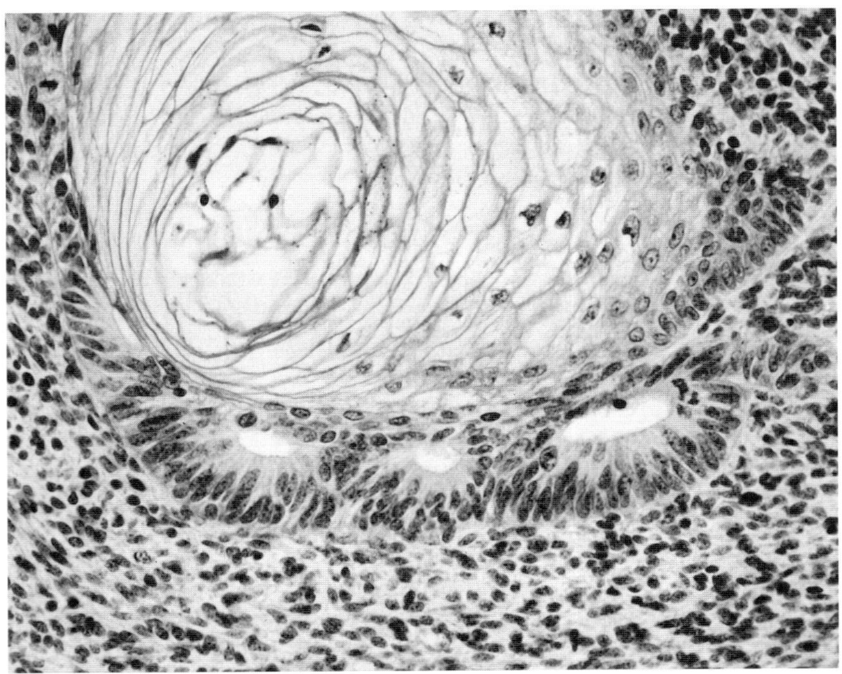

FIGURE 10.31. Vaginal adenosis after exposure to DES. Three adenotic glands, which are characterized by immature columnar cells lacking cilia and intracytoplasmic mucin, are located at the base of highly glycogenated, vaginal squamous epithelium. Reprinted with permission from Robboy SJ, Taguchi O, Cunha GR. Human Pathol 1982;13:190–198.

lining/covering the vagina and exocervix during fetal development. Our working hypothesis is that DES acts on the stroma of the uterine and vaginal wall rather than on the epithelial lining.

Ultrastructural studies on stromal epithelial interactions involving vaginal adenosis and the vaginal wall have shown that some epithelial cells are in direct contact with stromal cells, suggesting that the stroma may directly affect epithelial function (76).

As mentioned earlier in this chapter, in addition to affecting the development of the lower genital tract, prenatal exposure to DES affects development of the cervix and uterine corpus. The embryonic stromal components of the uterine wall do not segregate normally into the outer layers of smooth muscle and inner layers of endometrial stroma (54). The clinical correlates appear to be the gross structural changes in the human uterus and cervix. Another manifestation is a functionally imperfect uterus, which is sometimes unable to sustain fetal growth to term (76). These techniques offer the promise of entirely new investigative approaches for the study of human disease under controlled conditions.

REFERENCES

1. Herbst AL, Bern H. Developmental Effects of DES in Pregnancy. New York: Thieme Stratton, 1981.
2. Herbst AL. Problems of prenatal DES exposure. In: Herbst AL, Mishell DR Jr, Stenchever MA, Droegemueller W. Comprehensive Gynecology. St. Louis: Mosby-Year Book, 1992: 409–423.
3. Palmlund I, Apfel R, Buitendijk S, et al. Effects of diethylstilbestrol (DES) medication during pregnancy: report from a symposium at the 10th international congress of ISPOG. J Psychosom Obstet Gynaecol 1993;14:71–89.
4. Report of the recommendations of the 1985 DES Task Force of the U.S. Department of Health and Human Services. MMWR 1986;35:155–156,161–162.
5. Giusti RM, Iwamoto K, Hatch EE. Diethylstilbestrol revisited: a review of the long-term health effects. Ann Intern Med 1995;122:778–788.
6. Marselos M, Tomatis L. Diethylstilboestrol: I. Pharmacology, toxicology and carcinogenicity in humans. Eur J Cancer 1992;28A:1182–1189.
7. Marselos M, Tomatis L. Diethylstilboestrol: II. Pharmacology, toxicology and carcinogenicity in experimental animals. Eur J Cancer 1992;28A:149–155.
8. Mascaro ML. Preconception tort liability: recognizing a strict liability cause of action for DES grandchildren. Am J Law Med 1991;17:435–455.
9. Fern FH, McHugh LS. Market share liability for pharmaceuticals. The distinction between DES and DPT. J Leg Med 1990;11:391–426.
10. Brahams D. Diethylstilboestrol: third-generation injury claims. Lancet 1991;337:785.
11. Walker BE. Animal models of prenatal exposure to diethylstiboestrol. In: Napalkov NP, Rice JM, Tomatis L, et al. Perinatal and Multigeneration Carcinogenesis. Lyon: Intl Agency Res Cancer, 1989:349–364.
12. Johnson LD. Lesions of the female genital system caused by diethylstilbestrol in humans, subhuman primates, and mice. In: Jones TC, Mohr U, Hunt RD, eds. Monographs on Pathology of Laboratory Animals: The Genital System. New York: Springer-Verlag, 1987: 84–109.
13. Cunningham A, Klopman G, Rosenkranz HS. The carcinogenicity of diethylstilbestrol: Structural evidence for a non-mechanism. Arch Toxicol 1996;70:356–361.
14. Huff J, Boyd J, Carrett JC. Cellular and Molecular Mechanisms of Hormonal Carcinogenesis. Environmental Influences. New York: Wiley-Liss Pub, 1996.

15. Berendes HW, Lee YJ. Suspended judgment. The 1953 clinical trial of diethylstilbestrol during pregnancy: could it have stopped DES use? Control Clin Trials 1993;14:179–182.

16. Potter EL. A historical view: diethylstilbestrol use during pregnancy: a 30-year historical perspective. Pediatr Pathol 1991;11:781–789.

17. Robboy SJ, Noller KL, Kaufman RH, et al. An atlas of findings in the human female after intrauterine exposure to diethylstilbestrol. DHEW publication 84-2344, 1984.

18. Wilcox AJ, Baird DD, Weinberg CR, et al. Fertility in men exposed prenatally to diethylstilbestrol. N Engl J Med 1995;332:1411–1416.

19. Colton T, Greenberg ER, Noller K, et al. Breast cancer in mothers prescribed diethylstilbestrol in pregnancy. Further follow-up. JAMA 1993;269:2096–2100.

20. Leary FJ, Resseguie LJ, Kurland LT, et al. Males exposed in utero to diethylstilbestrol. JAMA 1984;252:2984–2989.

21. Proc NIH Workshop. Long Term effects of exposure to diethylstilbestrol (DES), April 22-24, Falls Church, VA, 1992 1–94.

22. Noller KL. DES Update. Clin Prac Gynecol 1990;2:144–149.

23. Trimble EL, Rubinstein LV, Menck HR, et al. Vaginal clear cell adenocarcinoma in the United States. Gynecol Oncol 1996;61:113–115.

24. Hanselaar AG, Van Leusen ND, De Wilde PC, et al. Clear cell adenocarcinoma of the vagina and cervix. A report of the Central Netherlands Registry with emphasis on early detection and prognosis. Cancer 1991;67:1971–1978.

25. Sharp GB, Cole P. Vaginal bleeding and diethylstilbestrol exposure during pregnancy: relationship to genital tract clear cell adenocarcinoma and vaginal adenosis in daughters. Am J Obstet Gynecol 1990;162:994–1001.

26. Waggoner SE, Mittendorf R, Biney N, et al. Influence of in utero diethylstilbestrol exposure on the prognosis and biologic behavior of vaginal clear-cell adenocarcinoma. Gynecol Oncol 1994;55:238–244.

27. Sharp GB, Cole P, Anderson D, et al. Clear cell adenocarcinoma of the lower genital tract. Correlation of mother's recall of diethylstilbestrol history with obstetrical records. Cancer 1990;66:2215–2220.

28. Melnick S, Cole P, Anderson D, et al. Rates and risks of diethylstilbestrol-related clear-cell adenocarcinoma of the vagina and cervix. An update. N Engl J Med 1987;316:514–516.

29. Meara J, Vessey M, Fairweather DV. A randomized double-blind controlled trial of the value of diethylstilboestrol therapy in pregnancy: 35-year follow-up of mothers and their offspring. Br J Obstet Gynaecol 1989;96:620–622.

30. Vessey MP. Epidemiological studies of the effects of diethylstilboestrol. In: Napalkov NP, Rice JM, Tomatis L, et al, eds. Perinatal and Multigenerational Carcinogenesis. Lyon: Intl Agency Res Cancer 1989;96:335–348.

31. Noller KL. Cancer in DES-exposed offspring. In: Proc NIH Workshop: Long term effects of exposure to diethylstilbestrol (DES), April 22-24, Falls Church, VA, 1992:10-11.

32. Horwitz RI, Viscoli CM, Merino M, et al. Clear cell adenocarcinoma of the vagina and cervix. Incidence, misclassified disease, and diethylstilbestrol. J Clin Epidemiol 1988;41:593–597.

33. Sander R, Nuss RC, Rhatigan R. Diethylstilbestrol-associated vaginal adenosis followed by clear cell adenocarcinoma. Intl J Gynecol Pathol 1986;5:362–370.

34. Emens JM. Continuing problems with diethylstilboestrol. Br J Obstet Gynaecol 1994;101:748–750.

35. Sharp GB, Cole P. Identification of risk factors for diethylstilbestrol-associated clear cell adenocarcinoma of the vagina: similarities to endometrial cancer. Am J Epidemiol 1991;134:1316–1324.

36. Herbst AL, Anderson S, Hubby MM, et al. Risk factors for the development of diethylstilbestrol-associated clear cell adenocarcinoma: a case-control study. Am J Obstet Gynecol 1986;154:814–822.

37. Senekjian EK, Hubby M, Bell DA, et al. Clear cell adenocarcinoma (CCA) of the vagina and cervix in association with pregnancy. Gynecol Oncol 1986;24:207–219.

38. Burks RT, Schwarz AM, Wheeler JE, et al. Late recurrence of clear cell adenocarcinoma of the cervix. Case report. Obstet Gynecol 1990;76:525–527.
39. Palefsky JM, Holly EA. Molecular virology and epidemiology of human papillomavirus and cervical cancer. Cancer Epidemiol Biomark Prevent 1995;4:415–428.
40. Waggoner SE, Anderson SM, Van Eyck S, et al. Human papillomavirus detection and p53 expression in clear-cell adenocarcinoma of the vagina and cervix. Obstet Gynecol 1994; 84:404–408.
41. Boyd J, Takahashi H, Waggoner SE, et al. Molecular genetic analysis of clear cell adenocarcinomas of the vagina and cervix associated and unassociated with diethylstilbestrol in utero. Cancer 1996;77:507–513.
42. Robboy SJ, Welch WR. Microglandular hyperplasia in vaginal adenosis associated with oral contraceptives and prenatal diethylstilbestrol (DES) exposure. Obstet Gynecol 1977; 49:430–434.
43. Kaufman RH, Adam E, Noller K, et al. Upper genital tract changes and infertility in diethylstilbestrol-exposed women. Am J Obstet Gynecol 1986;154:1312–1318.
44. Jefferies JJ, Robboy SJ, O'Brien PC, et al. Structural anomalies of the cervix and vagina in women enrolled in the diethylstilbestrol adenosis (DESAD) project. Am J Obstet Gynecol 1984;148:59–66.
45. van Gils AP, Tham RT, Falke TH, et al. Abnormalities of the uterus and cervix after diethylstilbestrol exposure: correlation of findings on MR and hysterosalpingography. Am J Roentgenol 1989;153:1235–1238.
45. Anderson MC, Jordan JA, Morse A, et al. Diethylstilbestrol exposure. In: A Text and Atlas of Integrated Colposcopy. Edition 2. London: Chapman & Hall Medical, 1996:240-242.
46. Follen MM, Fox HE, Levine RU. Cervical vascular malformation as a couse of antepartum and intrapartum bleeding in three diethylstilbestrol-exposed progeny. Amer J Obstet Gynecol 1985;153:890–891.
47. Antonioli DA, Burke L, Friedman EA. Natural history of diethylstilbestrol associated genital tract lesions: cervical ectopy and cervicovaginal hood. Amer J Obstet Gynecol 1980;137:847–853.
48. de Virgiliis G, Sideri M, Rossi A, et al. "DES-like" anomalies. I. Biological and clinical problems. A study on 12,285 cases. Cervix Low Female Genital Tract 1985;3:297–312.
49. Robboy SJ, Hill EC, Sandberg EC, et al. Vaginal adenosis in women born prior to the diethylstilbestrol (DES) era. Human Pathol 1986;17:488–493.
50. Singer A, Mansell ME, Neill S. Symptomatic vaginal adenosis. Brit J Obstet Gynaecol 1994; 101:633–635.
51. Robboy SJ. A hypothetic mechanism of diethylstilbestrol (DES)-induced anomalies in prenatally exposed women. Human Pathol 1983;14:831–833.
52. Kurman RJ, Scully RE. The incidence and histogenesis of vaginal adenosis: an autopsy study. Human Pathol 1974;5:265–276.
53. Johnson LD, Driscoll SG, Hertig AT, et al. Vaginal adenosis in stillborns and neonates exposed to diethylstilbestrol and steroidal estrogens and progestins. Obstet Gynecol 1979; 53:671–679.
54. Robboy SJ, Taguchi O, Cunha GR. Normal development of the human female reproductive tract and alterations resulting from experimental exposure to diethylstilbestrol. Human Pathol 1982;13:190–198.
55. Noller KL. Role of colposcopy in the examination of diethylstilbestrol-exposed women. Obstet Gynecol Clin North Am 1993;20:165–176.
56. Robboy SJ, Young RH, Welch WR, et al. Atypical (dysplastic) adenosis: forerunner and transitional state to clear cell adenocarcinoma in young women exposed in utero to diethylstilbestrol. Cancer 1984;54:869–875.
57. Robboy SJ, Welch WR, Young RH, et al. Topographic relation of adenosis, clear cell adenocarcinoma and other related lesions of the vagina and cervix in DES exposed progeny. Obstet Gynec 1982; 60:546–551.

58. Robboy SJ, Szyfelbein WM, Goellner JR, et al. Dysplasia and cytologic findings in 4,589 young women enrolled in diethylstilbestrol adenosis (DESAD) project. Am J Obstet Gynecol 1981;140:579–586.

59. Welch WR, Robboy SJ, Kaufman RH, et al. Pathology of colposcopic findings in 2,635 diethylstilbestrol exposed young women. Gynecol Oncol 1985;21:277–286.

60. Robboy SJ, Noller KL, O'Brien P, et al. Increased incidence of cervical and vaginal dysplasia in 3,980 diethylstilbestrol (DES) exposed young women: experience of the National Collaborative DES-Adenosis (DESAD) Project. J Amer Med Assoc 1984;252: 2979–2983.

61. Faber K, Jones M, Tarraza HM Jr. Invasive squamous cell carcinoma of the vagina in a diethylstilbestrol-exposed woman. Gynecol Oncol 1990;37:125–128.

62. Piver MS, Lele SB, Baker TR, et al. Cervical and vaginal cancer detection at a regional diethylstilbestrol (DES) screening clinic. Cancer Detect Prevent 1988;11:197–202.

63. Bornstein J, Adam E, Adler-Storthz K, et al. Development of cervical and vaginal squamous cell neoplasia as a late consequence of in utero exposure to diethylstilbestrol. Obstet Gynecol Survey 1988;43:15–21.

64. Richart RM. The incidence of cervical and vaginal dysplasia after exposure to DES. JAMA 1986;255:36–37.

65. DeMars LR, Van Le L, Huang I, et al. Primary non-clear-cell adenocarcinomas of the vagina in older DES-exposed women. Gynecol Oncol 1995;58:389–392.

66. Barter JF, Austin M Jr, Shingleton HM. Endometrial adenocarcinoma after in utero diethylstilbestrol exposure. Obstet Gynol 1986;67:84S–85S.

67. Lazarus KH. Maternal diethylstilboestrol and ovarian malignancy in offspring. Lancet 1984;I:53.

68. Haney AF, Newbold RR, Fetter BF, et al. Paraovarian cysts associated with prenatal diethylstilbestrol exposure: Comparison of the human with a mouse model. Am J Pathol 1986;124:405–411.

69. Seoud MA, Tawfik O, Hunter V. Peritoneal papillary serous carcinoma in a woman with a history of utero DES exposure. Gynecol Oncol 1993;50:371–373.

70. Taguchi O, Cunha GR, Lawrence WD, et al. Timing and irreversibility of Mullerian Duct inhibition the embryonic reproductive tract of the human male. Develop Biol 1984;106: 394–398.

71. Robboy SJ, Bernhardt PF, Parmley T. Embryology of the female genital tract and disorders of abnormal sexual development. In: Kurman RT, ed. Blaustein's Pathology of the Female Genital Tract. 4th ed. New York: Springer-Verlag, 1994:3–31.

72. Taguchi O, Cunha GR, Robboy SJ. Expression of nuclear estrogen binding sites within developing human fetal vagina and urogenital sinus. Amer J Anat 1986;177:473–480.

73. Taguchi O, Cunha GR, Robboy SJ. Experimental study of the effect of diethylstilbestrol (DES) on the development of the human female reproductive tract. Biol Res Pr 1983;4: 56–70.

74. Cunha GR, Taguchi O, Namikawa R, et al. Teratogenic effects of clomiphene, tamoxifen, and diethylstilbestrol on the developing human female and genital tract. Hum Path 1987; 18:1132–1143.

75. Cunha GR, Taguchi O, Sugimura Y, et al. Absence of teratogenic effects of progesterone on the developing genital tract of the human female fetus. Hum Path 1988;19:777–783.

76. Roberts DK, Walker NJ, Parmley TH, et al. Interaction of epithelial and stromal cells in vaginal adenosis. Hum Path 1988;19:855–861.

77. Herbst AL, Scully RE. Adenocarcinoma of the vagina in adolescence. A report of 7 cases including 6 clear-cell carcinomas (so-called mesonephromas). Cancer 1970;25:745–757.

78. Scully RE, Robboy SJ, Herbst AL. Vaginal and cervical abnormalities, including clear-cell adenocarcinoma, related to prenatal exposure to stilbestrol. Ann Clin Lab Sci 1974;4: 222–233

79. Dickersin GR, Welch WR, Erlandson R, et al. Ultrastructure of 16 cases of clear cell

adenocarcinoma of the vagina and cervix in DES exposed young women. Cancer 1980;45: 1615–1624.
80. Zaino R, Robboy SJ, Bentley R, et al. Vagina. In: Kurman RT, ed. Blaustein's Pathology of the Female Genital Tract. 4th ed. New York: Springer-Verlag, 1994: 131–185.
81. Taft PD, Robboy SJ, Herbst AL, et al. Cytology of the clear-cell adenocarcinoma of the genital tract in young females: analysis of 95 cases from the Registry. Acta Cytol 1974;19: 279–290.
82. Robboy SJ, Scully RE, Herbst AL. Pathology of vaginal and cervical abnormalities associated with prenatal exposure to diethylstilbestrol (DES). J Reprod Med 1975;15:13–18.
83. Herbst AL, Kurman RJ, Scully RE, et al. Clear cell adenocarcinoma of the genital tract in young females. Registry report. New Eng J Med 1972;287:1259–1264.
84. Herbst AL, Robboy SJ, MacDonald GJ, et al. The effects of local progesterone on stilbestrol-associated vaginal adenosis. Amer J Obstet Gynec 1974;118:607–615.
85. Herbst AL, Robboy SJ, Scully RE. Malignant and non-malignant changes in the female genital tract associated with maternal DES ingestion. Hosp Practice 1975;10:51–57.
86. Robboy SJ, Kaufman RH, Prat J, et al. Pathologic findings in young women enrolled in national cooperative diethylstilbestrol adenosis (DESAD) project. Obstet Gynecol 1979;53: 309–317.

11

THE ROLE OF MOLECULAR PATHOLOGY IN DISEASES OF THE LOWER FEMALE GENITAL TRACT

Tamara Kalir, MD, PhD

■

Basic Principles of Cell Function
DNA Analysis Techniques
RNA Analysis Techniques
Protein Analysis Techniques
Molecular Model of Carcinogenesis

The past several decades have witnessed the development of many powerful techniques in the field of molecular biology, which include sophisticated methods—some qualitative, others quantitative—of DNA, RNA, and protein analysis. Many of these techniques are being used in diagnostic pathology laboratories. Applicable to many areas of clinical investigation, these techniques are being used to further our understanding of numerous problems, ranging from causes of disease, to therapy and new therapeutic modalities.

The purpose of this chapter is not to give an exhaustive review of all the techniques that are currently being used in molecular biology, but rather to give a simplified overview of some of the methods employed in both the diagnostic and research pathology laboratories as they apply to diseases of the lower gynecologic tract. Some basic principles first need to be reviewed.

BASIC PRINCIPLES OF CELL FUNCTION

The cell's nucleus might be thought of as its control center. Directions for day-to-day cell operations are blueprinted in the DNA, in the form of genes, which constitute a cell's chromosomes. Genes contain the information for proper construction of proteins, which in turn serve a multitude of purposes, including the following: structural (helping

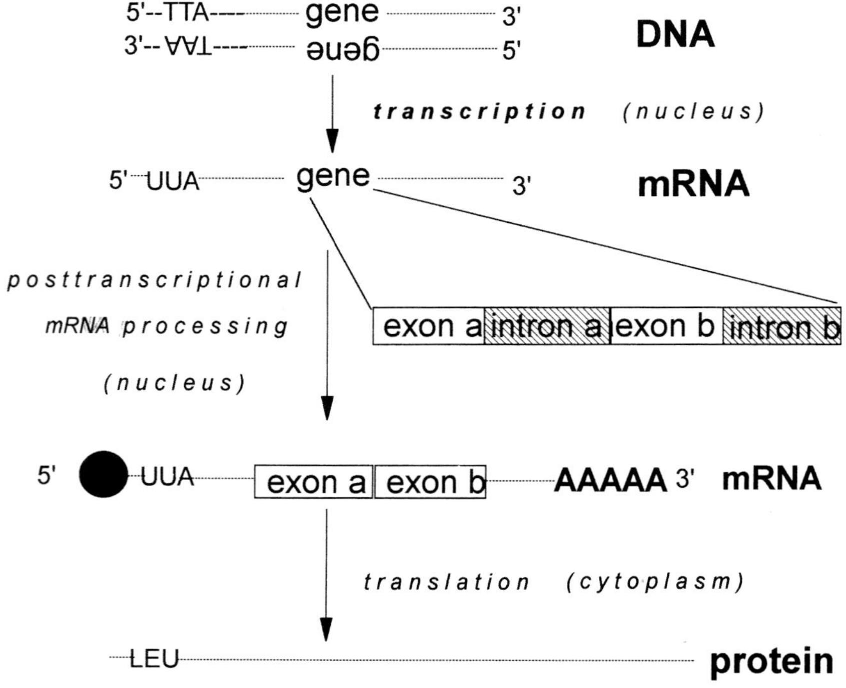

FIGURE 11.1. How a Protein Derives from a Gene.

form the cell membrane and cytoskeleton), functional (enzyme proteins), and regulatory (histone and nonhistone DNA-binding proteins, involved in regulating gene expression).

The human genome consists of 46 chromosomes. Each cell contains a set of 23 chromosomes from each biological parent. Every chromosome encodes several thousand genes (1), so the total number of genes in the human genome is an estimated one hundred thousand. All cells within the body contain the same genes. What makes a heart cell different from a toe cell is the differential expression of their genes.

Figure 11.1 illustrates how information contained in a gene becomes a protein (2). DNA is comprised of four types of phosphorylated deoxyribonucleotide base subunits: thymine, adenine, guanine, and cytosine. The deoxyribose phosphate portions of the subunits can be considered a backbone along which the bases lie. Each gene contains a specific sequence of these phosphorylated deoxyribonucleotide bases. Surrounding the genes are regulatory DNA sequences, as well as histone and nonhistone proteins. A special protein, RNA polymerase, transcribes the DNA into messenger RNA (mRNA). The so-called noncoding strand of DNA is copied (the upside down gene in Fig. 11.1). Each base in the noncoding DNA segment is faithfully copied into the corresponding position in the RNA macromolecule. What results is an RNA copy of the coding segment of the DNA. What makes RNA different from DNA is that, in RNA, the base uracil is substituted for thymidine, and ribose is the sugar instead of deoxyribose. The mRNA that is transcribed from the DNA then undergoes posttranscriptional processing. Certain segments of the transcribed RNA are removed (introns), and the remaining segments (exons) are spliced together. Then a methylated guanine "head" and a polyadenosine tail are added. The head is thought to guide the mRNA to the protein synthetic machinery (ribosomes), and the tail protects the mRNA from degradation. The processed mRNA is then transported to the cell's cytoplasm, where, in ribosomes, it is translated into a protein. Within the mRNA, groups of three nucleotides, called nucleotide triplets, code for specific amino acids. In Fig. 11.1, UUA means that amino acid leucine is to be inserted into the newly forming protein at this site. A mutation, or change in a nucleotide, can change the amino acid in a protein. This may affect the normal structure and/or function of the protein, and can be the etiology of a given disease. In addition to abnormalities in protein structure causing disease, there may alternatively be abnormalities in quantity of certain proteins. This type of problem stems from defects in one or more of the steps outlined earlier that lead to protein synthesis, including gene expression.

Differential gene expression, seen in different cells in the body, occurs through controls at the DNA level—called transcriptional controls—as well as through controls at the RNA and protein levels. Changes in these controls are necessary for normal growth and development, but such changes may also cause disease. Changes that have been documented in various tumors include gene amplification, rearrangement, deletions, point mutations, and insertions (3, 4).

As an example, Figure 11.2 illustrates one of the several ways in which human *Papillomavirus* (HPV) is involved in cervical dysplasia and possibly carcinogenesis. The mechanism involves insertion of the viral DNA into the host's DNA. After infecting a cell, HPV may remain in the cell's cytoplasm in so-called episomal form, or the DNA

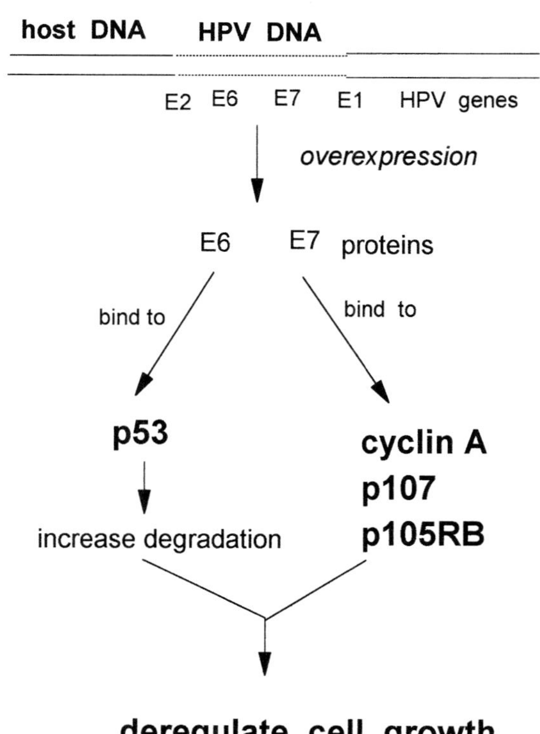

FIGURE 11.2.   Role of Human *Papillomavirus* in Cervical Dysplasia and Carcinogenesis.

can integrate into the host's DNA. The low-risk viruses, such as HPV strains 6 and 11, tend to be episomal, while the high-risk viruses, strains 16 and 18, tend to integrate into the host DNA. When the virus integrates into the host DNA, viral regulatory genes E1 and E2 are disrupted. These genes regulate the expression of viral genes E6 and E7. As a result of disruption of regulatory genes E1 and E2, overexpression of viral E6 and E7 genes occurs, with subsequent overproduction of their proteins. These proteins bind to, and interfere with, function of cellular regulatory proteins. Specifically, cellular protein p53 regulates cell growth and differentiation. E6 promotes degradation of p53 (5). Other cell proteins, cyclin A, p107, and p105RB regulate progression of cells from G1 to S phase of the cell cycle (6, 7), and E7 interferes with these constraints. The result is unrestrained cell growth. Although a number of studies have indicated a strong association between HPV, cervical dysplasia, and cancer, only a small fraction of women exposed to HPV actually develop cervical disease. One must remember that additional cofactors, other than HPV, are involved in the pathogenesis of cervical squamous disease.

The molecular biology techniques used to study HPV and other problems in medicine range from detection of proteins (immunohistochemistry) to DNA and RNA analysis. Descriptions of these techniques follow.

DNA ANALYSIS TECHNIQUES
SOUTHERN BLOTTING

This technique (8) allows for the detection of changes as small as single base mutations. Figure 11.3 illustrates the method. Sample DNA is obtained by protein digestion of the tissue, which is followed by DNA isolation. The DNA is broken up into smaller fragments using specific bacterial DNA digesting enzymes, called endonucleases, that degrade foreign DNA. The resulting DNA fragments are subjected to gel electrophoresis, in which the negatively charged DNA molecules travel toward the positively charged pole in the gel. DNA fragments of different sizes travel at different speeds—the largest get detained in the gel matrix and travel at slower rates. After completion of electrophoresis, DNA from the gel is transferred to a positively charged membrane filter by adsorption. Since the DNA is invisible, a detection step ensues. The membrane is placed in a solution containing radioactively labeled probe DNA. After incubation and washing off the unbound probe, the filter is placed adjacent to x-ray film and, following an appropriate exposure period, the film is developed.

Figure 11.4 gives an example of results. Each small horizontal line represents DNA fragments of a certain length (in some cases these may represent specific genes), which were complementary to a given gene probe. Normal (wild type) and tumor DNA from patient 1 both have two allelic forms of the gene. The patient is heterozygous for the gene, and the tumor does not show a detectable change from normal tissue for this gene. Normal and tumor DNA from patient 2 were identical and showed one allele for this gene. This patient is homozygous for the gene, and again, the tumor does not show a detectable change from normal for this gene. For patient 3, normal tissue is heterozygous for the gene, but tumor tissue is homozygous. The mutation in this patient's tumor involved loss of one allele, so-called loss of heterozygosity. This phenomenon has been reported, in a number of cancers, with putative tumor suppressor genes (9).

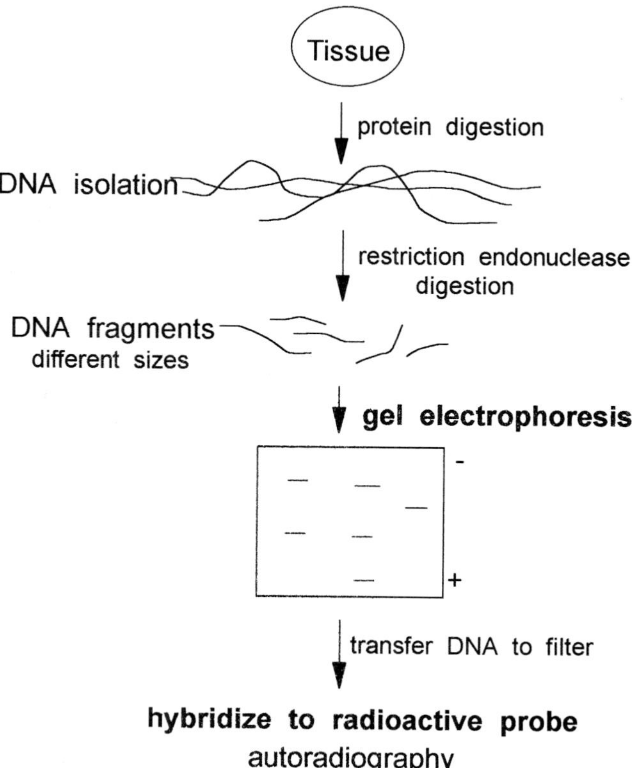

FIGURE 11.3. Southern Blotting Method.

DNA CLONING

This technique is used to increase the amount of DNA present in too limited a quantity for analysis. The procedure is time-consuming and difficult. As illustrated in Figure 11.5, DNA cloning involves placing a DNA segment, which one hopes to increase in amount, into a vector, usually a virus or plasmid—an autonomously replicating DNA—also containing an antibiotic resistance gene. The virus or plasmid is then introduced into a culture of bacteria. Once inside the bacteria, viruses and plasmids may replicate, creating multiple copies of their DNA, including the investigator's gene and the antibiotic resistance gene. Such bacteria are detected by their ability to grow in the presence of the antibiotic, to which their nontransformed neighbors are susceptible. Growing colonies are removed, bacteria are lysed, and all DNA is collected. The gene of interest can be isolated by restriction digestion, gel electrophoresis, and elution from the gel, as previously described.

POLYMERASE CHAIN REACTION

Like DNA cloning, this procedure can yield large amounts of a specific DNA segment. Easier to perform and less time-consuming than cloning, this procedure uses an automated system of heating and cooling, repeated for several cycles, to amplify the DNA.

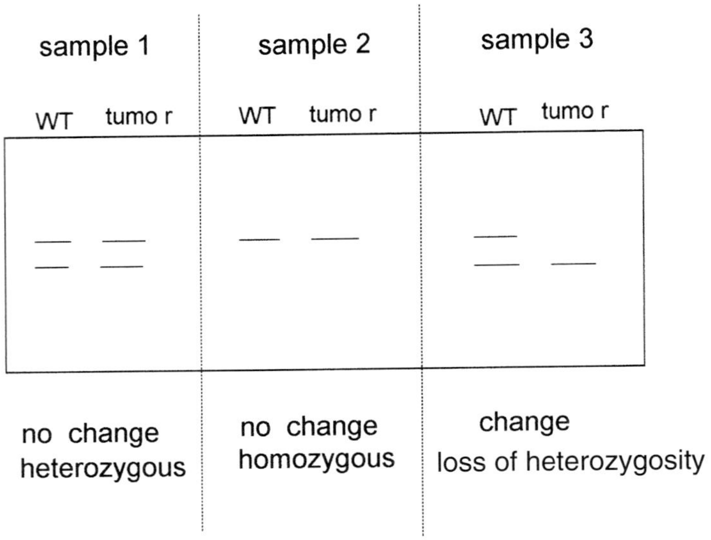

FIGURE 11.4.   Southern Blotting Results.

As shown in Figure 11.6, the DNA is first denatured by heating. Then priming DNA, a thermostable DNA polymerase, and the four deoxyribonucleotide triphosphates are added (dATP, dGTP, dTTP, and dCTP). Two sequences of DNA are replicated into four. Another cycle of heating and cooling occurs. Four sequences are replicated into eight. Another cycle of heating and cooling may be repeated, such that at the end of n cycles, there are 2^n double-stranded DNA molecules of the sequence that was amplified.

Some drawbacks include an occasional replication error by DNA polymerase, non-specific priming from other DNA segments that are complementary to the primer, and easy contamination of the samples due to the sensitivity of this technique.

DNA SEQUENCING

DNA sequencing elucidates the order of the deoxyribonucleotide bases comprising a segment of DNA in question. This is a sensitive technique that can detect a change as small as a single nucleotide mutation.

As shown in Figure 11.7, sample DNA, obtained either from cloning or PCR, is heated to denaturation. The sample is cooled; then primer DNA is added. The sample is split into four tubes, to which are added DNA polymerase, radioactively labeled dATP, and nonradioactive deoxyribonucleotide triphosphates. Each tube also contains a different terminator deoxynucleotide (di-deoxy A, C, G, or T). When a terminator base is added to a lengthening DNA fragment, replication will stop. For example, the tube containing di-dATP will have, at reaction's end, DNA strands of different lengths, each terminated at an A residue, at the point where di-deoxy ATP was added. DNAs are analyzed on a gel. Visualization is possible via x-ray film exposure because of the presence of radioactive deoxyadenosine. A sample of the result that may be obtained is shown in Figure 11.8. The film has been turned upside down to facilitate reading. Comparison of patient's normal tissue with their tumor would show if sequence changes have occurred in the specific DNA analyzed.

Drawbacks of this technique are that it is tedious and contaminating normal cells may be represented in a sample of tumor tissue, possibly masking a subtle mutation.

IN-SITU HYBRIDIZATION

In tissues used in the preceding techniques, DNA is analyzed in bulk; thus, the tissue sample includes an admixture of blood cells, blood vessel cells, and tissue parenchymal cells. In in-situ analysis, in contrast, the tissue is preserved so that individual cells can be examined and tumor cells can be compared with adjacent normal cells.

Figure 11.9 shows that the technique uses a tissue section or cell smear on a glass slide. DNA probe is added. For visualization, the probe may be labeled with a radioactive substance—or biotin or digoxigenin—to which fluorescent or colorimetric compounds can be added. The sample area, containing test tissue and probe, is covered with a coverslip and sealed. The slides are heated to codenature the sample and probe DNAs and then cooled to 37°C, at which temperature they are incubated for several hours to allow the DNAs to reanneal. To remove nonspecifically bound probe, slides are then heated and washed. Then color, fluorescence, or radioactivity is detected. The probe signal will be seen at the site where the probe DNA has annealed to the host's DNA.

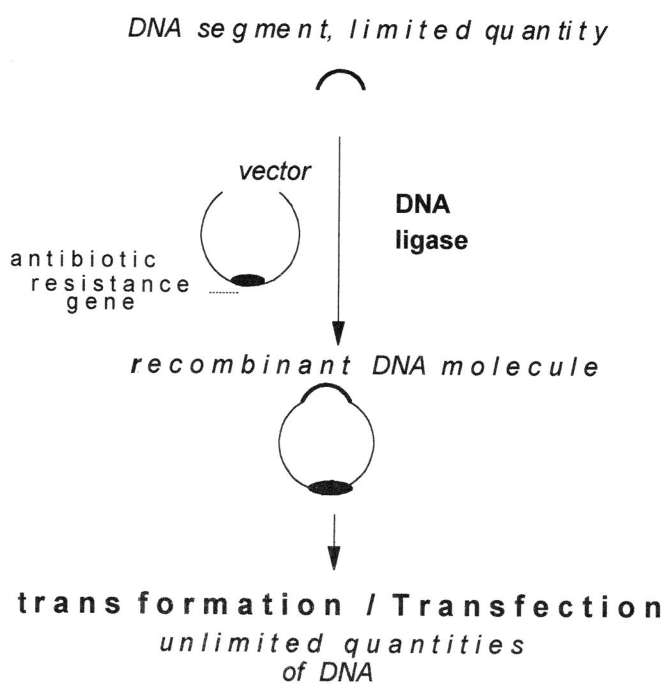

FIGURE 11.5.   DNA Cloning.

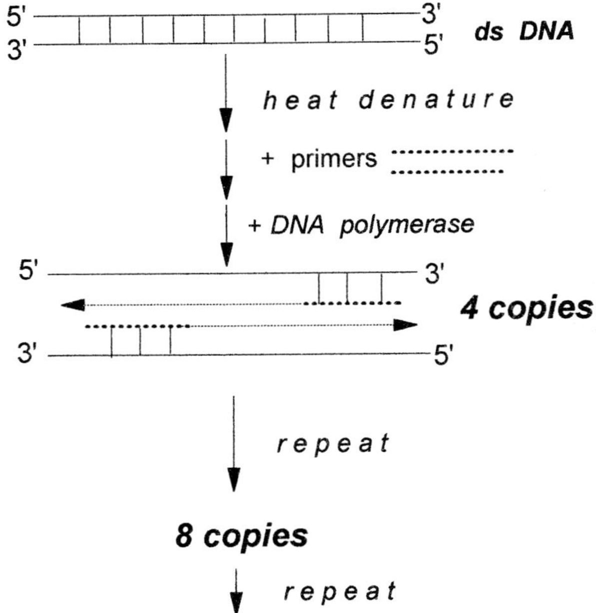

FIGURE 11.6.   Polymerase Chain Reaction (PCR).

This technique is one of several used for detection of human *Papillomaviruses* in cervical biopsy samples or Pap smears. The assays used in many pathology labs employ one of several commercially available kits, which use DNA or RNA HPV probes and detect the seven most common anogenital HPV types. In a standard assay, three tissue sections are made from the cervical biopsy specimen. After they are placed in separate slide wells, each is hybridized with one of the following sets of HPV DNA probes:

1. combined HPV types 6 and 11—some of the low-risk viruses
2. combined HPV types 16 and 18—the high-risk viruses
3. combined HPV types 31, 33 and 51—some of the intermediate-risk viruses.

Drawbacks of this technique are that if viral copy number in the tissue is low, as in recent or in old infections, virus may not be detected. Additionally, if other HPV types are causing infection, such as types 42, 43, 44, 45, 52, 56, or others, they will not be detected. Additional assays have been, and are being developed, with the intent of improving detection of HPV types. Some of these assays include the following:

1. In-situ PCR (10). This technique involves a combination of amplifying the virus DNA by use of the polymerase chain reaction, with subsequent in-situ hybridization. The technique shows increased sensitivity in detecting trace amounts of viral DNA.
2. Hybrid capture (11). This is a relatively new technique in which the reaction is performed in solution in a test tube. Sample DNA is exposed to RNA HPV probes. Complementary sample DNA:RNA probe hybrids are captured onto the

surfaces of test tubes coated with anti-DNA:RNA-hybrid antibodies. This is a technique partially similar in theory to that shown in Figure 11.10. The bound hybrids are then detected by a special colorimetric reaction using alkaline phosphatase and a chemiluminescent substrate. Measurement of the color intensity, using a luminometer, can give a quantitative measure of the HPV DNA. The following two probe mixtures are used:
- Low-risk HPV types, including 6, 11, 42, 43, 44
- High-risk HPVs and intermediate-risk HPVs, including 16, 18, 31, 33, 35, 45, 51, 52, and 56

Advantages of this technique are that it allows for quantifying the amount of HPV DNA, and it is fast and not subject to contamination as with PCR techniques. Drawbacks are that detection rate is lower than with PCR, and that amount of HPV DNA does not correlate with the grade of the cervical lesion. Although HPV infection is considered to be a risk factor in cervical dysplasia and carcinogenesis, one must remember that only a small percentage of women infected with HPV develop cervical disease. Other factors are clearly required (12). Thus, while good tests for HPV detection exist and more sensitive tests are being developed, the exact role of HPV DNA testing in women's health care remains to be delineated.

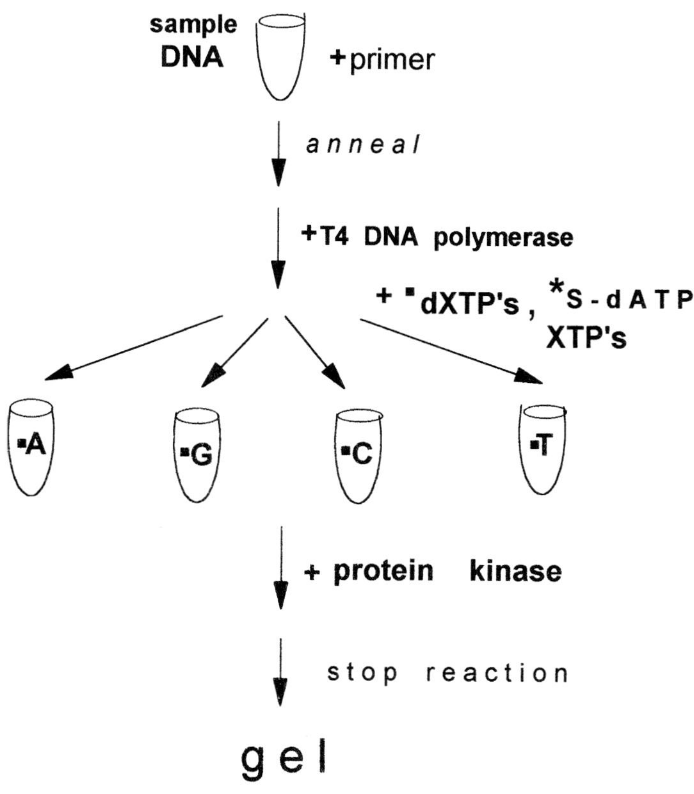

FIGURE 11.7.   DNA Sequencing Method.

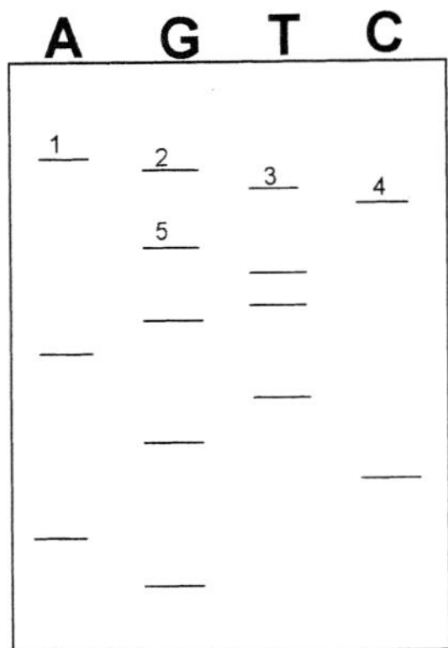

Sequence is: A G T C G T T G A T G C A G

FIGURE 11.8. DNA Sequencing Results.

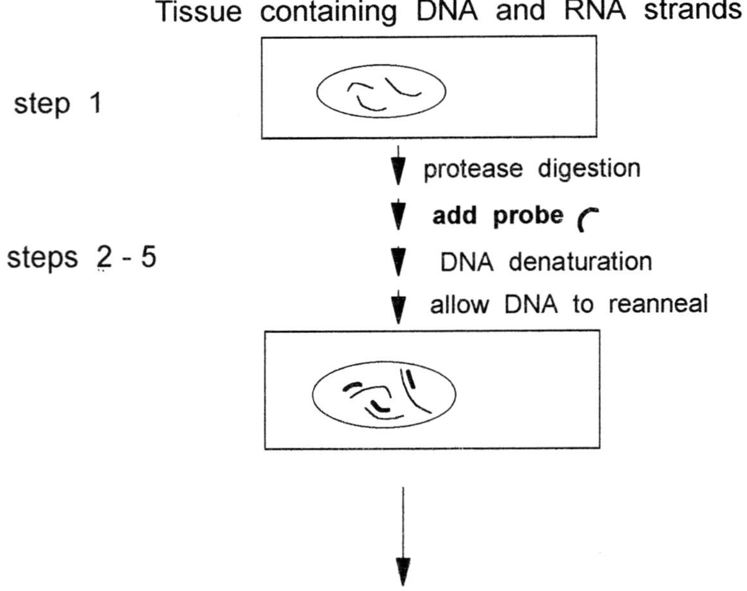

FIGURE 11.9. In-Situ Hybridization.

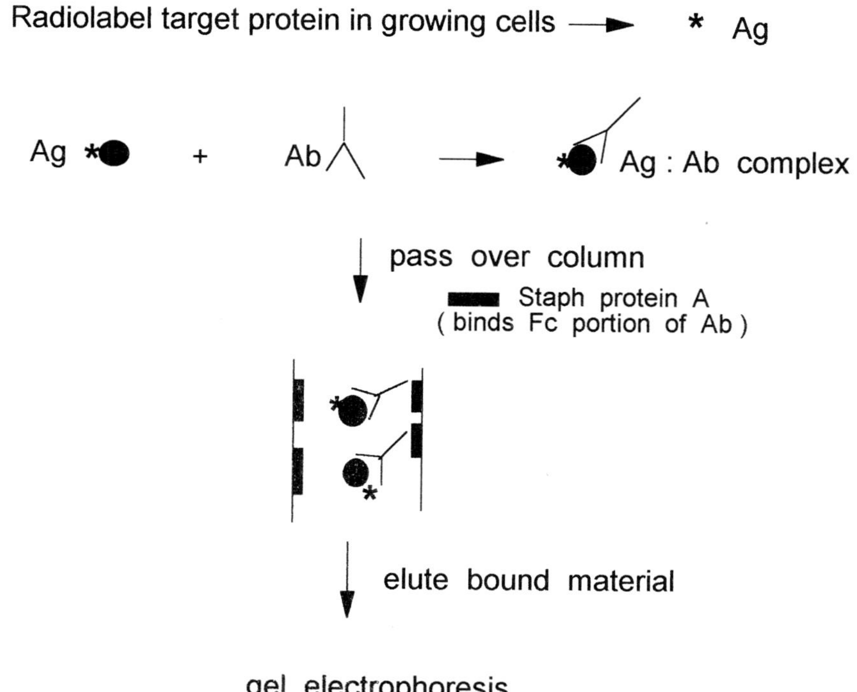

FIGURE 11.10.   Immunoprecipitation.

RNA ANALYSIS TECHNIQUES

RNAs, particulary mRNAs, are difficult to study because they are more labile than DNA. This means that RNA analysis techniques usually require fresh or frozen tissue. The techniques for RNA analysis are basically similar to those for DNA analysis.

NORTHERN BLOTTING

This technique is for RNA detection what Southern blotting is for DNA detection. Drawbacks of the technique are that fresh tissue is required, and in large amounts. Thus, analysis is further limited to RNAs from genes with high levels of expression.

REVERSE TRANSCRIPTASE PCR

In this technique, a DNA copy of total RNA is made using reverse transcriptase. Then, the complementary DNA (cDNA) is used as a template for PCR using primer DNAs to areas of interest. Cells are analyzed in bulk; thus, the drawbacks of using pooled samples apply.

PROTEIN ANALYSIS TECHNIQUES

Gene mutations result in altered RNA expression, either as a result of changes in the amount of RNA expressed or through changes in the nucleotide sequences comprising the RNAs. These changes, in turn, affect the proteins encoded by the RNAs, either as overexpression, underproduction, or as mutated proteins having altered function. Some of the techniques for analyzing proteins are discussed in the following.

WESTERN BLOTTING

This technique is somewhat similar to the Southern and Northern blotting techniques for DNA and RNA analysis in that individual proteins are separated via gel electrophoresis. A given protein is detected by application of a tagged antibody. This type of technique allows for determination of presence, quantity, and size of a given target protein. Limitations of the technique are its relative insensitivity, that only undenatured antibody binding sites (epitopes) are recognized by antibodies, and that the procedure evaluates protein expression from a pooled cell suspension.

IMMUNOPRECIPITATION

In this technique, target protein is radioactively labeled in vivo, by growing cells in the presence of radioactively labeled amino acid. Cells are then lysed, proteins extracted, and exposed to specific antibody, as illustrated in Figure 11.10. Radioactive antigen binds to specific antibody, to form antigen-antibody complexes. This solution is poured into a special column that contains Staphylococcal protein A. The protein A binds to the Fc portion (non-antigen-binding end) of antibodies, so that antibodies and antibody-antigen complexes are retained in the column. Unbound proteins pass through the column. The bound material can then be eluted by the use of a different buffer solution. The eluate is then subjected to gel electrophoresis, in which proteins are separated according to size and electrical charge.

This method allows for determination of protein size, presence, and quantity, and additionally may allow for an assessment of rate of synthesis or degradation of protein, interactions with other macromolecules, and presence or absence of posttranslational modifications. The prior two techniques assess a given protein pooled from a group of cells.

IMMUNOHISTOCHEMISTRY

Assessment of specific proteins in individual cells can be made using immunohistochemistry. This technique is somewhat similar to in-situ hybridization in that the cell smear or tissue section is exposed to a specific binding agent, which is, in this case, an antibody. Unbound and nonspecifically bound antibodies are washed away. The antigen:antibody complex is invisible by light microscopy, thus making colorimetric detection necessary. One common detection method is the avidin-biotin complex, illustrated in Figure 11.11. In this example, the antibody has been biotinylated. The avidin molecule complex contains four biotin binding sites and binds to the antigen-biotinylated antibody complex. Peroxidase molecules, attached to the avidin complex, are capable of oxidizing certain colorless chromogenic molecules—such as diaminobenzidine—which, when added, form an insoluble color product that can be visualized at the site of the bound antibody and thus clarify the protein.

A qualitative and, at best, semiquantitative technique, immunohistochemistry is limited by the quality and availability of antibodies, which may lack sensitivity or specificity and show limited binding in formalin-fixed tissues as compared with fresh or

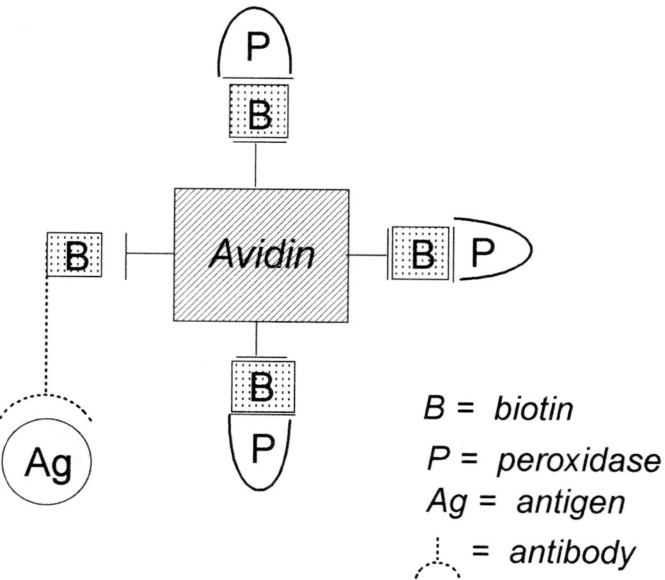

FIGURE 11.11.   Avidin-Biotin Complex Detection Method in Immunohistochemistry.

frozen tissues. The advantage of the technique is that it allows visualization of the precise intracellular location of a given protein.

Immunohistochemistry can be used in diagnostic surgical pathology because different types of normal tissues produce different tissue-specific proteins. Tumors from these tissues also may produce the tissue-specific proteins. Sometimes a tumor may be so poorly differentiated that determination of whether it is a carcinoma, lymphoma, sarcoma, or melanoma may be impossible without the use of immunohistochemistry. Occasionally, different types of differentiated tumors may histologically resemble each other. Again, the presence or absence of tissue-specific antigens may be helpful in the diagnosis. For example, vulvar dysplasia may histologically be difficult to distinguish from Paget's disease and malignant melanoma. These three diseases can be differentiated by use of immunohistochemistry because of the presence in each of different cellular proteins, as shown in the table below.

	HPV antigen	CEA	HMB 45 protein
VIN	$+/-$	$-$	$-$
Paget's disease	$-$	$+$	$-$
Melanoma	$-$	$-$	$+$

As another example, occasionally a patient will have adenocarcinoma in the form of one tumor mass in the endometrium with local extension and a second mass in the cervix with local extension. The question arises as to whether there is one primary site, or two. Some stains that are used to help resolve the question are the following:

	Vimentin	**Keratin**	**CEA**
Endocervix	−	+/−	+
Endometrium	+	+	+/−

Vimentin is a protein normally produced by mesenchymal cells (fibroblasts, muscle cells, lymphocytes, etc.). Notice that its differential staining in uterine corpus and cervix adenocarcinomas may help distinguish between the two. Keratins are a family of proteins produced by epithelial cells and by tumors showing epithelial differentiation.

Antigens are being used in numerous additional ways in immunohistochemistry, and new antibodies are being developed. The basic problem in immunohistochemistry is that no single stain is 100% sensitive and specific for a given target tissue. Some degree of overlapping of staining between different types of tissues may occur. Sometimes the staining results can be equivocal. The results must be interpreted in conjunction with the histologic findings and clinical history and findings. The previously mentioned molecular biology techniques, as well as other techniques, are also being used in research to further our knowledge of the molecular events in tumorigenesis.

MOLECULAR MODEL OF CARCINOGENESIS

Tumors are thought to arise as a result of the ability of a mutated (malignant) cell to overcome the multiple regulatory mechanisms that ensure normal cell growth. The mutated cell has a growth advantage over normal cells. Normal cell growth is regulated by signaling proteins or molecules or by growth factors. A growth factor exerts its effect by binding to a cell receptor. Attachment of the growth factor to the cell receptor may set off a cascade of reactions, including activation of phosphorylating enzymes, the protein kinases (13). The cascade of events eventually triggers histone and nonhistone proteins in the nucleus to allow the transcription of certain genes that, when translated into proteins, cause growth. Mutations allowing activation at any of these steps could give a mutant cell a growth advantage. The four types of proteins that, when mutated, confer a growth advantage on cells include the following:

1. Growth factors
2. Growth factor receptors
3. Cytoplasmic signal transduction molecules
4. Nuclear transcription factors

These are the types of proteins encoded by proto-oncogenes, the cell analogs of the oncogenes, and are normally involved in cell growth regulation. An illustration of the sites of action of these proteins is shown in Figure 11.12. A mutated protein at steps 2, 3, or 4 could act independently of preceding signals to give the cell a constant growth signal. A mutated protein results from a mutated gene. Three types of mutant genes thought to be involved in carcinogenesis are as follows:

1. *Proto-oncogenes:* These are genes normally involved in growth regulation and, in

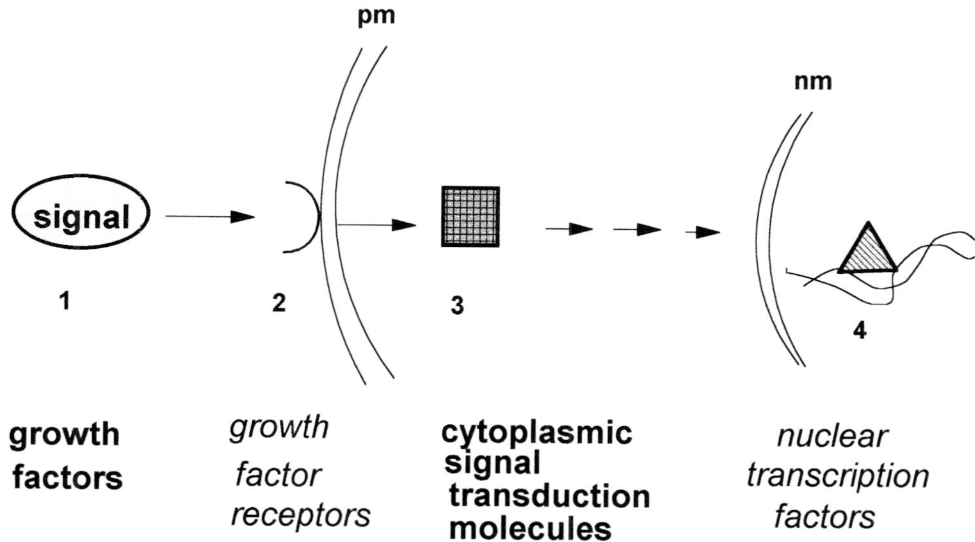

FIGURE 11.12. Types of proteins encoded by proto-oncogenes.

tumors, have been found to be present in increased amounts or have been amplified (14).

2. *Tumor suppressor genes:* These genes normally negatively regulate cell growth and differentiation and, in some tumors, are found to be deleted (15).

3. *Mutator genes:* These genes are involved in repairing errors in DNA synthesis.

Various gene mutations have been shown to arise either from loss of DNA, insertion of DNA, including viral DNAs, or changes in single nucleotide bases (point mutations). A tremendous amount of scientific information has been obtained through the use of the various techniques mentioned above. An additional and crucial use involves applying the knowledge toward newer and better therapies, which include the following:

1. Replacing defective tumor suppressor genes
2. Using blocking oligonucleotides to decrease expression of overexpressed oncogenes
3. Creating drugs that interfere with viral interaction with cell regulatory proteins

The combined skills of the clinician, the pathologist, and the scientist will be needed to help solve these problems.

REFERENCES

1. Cho KR, Hendrick L. Molecular biology. In RJ Kurman, ed. Blaustein's Pathology of the Female Genital Tract. 4th ed. Springer-Verlag, New York 1994:1174.

2. Alberts B, Bray D, Lewis J, et al. Molecular Biology of the Cell. New York: Garland. 1989: 201–219.
3. Pejovic T, Heim S, Mandahl N, et al. Bilateral ovarian carcinoma: cytogenetic evidence of unicentric origin. Int J Cancer 1991;47:358–361.
4. Bishop JM. Molecular themes in oncogensis. Cell 1991;64:235–248.
5. Moreau F, Matlashewski F. Molecular analysis of different allelic variants of wild-type human p53. Biochem Cell Biol 1992;70:1014–1019.
6. Dyson N, Howlet PM, Munger K, et al. The human *Papillomavirus* 16 E7 oncoprotein is able to bind to the retinoblastoma gene product. Science 1989;243:934–937.
7. Munger K, Werness BA, Dyson N, et al. Complex formation of human *Papillomavirus* E7 proteins with the retinoblastoma tumor suppressor gene product. EMBO J 1989;8: 4099–4105.
8. Alberts B, Bray D, Lewis J. et al. Molecular Biology of the Cell. New York: Garland, 1989: 189–191.
9. Sato T, Tanigami A, Yamakawa K, et al. Allelotype of breast cancer: cumulative allele losses promote tumor progression in primary breast cancer. Cancer Res 1990;50:7184–7189.
10. Smits HL, Bollen LJ, Tjong-A-Hung SP, et al. Intermethod variation in detection of human *Papillomavirus* DNA in cervical smears. J Clin Microbiol 1995;33:2631–2636.
11. Sun XW, Ferenczy A, Johnson D, et al. Evaluation of the hybrid capture human *Papillomavirus* deoxyribonucleic acid detection test. Am J Obstet Gynecol 1995;173: 1432–1437.
12. Wright TC, Kurman RJ, A Ferenczy. Precancerous lesions of the cervix. In: Kurman RJ, ed. Blaustein's Pathology of the Female Genital Tract. 4th ed. New York: Springer-Verlag 1994:241.
13. Amano M, Mukai H, Ono Y, et al. Identification of a putative target for Rho as the serine-threonine kinase protein kinase N. Science 1996;271:6488–6650.
14. Yang-Feng TL, Li S, Leung W-Y, et al. Trisomy 12 and K-ras-2 amplification in human ovarian tumors. Int J Cancer 1991;48:678–681.
15. Hahn SA, Schutte M, Hoque ATM, et al. DPC4, a candidate tumor suppressor gene at human chromosome 18q21.1. Science 1996;271:350–353.

Index

Note: Page numbers in italics denote figures. Those followed by "t" denote tables.